Advances in
Peptic Ulcer Pathogenesis

Advances in Peptic Ulcer Pathogenesis

EDITED BY

W. D. W. Rees

MD, MRCP

Consultant Physician and Gastroenterologist
Department of Gastroenterology
Hope Hospital
Salford, Lancs, UK

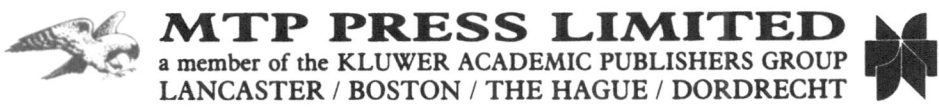

MTP PRESS LIMITED
a member of the KLUWER ACADEMIC PUBLISHERS GROUP
LANCASTER / BOSTON / THE HAGUE / DORDRECHT

Published in the UK and Europe by
MTP Press Limited
Falcon House
Lancaster, England

British Library Cataloguing in Publication Data

Advances in peptic ulcer pathogenesis.
   1. Peptic ulcer—Etiology
   I. Rees, W.D.W.
   616.3'43071   RC821

Published in the USA by
MTP Press
A division of Kluwer Academic Publishers
101 Philip Drive
Norwell, MA 02061, USA

Library of Congress Cataloging-in-Publication Data

Advances in peptic ulcer pathogenesis.

   Includes bibliographies and index.
   1. Peptic ulcer—Pathophysiology.   2. Peptic
ulcer—Etiology.   I. Rees, W. D. W.   [DNLM: 1. Gastric
Mucosa—physiology.   2. Peptic Ulcer—etiology.
W1 350 A244]
RC821.A37   1988   616.3'43071   87–31067

ISBN-13: 978-94-010-7052-2   e-ISBN-13: 978-94-009-1245-8
DOI: 10.1007/978-94-009-1245-8

Copyright © 1988 MTP Press Limited

Softcover reprint of the hardcover 1st edition 1988

Contents

List of contributors

A. Allen
Department of Physiological Sciences
Medical School
University of Newcastle upon Tyne
Framlington Place
Newcastle upon Tyne NE2 4HH

P. Bauerfeind
Division de gastroentérologie
Départment de médecine interne
Centre hospitalier universitaire Vaudois
  (CHUV)
CH–1011 Lausanne
Switzerland

J. R. Crampton
Department of Medicine
University of Cambridge School of Clinical
  Medicine
Addenbrooke's Hospital
Hills Road
Cambridge CB2 2QQ

I. A. Eyre-Brook
University Surgical Unit
Royal Hallamshire Hospital
Glossop Road
Sheffield S10 2JF

A. Garner
Bioscience Deopartment
ICI Pharmaceuticals Division
Alderley Park, Macclesfield
Cheshire SK10 4TG

R. V. Heatley
Department of Medicine
St James's University Hospital
Leeds LS9 7TF

A. G. Johnson
University Surgical Unit
Royal Hallamshire Hospital
Glossop Road
Sheffield S10 2JF

E. R. Lacy
Department of Anatomy and Cell Biology
Medical University of South Carolina
171 Ashley Avenue
Charleston
SC 29425
USA

M. J. S. Langman
Department of Internal Medicine
Queen Elizabeth Hospital
Birmingham B15 2TH

LIST OF CONTRIBUTORS

P. E. O'Brien
Department of Surgery
Monash University
Alfred Hospital
Prahan, Victoria 3181
Australia

R. E. Pounder
Academic Department of Medicine
Royal Free Hospital School of Medicine
Pond Street
London NW3 2QG

B. J. Rathbone
Department of Medicine
St James's University Hospital
Leeds LS9 7TF

W. D. W. Rees
Department of Gastroenterology
Hope Hospital
Eccles Old Road
Salford M6 8HD

L. A. Sellers
Department of Physiological Sciences
Medical School
University of Newcastle upon Tyne
Framlington Place
Newcastle upon Tyne NE2 4HH

A. Sengupta
Gastroenterology Division
Department of Medicine
Beth Israel Hospital and Harvard Medical
   School
330 Brookline Avenue
Boston, MA 02215
USA

A. Sonnenberg
Division of Gastroenterology
Department of Medicine
VA Medical Center and The Medical College
   of Wisconsin
5000 West National Avenue
Milwaukee, WI 53296
USA

J. L. Wallace
Department of Mediator Pharmacology
Wellcome Research Laboratories
Langley Court, Beckenham
Kent BR3 3BS

B. J. R. Whittle
Department of Mediator Pharmacology
Wellcome Research Laboratories
Langley Court, Beckenham
Kent BR3 3BS

J. I. Wyatt
Department of Medicine
St James's University Hospital
Leeds LS9 7TF

Foreword

Over the past decade a great deal of research activity has occurred on either side of the gastroduodenal epithelial interface, with the common goal of elucidating the mechanisms of mucosal protection and how these may be compromised in peptic ulcer disease. A prime stimulus to such research has been the realization that abnormal acid secretion or its delivery into the duodenum in excessive amount cannot fully explain ulcer pathogenesis in the majority of patients.

One may envisage the stomach and proximal duodenum as being in a dynamic equilibrium, with aggressive luminal factors, such as acid and pepsin, being counteracted by protective mucosal mechanisms. Until recently, the mechanisms involved in mucosal protection had been poorly defined while the physiology and pathophysiology of acid and pepsin secretion had been elucidated. The impression that gastroduodenal mucosa was protected by a single mechanism has at last been replaced by a more realistic view, suggesting a number of protective zones acting in series. Some of these zones may act as first or second line defences against aggressive factors while certain zones may specifically protect against certain aggressors.

This text discusses recent developments which have improved our under-standing both of aggressors in the lumen and protective zones within the mucosa. Since there is marked geographic and temporal variation in peptic ulcer prevalence, epidemiological studies may be helpful in detecting as yet undefined environmental or genetic factors. The dictum 'no acid, no ulcer' holds true for most benign ulcers and therefore no text would be complete without evaluating current ideas on acid pathophysiology. The importance of bile reflux in causing mucosal damage in the unoperated stomach remains contentious with many factors such as the magnitude of duodenogastric reflux in health and disease, relationship between reflux and antroduodenal motility, and the precise nature of the damaging ingredient of refluxed duodenal content requiring careful and critical evaluation. There has been a re-awakening of interest in two other damaging factors: non-steroidal anti-inflammatory drugs and *Campylobacter pylori*. There is now evidence that non-steroidal anti-inflammatory drugs contribute significantly to the incidence, morbidity and mortality of peptic ulcer disease in elderly patients. This has led to a liaison between rheumatology and gastroenterology in order to define the mechanism of damage by these drugs and how this may be overcome in patients requiring such medication. *Campylobacter* remains somewhat of an enigma: is it a pathogen causing a certain form of mucosal disease, or is it an epiphenomenon?

Mucus gel has finally come of age! Often regarded as a mere lubricant this complex mucoprotein polymer acts as an ideal unstirred layer for confining acid–bicarbonate interaction to the epithelial cell surface. The idea that gastric mucosa secretes alkali remains alien to many clinicians, but there is now little doubt that the surface epithelial layer secretes both mucus gel and alkali, which complement each other as the most superficial of the protective zones – 'the mucus–bicarbonate' barrier. A further zone has been identified between the mucus gel layer and epithelial cell membrane consisting of a mono- or bi-molecular layer of surface-active phospholipids. These molecules repel water-containing hydrogen ions and the layer acts in a similar way to wax containers which were used to store acid and were the predecessors of modern-day batteries.

The apical membrane and intercellular junctions have received little attention during the past decade and it is still conceivable that these impede ionic movement into the mucosa, therefore conferring protection. Finally, epithelial cells have a remarkable capacity to migrate across superficially-damaged epithelium to cover defects within hours. Clearly, this impressive repair process must play a crucial role in mucosal defence.

The epithelium relies on blood flow for oxygen, bicarbonate, nutrients and hydrogen ion removal. Regional variation in blood flow may well explain the location of ulcers in the stomach and duodenum, while reduction in blood flow may play an important role in causing damage by certain exogenous agents. Ischaemia may also lead to the local production of damaging factors, such as oxygen-derived free radicals, when the tissue is reperfused. Neurohormonal agents generated within the mucosa may be important in modulating the protective mechanisms. Prostaglandins of the E, F and I series have been shown to protect against a variety of noxious substances and influence many of the protective zones outlined. Synthetic prostaglandin analogues have been developed as ulcer-healing agents, although there is a suggestion that ulcer healing may be more dependent on their acid inhibitory action rather than effects on mucosal protection. A number of other arachidonic acid metabolites may be important in mucosal physiology or in the pathogenesis of damage, such as thromboxane A_2 and the 'leukotrienes'. Clearly, these as well as other mucosal agents such as sulphydryls and platelet-activating factor require further investigation.

For the clinician this new-found enthusiasm into mucosal pathophysiology may, as yet, have yielded little dividend. The cause of peptic ulceration remains unknown although information is slowly accumulating on the integrity of the various protective zones in ulcer patients. Most of the currently-available ulcer healing drugs which do not inhibit acid secretion were developed irrespective of current knowledge about the protective zones and even today most new drugs in this category are 'tested' on animal models of mucosal damage rather than on their ability to enhance certain protective mechanisms. The 'targeting' of antisecretory drugs for defined receptors or hydrogen transport mechanisms within parietal cell still remains a remote dream for 'protective' drugs. Nevertheless, progress is being made and we can now view the future of ulcer research with far more optimism than a decade ago.

This book contains contributions from physicians, surgeons, bacteriologists, pathologists, physiologists, pharmacologists and cell biologists. Such a multi-disciplinary approach serves to illustrate the current climate of cooperation that exists between the specialities dedicated to ulcer research. I extend my gratitude to all the contributors, who despite heavy demands upon their time, strived to complete the text within a relatively short period of time.

W. D. W. Rees

1
Epidemiology of peptic ulcer disease

A. SONNENBERG, A. SENGUPTA and P. BAUERFEIND

INTRODUCTION

The epidemiology of both gastric and duodenal ulcer is characterized by marked geographic and temporal variations. The incidence, prevalence and mortality of gastric and duodenal ulcer vary four- to ten-fold among different European countries[1]. During the past 20–30 years the number of patients who died from peptic ulcer disease[2-5], who have been operated upon[5,6], who saw physicians[7,8] or were hospitalized for peptic ulcer disease[9-11] have decreased by more than 100 per cent. These changes occurred within so short a period that a genetic basis can be ruled out. Thus, it seems likely that they stem from changes in environmental risk factors. The geographic variability of ulcer prevalence among populations of similar ethnicity and comparable medical standards also hints at environmental influences. Judging from their effect, it appears that environmental factors are of sufficient magnitude to constitute a fertile ground for inquiry because such information would engender the development of potent measures for prevention and treatment of gastric and duodenal ulcer disease. In addition, knowledge of environmental risk factors could provide new insights and methods to study the pathophysiology of peptic ulcer.

Four environmental risk factors have been shown to contribute to the epidemiology of gastric and duodenal ulcer: smoking; chronic intake of aspirin and other non-steroidal anti-inflammatory drugs; occupational workload; and salt consumption. Although all four risk factors influence the occurrence of ulcer disease in individual patients, only the variations in occupational workload

1

and dietary salt intake have shaped the geographic and temporal characteristics of ulcer disease. The first two sections of the present chapter deal with the geographic and temporal variations in the occurrence of peptic ulcer disease. Its prevalence is high in industrialized countries and low among Third World countries, respectively. The geographic pattern is similar in age groups ranging from 15 years onward suggesting that the exposure to the environmental agents starts around the age of 15 years. The temporal variations, on the other hand, show that the risk of developing peptic ulcer disease was highest among those generations born at the turn of the century and that the risk declined for all consecutive generations. These changes occurred in different countries alike. In the subsequent sections, it is investigated which environmental risk factors display temporal and geographic distributions that match those of ulcer disease. Only the variations in workload and salt consumption are shown to run parallel to those of ulcer disease. In the final section, it is shown how knowledge about exogenous risk factors may lead to a better understanding of the natural history of peptic ulcer disease.

GEOGRAPHIC VARIATION

Mortality from gastric ulcer disease varies four-fold among different countries. The highest mortality occurs in Japan and Portugal, the lowest one in Canada and the United States (Table 1.1). Studies dealing with the incidence of gastric ulcer show a geographic pattern similar to that of mortality[12-16]. Mortality from duodenal ulcer is high in Scotland, England, Italy, and Portugal and low in Belgium and France. Again, the geographic variation in mortality is confirmed by studies dealing with the incidence of duodenal ulcer[12-16]. Both ulcer types are rare in Third World countries[17,18].

The same type of geographic variation of ulcer mortality applies to different age groups. For instance, mortality from gastric ulcer is high in all Japanese age groups, while it is low in all U.S. age groups. The ratio of ulcer mortality from two different countries remains the same for any two age groups compared. Hence, when the death rates of consecutive age groups from different countries are plotted versus one another, significant linear relationships emerge[19] (Figure 1.1). The age-specific death rates from different countries were standardized according to the method of indirect standardization for purposes of comparison[20,21]. (The standardized mortality ratio (SMR) of each country corresponds to the ratio of the observed over the expected number of deaths during the periods 1921–1980 or 1951–1980: SMR = Observed/Expected. The expected number of deaths in each individual country was calculated from the average age-specific death rates $(\bar{r})$ of all countries applied to the population of the individual country: Expected = $\bar{r} \times$ Population.) In Figure 1.1, the SMR of the age group 0–4 years was plotted versus the

2

Table 1.1   Death rates from gastric and duodenal ulcer*

Country	Gastric ulcer		Duodenal ulcer	
	Men	Women	Men	Women
Australia	29	21	36	14
Austria	49	29	48	24
Belgium	48	26	8	5
Canada	24	14	27	11
Denmark	41	34	27	13
England	32	25	45	20
Finland	35	23	16	9
France	42	18	9	3
West Germany	56	26	28	9
Greece	30	17	19	8
Iceland	17	25	13	10
Ireland	26	21	45	17
Italy	40	16	54	16
Japan	95	60	15	6
Netherlands	31	23	22	10
New Zealand	28	21	36	20
Northern Ireland	25	18	46	21
Norway	25	18	20	7
Poland	65	25	28	8
Portugal	84	31	58	15
Scotland	25	24	62	21
Spain	68	24	27	8
Sweden	60	44	32	16
Switzerland	32	26	28	16
U.S.A.	19	12	23	10

*The death rates refer to the average of 1971–1975 (Portugal 1966–1970), expressed per million living men or women per year. They are adjusted to the age distribution of the average population from all countries by the method of direct standardization[21].

SMR of the age group 5–9 years, 5–9 years versus 10–14 years, 10–14 years versus 15–19 years, etc. For both gastric and duodenal ulcer, there are significant linear relationships between all SMRs of each two successive age groups from 20 to over-80 years, the regression coefficients ranging between 0.87 and 0.99. In gastric ulcer, the linear regressions between two successive age groups include the age group 15–19 years, and possibly even younger age groups. For duodenal ulcer, however, the series of significant regressions between each pair of successive age groups stops below the age of 15 years. Similar results are obtained using either the SMR of 1921–1980 from 10 countries, as shown in Figure 1.1, or the SMR of 1951–1980 from 18 countries. The disadvantage of analysing data from only 10 rather than all countries is outweighed by higher and more variable death rates including the time period 1921–1950 when mortality from peptic ulcer used to be much greater[19]. The significant linear regressions among successive age groups 15–80+ years from different countries indicate that the age groups from one country had

3

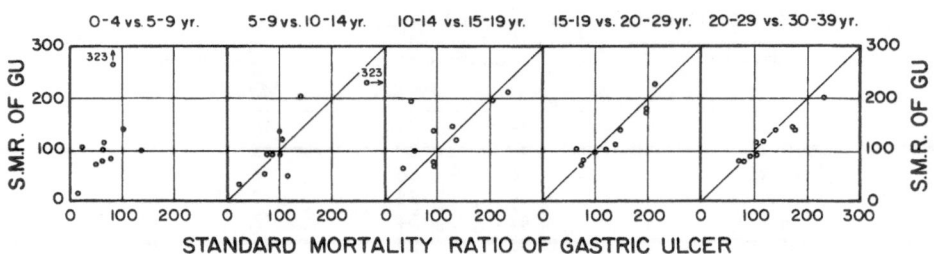

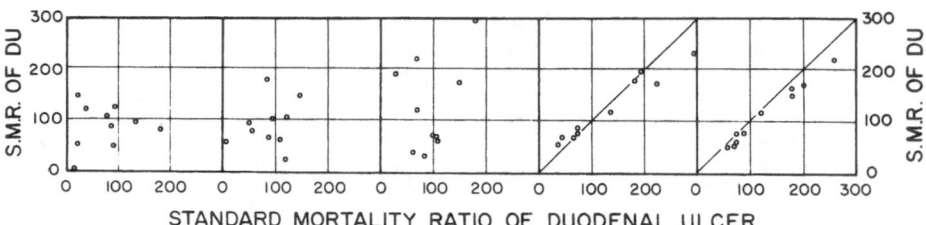

Figure 1.1 Linear regressions between the standardized mortality ratios (SMRs) of two consecutive age groups. Each point represents the data from one country. The SMR was calculated as the average of 1921–1980. The correlation coefficients for the subsequent regressions between two consecutive age groups older than 30 ranged between 0.8 and 1.0. Reproduced with permission from Ref. 19

been under the influence of the same environmental factor and that the environmental factors started exerting their effects before the age of 15 years. In the young age groups, whose geographic pattern does not correlate with the older age groups, other factors or random influences must have shaped the geographic distribution.

Figure 1.2 is shown to illustrate the same point. The mortality from duodenal ulcer in five exemplary countries was plotted versus the age of death. The age-specific death rates were calculated as the number of deaths per age group during 1921–1980 divided by the total population of the same age living at the same time. Each line joins the rates of residents from the same country having died at a different age. Between the age of 15 and over-80 years, the lines are fairly parallel and continuous. In different age groups over 15, the ranks between Norway with the lowest and Scotland with the highest death rates are distributed in the same manner. The parallel course indicates that, if mortality from duodenal ulcer is related to some environmental risk factor, the geographic distribution of this risk factor must be similar in different age groups 15 years and over. The continuity and parallelism of the lines are also represented by the significant linear regressions between any two age groups 15–80 + as shown in Figure 1.1. The curves joining the age groups 0–4 to

4

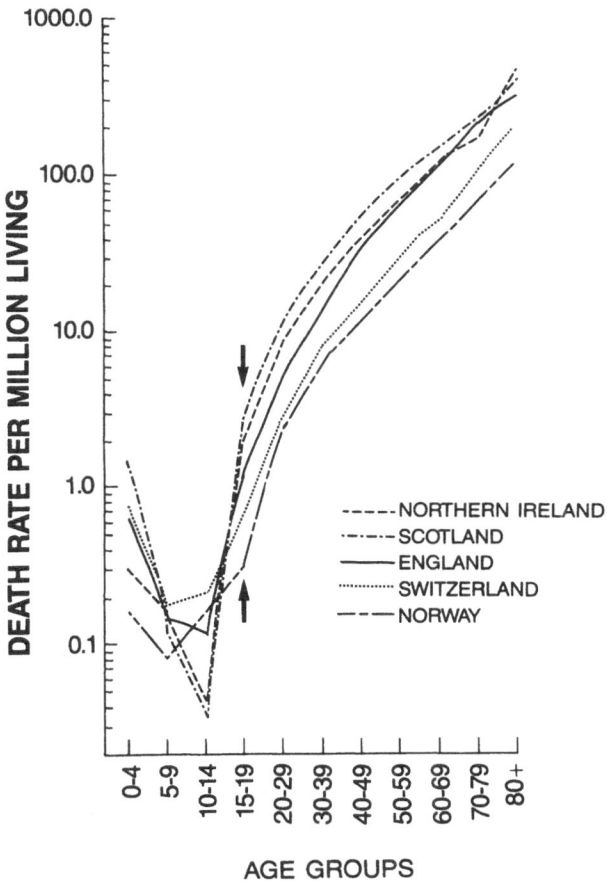

Figure 1.2 Duodenal ulcer mortality from five different countries plotted versus the age at death. The age-specific death rates were calculated as the average of 1921–1980. The parallelism and continuity of the curves break off below the age of 15 years

15–19 years, on the other hand, run zig-zag with multiple crossovers. The discontinuity indicates the influence of varying factors affecting different countries and age groups or the lack of any environmental influence and random variation only.

The marked geographic patterns of both gastric and duodenal ulcer lead one to believe that environmental factors must play a role in the development of the two diseases. The consistency in the geographic distribution of the SMRs of successive age groups shows that the same geographic variation of one or several of the environmental factors was effective in different age groups. The reverse is also true: the absence of consistency implies diversity in geographic variation or the absence of a common factor acting on consecutive age groups. Hence it appears that the exposure to the exogenous risk factors starts around the age of 15 years.

TEMPORAL VARIATION

Peptic ulcer was a rare disease before 1800[22]. In the 1830s acute perforations of gastric ulcers suddenly started to occur in young girls. Later in the 19th century, peptic ulcer also became more frequent in men. By the end of the century the incidence of duodenal ulcer had surpassed that of gastric ulcer. In the following decades peptic ulcer changed from a disease of young age to a disease of the middle and old ages[22]. In the last 20–30 years, prevalence of ulcer disease fell once again, fewer patients were admitted to hospitals for acute gastric and duodenal ulcer disease[9-11], and surgical operations for peptic ulcer became less common[5,6,8]. Fewer patients died of peptic ulcer[2-5]. The changes cannot be attributed to the introduction of H_2-receptor antagonists in 1977, since the fall started 10–20 years earlier and shows only a small discontinuity, if any, owing to changes in medical treatment.

The temporal changes of both gastric and duodenal ulcer have first been interpreted by Susser and Stein in terms of a birth-cohort phenomenon[23,24]. The age- and sex-specific death rate corresponds to the annual number of deaths per 100 000 or 1 million living population of the same age and sex. The age-specific death rates from peptic ulcer disease plotted versus the period of death show a fan-like pattern (Figure 1.3). Over the last 60 years the death rates increased in the old age groups, but decreased in the young age groups at the same time. If the age-specific death rates are re-plotted versus the year of birth rather than year of death, the individual curves of successive age groups add to one hyperbola. This pattern is suggestive of an underlying birth-cohort pattern of ulcer disease. The death rates from peptic ulcer increased in successive generations, that is birth-cohorts, born between 1840 and 1900 and declined in all subsequent generations.

For the cohort analyses shown in Figures 1.4 and 1.5, the average age-specific death rates of consecutive 5-year periods were plotted versus the year of birth. Mortality data of the period 1951–1980 were available for the twelve countries shown on the right side (Portugal–Belgium). It will be obvious that the length of this period permitted the calculation of the average death rates of only six consecutive 5-year periods. The six death rates were plotted versus the year of birth. Those who died during 1951–1955 aged 70–79 were born 1871–1885, their central year of birth being 1878. Those who died during the next period of 1956–1960 aged 70–79 were born 1876–1890, their central year of birth being 1883. Those who died during 1961–1965 aged 70–79

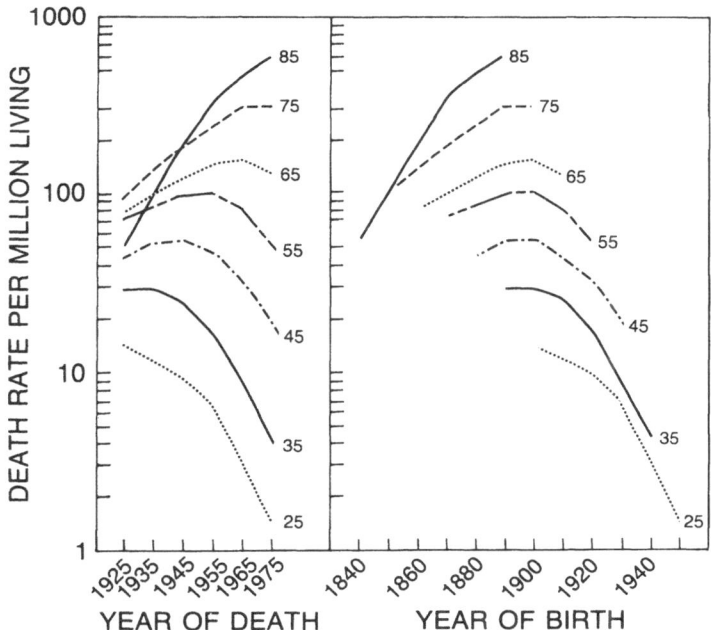

Figure 1.3 Scheme of the age-specific death rates from peptic ulcer plotted versus the year of death (left) and versus the year of birth (right). Logarithmic graphs, each curve named by the average age at death. The fan-like pattern of the period-age contours (left) changes to a hyperbola of the cohort-age contours (right). In the average death rates of all ages taken together the decline in the young age groups from 1925 to 1975 is masked by the simultaneous logarithmic increase in the old age groups

were born 1881–1895, their central year of birth being 1888, etc. The death rates of each 10-year age group plotted versus the year of birth can contribute data points to only six consecutive birth-cohorts. (The age-specific curves are represented by less than six points in those countries where ulcer mortality had been followed for shorter periods than 1951–1980.) Each birth-cohort in the graphs of Figures 1.4 and 1.5 is represented by only three age-specific death rates rather than by the total range from all age groups. However, the short individual curves add up to give a more comprehensive picture of the overall cohort pattern. For the four countries shown on the right side of Figures 1.4 and 1.5, mortality data since 1921–1930 (or 1931–1940) were available. For these, the death rates were calculated as averages of 10-year periods, e.g. 1921–1930, 1931–1940, etc.; for the age group 70–79, the corresponding birth-cohorts relate to 1841–1860, 1851–1870, etc.

In most countries, mortality from gastric ulcer in the over-80 age group increased for successive cohorts born between 1868 and 1893. In the 70–79 and 60–69 age groups, mortality from gastric ulcer increased for successive

7

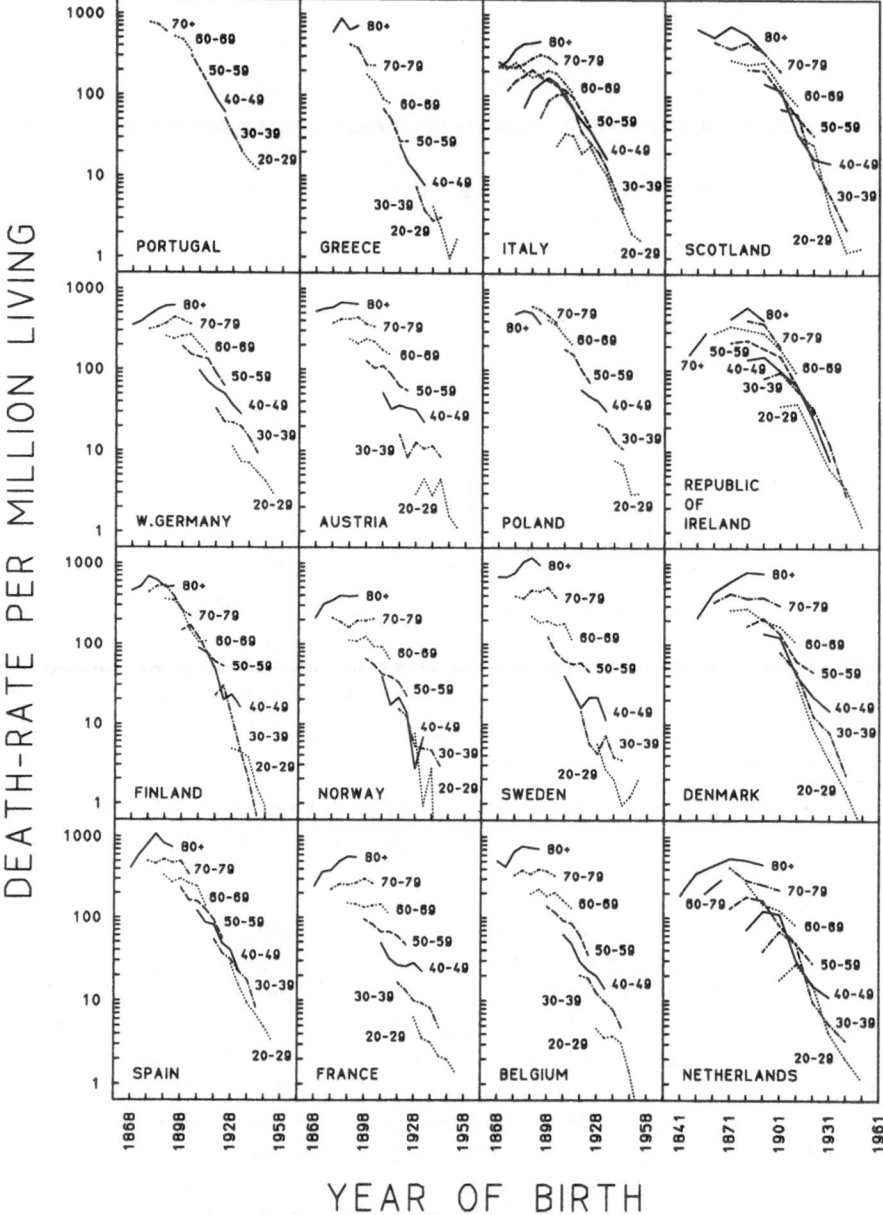

Figure 1.4 Age-specific death rates from gastric ulcer in men by year of birth. Cohorts named by central year of birth (logarithmic graphs). Each point is the mean rate of 5 or 10 consecutive years

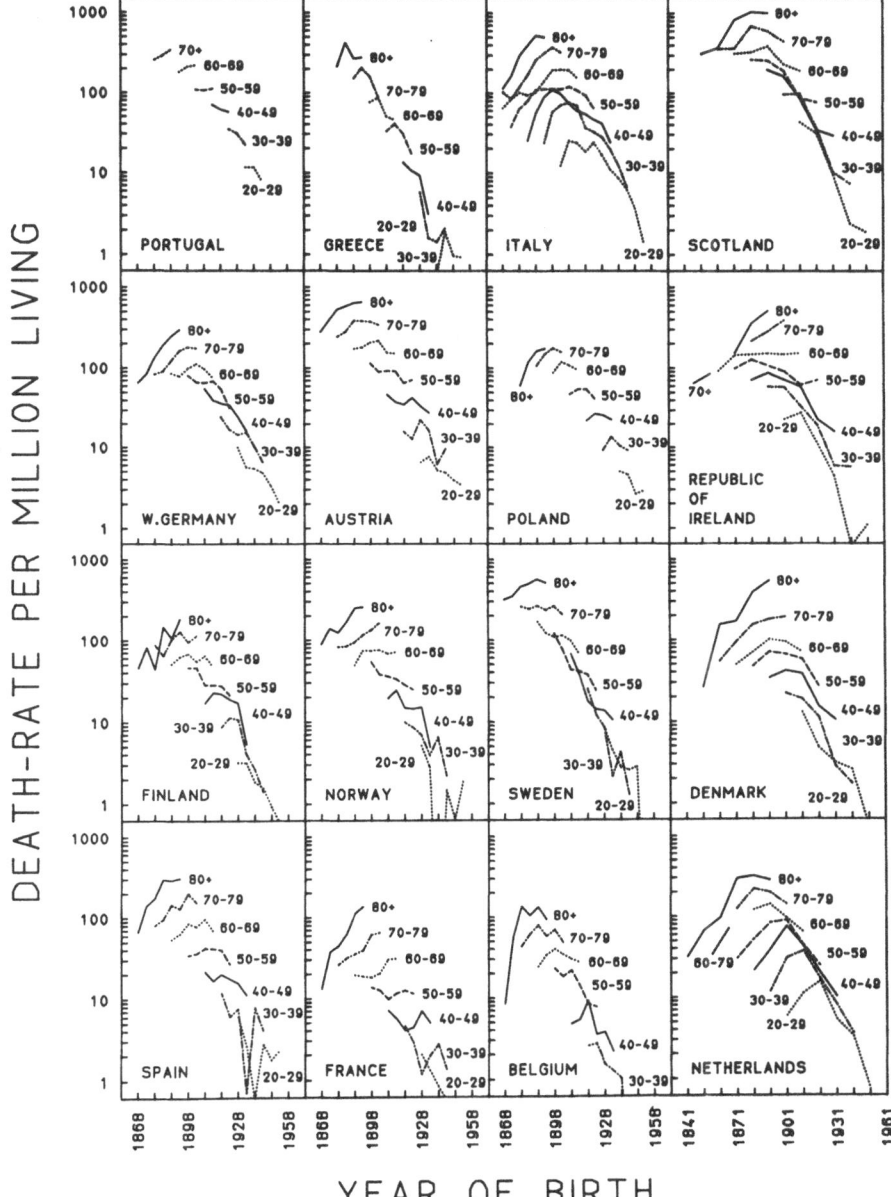

Figure 1.5 Age-specific death rates from duodenal ulcer in men by year of birth. Cohorts named by central year of birth (logarithmic graphs). Each point is the mean rate of 5 or 10 consecutive years

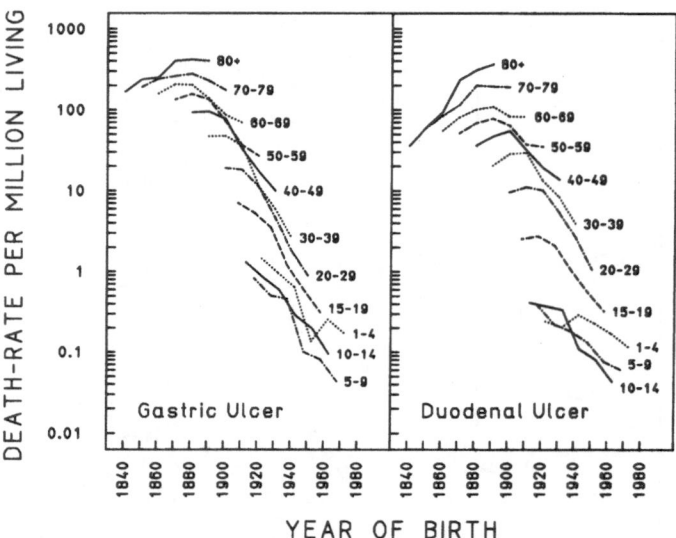

Figure 1.6 Age-specific death rates from peptic ulcer in men and women by year of birth. The curves represent the average of nine European countries where vital statistics covered the period from 1921 to 1980. Reproduced with permission from Ref. 19

cohorts until 1898 and then declined. The subsequent age groups exhibit a continuous fall of ulcer mortality. For duodenal ulcer, the age-specific death rates exhibit a rise among the cohorts born between 1868 and 1908 and a fall in all subsequent birth-cohorts. It is of interest that although the birth-cohorts with the highest risk of dying from peptic ulcer may vary among different countries, the peak mortality from duodenal ulcer lagged about 10 years behind that of gastric ulcer in all countries[24-27]. A birth-cohort pattern is present in female death rates and parallels that of male death rates shown in Figures 1.4 and 1.5, and in each country male and female cohorts with the highest risk were born at the same time[24-27]. Furthermore, a birth-cohort pattern similar to that of the European countries was found for the death rates from gastric and duodenal ulcer from Japan[27] and the United States[1].

By superimposition of the cohort-age contours from the individual countries of Figures 1.4 and 1.5, average cohort-age contours can be calculated which allow to follow ulcer mortality in those aged less than 15 years[19] (Figure 1.6). The fall of gastric ulcer mortality related to successive birth-cohorts is preserved in the age groups 10–14 years and 15–19 years. In duodenal ulcer, only the age group 15–19 years follows the temporal pattern of the older age groups. The cohort-age contours in younger children do not participate in the birth-cohort pattern of peptic ulcer mortality. As with the geographic variations, the pattern of temporal variation within different age groups suggests that the

10

determinants for the risk of dying from gastric and duodenal ulcer begin to act at an age lower than 15 years.

The concept of a birth-cohort phenomenon is further corroborated by data relevant to the incidence of gastric and duodenal ulcer. Monson and MacMahon[28] analysed the incidence of peptic ulcer disease in physicians from Massachusetts. The two cohorts of physicians born in 1870–1901 and in 1922–1943 exhibited a lower incidence of duodenal ulcer than the cohorts born in 1902–1921. The frequency of perforated ulcers has been claimed to represent true changes in ulcer incidence, since any perforated ulcer requires medical treatment and is hardly likely to be miscoded. Coggon et al.[9] have analysed the number of hospital admissions for perforated gastric and duodenal ulcer in England and Wales during 1958–1977. When their data are plotted in terms of a birth-cohort analysis, the curves support the contention that besides mortality, the incidence of gastric and duodenal ulcer in men also occurs in a fashion characteristic of birth-cohort risks[1]. The increase of peptic ulcer incidence parallel to age can also be explained as arising from an underlying cohort phenomenon. Instead of plotting the death rates versus the year of birth (as shown in Figures 1.4 and 1.5), Figure 1.7 shows the death rates plotted versus the age of death. The same statistics as in Figure 1.4 were used[29]. For instance, the curve of duodenal ulcer mortality from 1952–1954 rises until the age of 50, levels off, and then shows a decline in the oldest age groups. In 1952–1954 these age groups represented the generations born shortly before the high-risk cohorts. Interestingly, the age-specific incidence of gastric and duodenal ulcer shows a rather similar pattern[30,31]. The curves of ulcer incidence from Copenhagen County in 1963–1968 rose steadily from the age 15 to 70 and declined in the oldest age groups corresponding to those generations born before the turn of the century. Finally, temporal changes compatible with an underlying cohort phenomenon were found in the rates of disability pension granted to German employees between 1956 and 1983 because of gastric and duodenal ulcer[32].

The mainstay of present theory about the development of peptic ulceration is based on the balance of aggressive and protective factors at the mucosal level[33]. The aggressive factors include hydrochloric acid, pepsin, bile salts, aspirin, and smoking, all of which help to disrupt the 'mucosal barrier'. Their effects are counteracted by the protective influence of mucus and bicarbonate secretion, mucosal blood flow, and cell renewal possibly mediated by local prostaglandins. The momentary dominance of either side determines whether the mucosa ulcerates or remains intact. The long-lasting importance of the year of birth for contracting peptic ulcer disease seems to contradict this model of a constantly varying interaction of aggressive and protective factors. Apart from conceptual difficulties with the cohort analysis, this might have been the main reason why the original observation by Susser and Stein[23] has remained

11

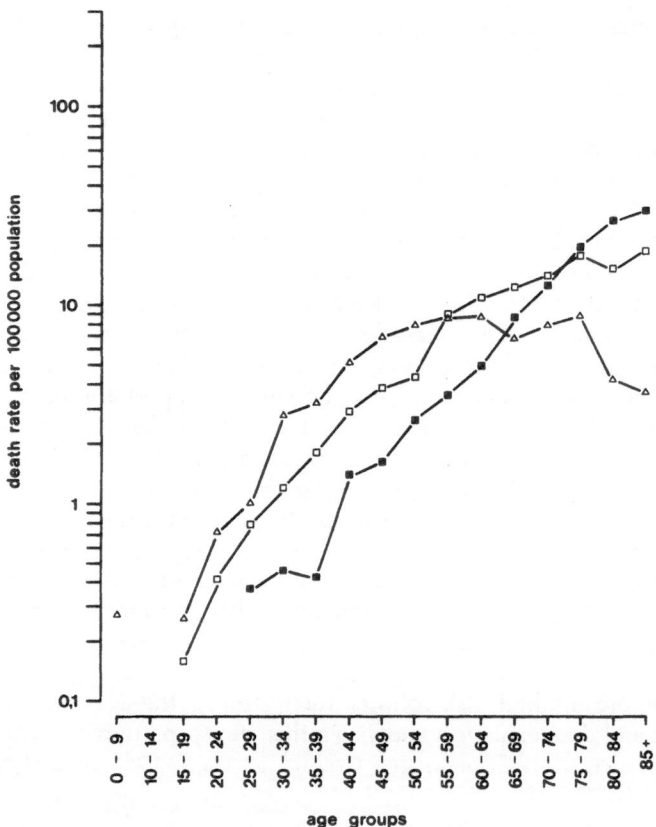

Figure 1.7 Age-specific death rates from duodenal ulcer in men from West Germany: △, 1952–1954; □, 1965–1967; ■, 1978–1980

little appreciated. However, the birth-cohort pattern of ulcer disease does not mean that acute changes in mucosal physiology are irrelevant and overridden for a lifetime by some harmful influence experienced in childhood or adolescence 10–70 years before the ulcer develops. The chances of being exposed during a lifetime to a specific environmental risk factor may well depend upon the year of birth. On a population level, dietary habits, consumption of alcohol, smoking, social behaviour, educational and occupational status relate to the time of birth. Any risk factor associated with these can influence ulcer prevalence in a fashion characteristic of a birth-cohort pattern. In the individual patient, nevertheless, present patterns of behaviour and exposure may still determine the likelihood of acute ulceration of the mucosa.

To sum up: The ubiquitous occurrence of the birth-cohort pattern suggests that worldwide, at the same time, similar environmental factors precipitated the risk of developing gastric and duodenal ulcer. The temporal pattern implies that the risk factors occurred early in the life of a cohort and that these factors were changing with time. They must have started to operate before the cohort pattern became evident[34]. Both the geographic and temporal variation indicate that the exposure to these factors started before the age of 15 years in both gastric and duodenal ulcer. In the following section it will be shown how changes in occupational workload meet those criteria for an exogenous risk factor in peptic ulcer disease.

OCCUPATIONAL WORKLOAD AND ENERGY EXPENDITURE

The uniform and worldwide decline in peptic ulcer prevalence and mortality led to the hypothesis that it might be related to a general decline of workload in the industrialized countries. The Industrial Revolution at the beginning of the 19th century started with an increase in the number of people employed in factories, with a rise of work discipline, and a decrease in resting and leisure time during work. A larger fraction of the population came to bear a harder workload than in pre-industrialized society. Owing to legislative intervention and technological advancement, the amount of working hours and the extent of occupational energy expenditure have declined since the turn of the century[35-37]. These temporal changes might have helped to shape the secular trends of ulcer disease.

To investigate whether the temporal patterns of occupational workload show the same birth-cohort phenomenon as ulcer mortality, the historic changes in the number of German industrial blue-collar workers and their energy expenditure between 1871 and 1984 were analysed[38]. German statistics were chosen, because in the occupational surveys of the German Statistical Office, the economically-active population had been listed according to different industries and occupational status, and because data regarding occupational energy expenditure were available for this country since 1882. The age-specific numbers of all residents and industrial blue-collar workers in Germany between 1871 and 1984 were taken from German census reports. Average occupational energy expenditure according to the type of work and the fractions of the German workforce engaged in light work, moderate, heavy, and very heavy work were taken from Wirths[39-41]. Average energy expenditure was converted from a daily to a yearly basis by multiplication by 300 work days. The rates of industrial blue-collar workers multiplied by annual energy expenditure gave a measure of industrial workload expressed as rate per hundred living population (Figure 1.8).

The average occupational energy expenditure fell from 770 calories per day in 1882 to 184 in 1984, the steepest decline occurring after 1925. The fraction

13

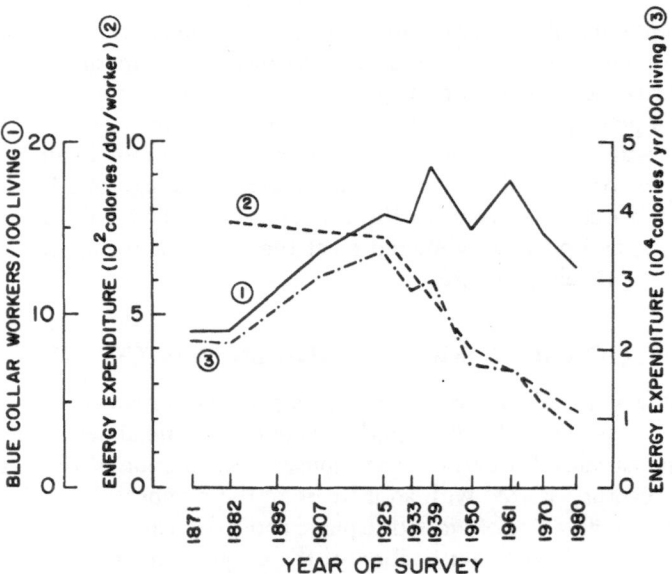

Figure 1.8   Temporal changes in the size of the industrial blue-collar workforce (1), daily occupational energy expenditure by the workforce (2), and yearly energy expenditure by industrial blue-collar workers per 100 living population (3). This last $(3) = (1) \times (2) \times 300$ work days

of blue-collar workers employed in mining, manufacturing, and construction increased during the period 1871–1939 and then started to fall off again. The rate of energy expenditure originating from industrial blue-collar work increased from 1871 to 1925 and has declined since then (Figure 1.8).

The age-specific rates of energy expenditure originating from blue-collar work during the period 1870–1984 can also be used to calculate accumulated energy expenditure over a lifetime for consecutive cohorts born between 1860 and 1955. The age-specific curves of cumulative energy expenditure show a peak for the cohorts born during the last quarter of the 19th century. A marked decline occurred in all cohorts born after 1905. The pattern resembled quite closely the birth-cohort pattern of ulcer mortality in Germany[38]. The correspondence in the two birth-cohort patterns does not necessarily indicate that it is really the cumulative rather than the acute workload which represents the relevant risk factor for the mortality or development of an ulcer. In each age group the rates of high occupational energy expenditure were highest for those born around 1880–1900. This means that the likelihood of being involved during a particular lifetime in an occupation demanding high energy expenditure was highest for those born at the turn of the century. As the

14

predominant occupations changed over the years, the cohorts born during these years had a higher probability of being blue-collar workers and spending high occupational energy. In general, a given person's energy expenditure is dependent upon his or her occupation, which in turn is dependent upon early training. The nature of this early training is likely to be linked to the year of birth. For instance, people born in 1900 were much more likely to be trained as miners compared with people born in 1950. This is how in the total population occupational energy expenditure at adult and old age may depend on the year of birth. In any individual case the development of an acute ulcer or of an ulcer relapse may, nevertheless, depend on recent changes in occupational energy expenditure.

Patients with gastric and duodenal ulcer have lower status occupations than healthy controls[42]. Lower status occupations are associated with increased occupational workload. In West Germany and in Switzerland, duodenal ulcer was observed twice as frequently in migrant workers from southern Europe as in the native population[43-46]. Migrant workers were predominantly employed in blue-collar jobs associated with heavy manual work, while the physically less-demanding sedentary occupations were mostly handled by the indigenous population. A similar phenomenon was observed in the north of the United States fifty years ago, when peptic ulcer became greatly increased in southern Blacks who had migrated from the predominantly rural south to the industrialized northern areas[47]. A review of the older literature on occupational factors in the etiology of gastric and duodenal ulcer shows a general agreement in that sedentary workers were less prone to develop peptic ulcer than industrial workers[48-50]. Unfortunately, the older publications did not differentiate between gastric and duodenal ulcer. Many of these publications were restricted to 3–10 occupational groups[48-52]. Studying the distribution of ulcer prevalence among different occupations, Ihre and Müller[53] noted an appreciably lower proportion of ulcers among intellectuals. The occupational survey carried out by Doll and his colleagues[54] revealed a high prevalence of peptic ulcer among unskilled labourers and a low incidence among agricultural workers and sedentary workers, that is civil servants, scientists, and draughtsmen. The data reported by Pulvertaft[55] and Langman[20] also suggested that duodenal ulcer is more common among unskilled workers. Emery and Monroe[56] noted that fatigue arising from overly long hours of work, exhausting work, or a poorly arranged schedule preceded an ulcer relapse in 334 out of 1279 of their patients who were studied in this regard.

In order to further substantiate the association between workload and the occurrence of peptic ulcer disease, we did three additional studies. In the first study, the number of disability pensions awarded to employees from West Germany between 1979 and 1983 because of ulcer diseases served as a marker of peptic ulcer morbidity[32,57]. Both ulcer types were more common among

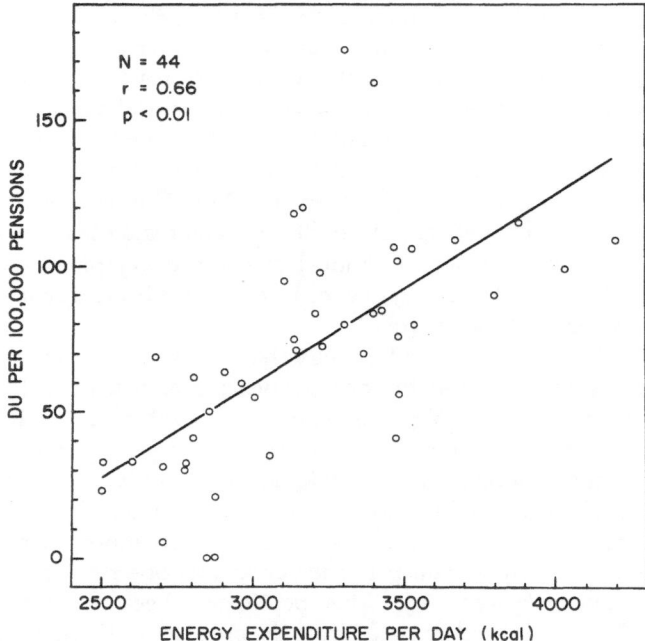

Figure 1.9 The relationship between daily energy expenditure and the proportion of disability pensions provided to men because of duodenal ulcer. Reproduced with permission from Ref. 57

occupations associated with manual work than among sedentary occupations. In men a significant linear correlation was found between the energy expenditure of different occupations and the occurrence of duodenal ulcer, but not gastric ulcer (Figure 1.9).

In a second study, the Registrar General's Decennial Supplement from England and Wales and the Vital Statistics Special Reports of the U.S. Department of Health, Education, and Welfare on occupational mortality were analysed for occupation-specific mortality from peptic ulcer[58]. The data from both countries disclosed a high mortality from both ulcer types among manual workers and a low mortality among sedentary occupations. This general pattern ran parallel to a low mortality from gastric and duodenal ulcer among the high social classes and a low mortality in the low social classes. Married women displayed a gradient of gastric ulcer mortality increasing from social class 1 to social class 5, but showed no evidence of social class correlation with respect to duodenal ulcer. In duodenal ulcer again, the varying extent of energy expenditure among differing occupations seemed to be responsible for the different risk of contracting duodenal ulcer and dying from it (Figure 1.10). The association between energy expenditure and peptic ulcer mortality was

16

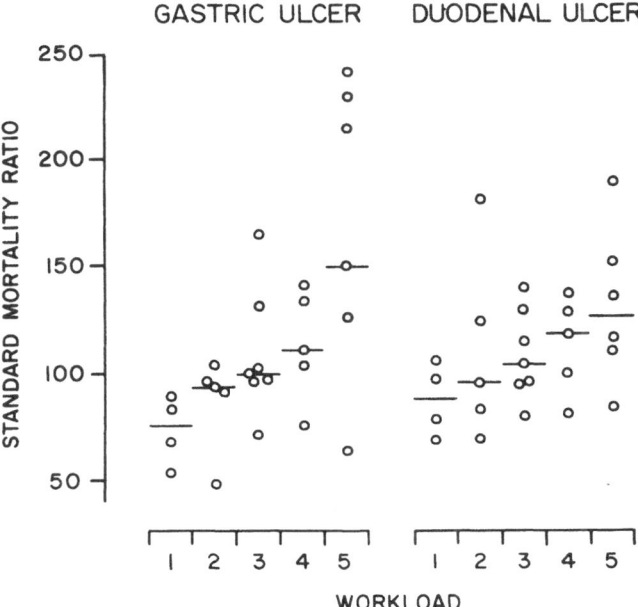

Figure 1.10 Standardized mortality ratio from gastric and duodenal ulcer plotted against workload of different occupations assigned a rank value between 1 (low) and 5 (high). Reproduced with permission from Ref. 58

less clear-cut for gastric ulcer, where additional factors associated with social class seemed to be in operation.

The joint effect of occupation and nationality on the prevalence of gastric and duodenal ulcer was studied in 73 000 active members of the German workforce who were considered healthy at the time of a medical interview conducted by occupational health authorities[59]. Gastric but not duodenal ulcer were found more frequently in migrant than in indigenous workers. Manual workers were more prone to develop gastric and duodenal ulcer and non-ulcer dyspepsia than sedentary workers. The seemingly increased prevalence of duodenal ulcer in migrant workers observed by other authors[78–81] might be owing to migrant workers having been employed predominantly as blue-collar workers, a factor which, according to this study carried a two-fold risk of contracting duodenal ulcer and a 1.5-fold risk of contracting gastric ulcer.

Several mechanisms are conceivable by which increased energy expenditure could lead to peptic ulcer disease. Physical stress alone has been reported to affect gastric secretion. Gastric basal acid secretion was studied during exercise and restitution in patients with duodenal ulcer disease and in healthy subjects[60]. In duodenal ulcer patients, exercise significantly increased acid output as compared to pre-exercise and restitution period[60]. No such exercise-induced increase was found in healthy subjects[61]. In contrast, Øktedalen and coworkers[62] reported that also in healthy subjects basal acid and pepsin output were three-fold increased after a 4-day period of physical stress as experienced during a military training program. It seems that physical exercise *per se* stimulates acid secretion. The stimulation may be more marked in subjects susceptible to develop duodenal ulcer. On the other hand, in order to maintain a balanced energy turnover, increased occupational energy expenditure must be met with an increased food consumption. A steady increase in food consumption (not just a temporary one as in gaining weight) may also induce structural changes in the upper gastrointestinal tract which could predispose to the development of duodenal ulcer, such as an increased capacity to generate acid.

DIETARY SALT CONSUMPTION

In our own studies the relationship between energy expenditure and ulcer disease showed to be more obvious for duodenal than for gastric ulcer. The similar birth-cohort pattern of both diseases, however, indicates that the temporal changes of both ulcer types are related to the same environmental agent, namely occupational workload. It was speculated that in gastric ulcer, factors additional to workload must play a role. Increased food consumption could be associated with increased consumption of some nutritional toxin leading to an increased vulnerability of the gastric mucosa. Epidemiologic studies have shown that dietary salt is a risk factor for gastric cancer, possibly by leading to chronic gastritis and intestinal metaplasia. Gastritis is also known to be a predisposing factor for gastric ulceration. The peculiar history of salt consumption resembles many aspects of the secular trends of gastric ulceration. Salt was a precious and highly-taxed commodity throughout the Middle Ages and the Renaissance[63,64]. Only after the French Revolution were the high state taxes on salt abolished or markedly reduced, and only since then did salt become available to all sections of the population. Latterly, refrigeration has replaced salting as a means of food preservation, and there has been a corresponding general decline in salt consumption.

To substantiate the suspected relationship between salt consumption and gastric ulcer, the literature was searched for reports that could confirm this hypothesis. In addition, data from the vital statistics and industry reports on gross national salt production were checked with regard to a possible relationship between salt consumption and gastric ulcer. Since mortality from cerebrovascular diseases is known to be partly related to hypertension and salt consumption, it was used as an additional epidemiologic marker for temporal and geographic variations of salt consumption. Mortality from cerebrovascular diseases is easy to diagnose and in most instances does not require elaborate techniques. The disease entity is hardly likely to be miscoded. It was introduced into the International Classification of Death (ICD) even before gastric and duodenal ulcer were listed as separate entities in 1921. It occurs quite frequently so that its large number of deaths gives a good estimate of its true incidence.

Stemmermann and coworkers[65] analysed the risk of gastric ulcer among Japanese from Hawaii in a case control study. The authors found a strong association between salt intake, gastric ulcer, and gastric metaplasia in 133 patients with gastric ulcer as compared to 244 controls. Salt was shown to be capable of inducing gastritis in experimental animals[66]. The epidemiologic relationship between mortality from gastric cancer and cerebrovascular diseases lends further evidence to the contention that salt consumption affects the gastric mucosa[67,68]. The geographic and temporal variations in the amount of urinary salt excretion are significantly correlated to those of mortality from gastric cancer[67,69,70], and within countries like Japan and England, regions with a high mortality from gastric cancer also show a conspicuously high mortality from cerebrovascular diseases[66,70]. In agreement with the temporal changes of gastric ulcer disease, the incidence of cerebrovascular disease and gastric cancer has declined in most countries during the past 20–30 years[67,69,71].

Close epidemiologic relationships are found between gastric ulcer on one hand, and gastric cancer and cerebrovascular disease on the other[67,72,73]. As with temporal variation, the geographic pattern of all three diseases varies in a parallel manner. There are significant linear regressions between the mortalities from any two of these diseases among different countries (Figures 1.11 and 1.12). In accordance with these relationships, significant linear regressions also exist between the geographic variation of each disease and salt consumption[73] (Figure 1.12). It is noteworthy that none of these epidemiologic relationships, however, applies to duodenal ulcer. Gastric cancer and gastric ulcer occur more frequently in patients with hypertensive diseases than could be expected from the overall distribution of the three diseases[74]. Again, duodenal ulcer was not associated with an increased risk for any disease related to hypertension.

Kang and coworkers[75] measured 24-hour urinary salt excretion in 24 and 13 patients with gastric and duodenal ulcer respectively, and compared their values with equal numbers of age- and sex-matched controls. No difference was found between ulcer patients and controls. At first sight, this finding seems to contradict the results presented above. However, urinary salt excretion needs to be measured over 7 days to give a reliable picture of salt intake. A group of 24 patients was too small to test the association between salt and gastric ulcer. Lastly, the salt consumption at the time of the ulcer did not necessarily reflect the dietary salt consumption that favoured the development of gastritis and ulceration anywhere between 1 to 20 years ago.

A hypertonic solution of 1mM sodium chloride is frequently used as a simple

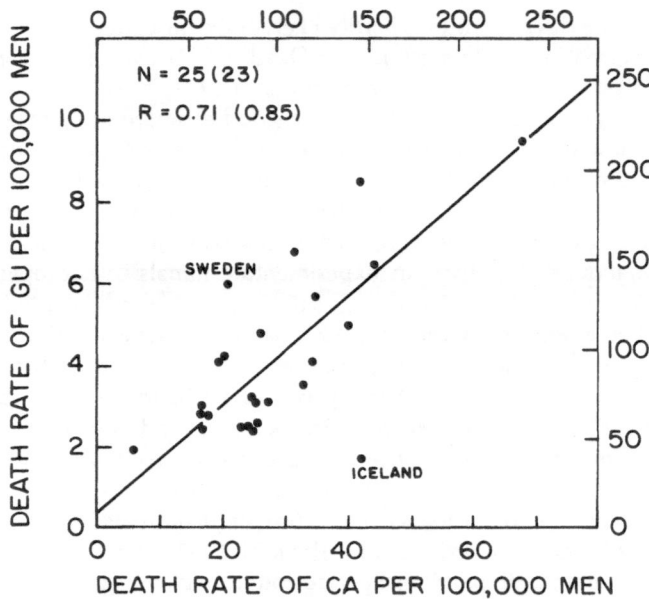

Figure 1.11 Correlation of death rates from gastric cancer (CA) with death rates from gastric ulcer (GU). Each point represents the annual average of 1971–1975 from one country. The age distribution of the total population from all 25 countries was used as the standard for age adjustment of the different countries according to the method of direct (lower and right axis) and indirect standardization (upper and right axis). Figures in parentheses refer to correlation without Sweden and Iceland

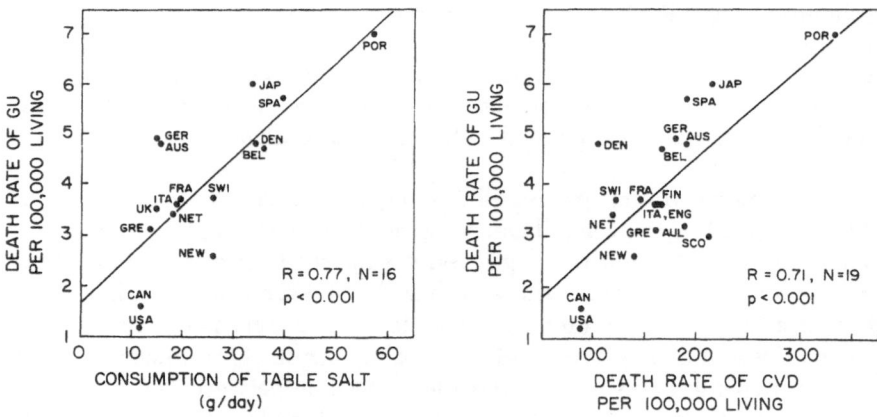

Figure 1.12 Correlation of death rates from gastric ulcer (GU) with average daily consumption of food grade salt (left) and death rates from cerebrovascular disease (CVD, right). Each point represents the annual average of 1971–1975 from one country. Reproduced with permission from Ref. 73

measure to disrupt the gastric mucosa in scientific experiments[76]. Salt is not ingested at such high concentrations in foodstuff, but becomes rapidly diluted by gastric juice. Nevertheless, some localized areas of the stomach may encounter unduly high concentrations of salt for short periods after a meal. Chronic ingestion of highly-salted food could increase the likelihood of localized damage. Disruption of the superficial cells may facilitate the entry of other nutritional toxins into the gastric mucosa. This type of challenge to the gastric mucosa once or several times daily over several years may eventually lead to gastritis and intestinal metaplasia[65,77]. Intestinalized gastric mucosa shows increased susceptibility to malignant transformation. Gastritis is also known to predispose the mucosa to gastric ulceration[78-83]. It probably renders the mucosa more vulnerable to the corrosive action of acid. Since gastritis appears to be the determinant mechanism in the pathogenesis of both gastric ulcer and gastric cancer, this could form the basis of the epidemiologic association between gastric ulcer and gastric cancer (Figure 1.11). The model does not preclude the etiologic influence of other environmental factors claimed to play a role in the pathogenesis of gastritis, gastric ulcer, and gastric cancer, respectively. For instance, the colonization and growth of bacteria possibly leading to gastritis[84,85] and nitrosation[86] may be facilitated by these mechanisms.

SMOKING AS RISK FACTOR FOR ULCER DISEASE

In addition to workload and salt consumption the influence of other environmental factors was tested. Initially cigarette consumption appeared to be a likely candidate for precipitating the cohort pattern of ulcer disease, since it occurs worldwide, is a habit acquired at a young age, and is continued for a lifetime. As will be shown below, cigarette smoking has actually decreased according to a birth-cohort risk, but the cohort pattern is different from that of peptic ulcer disease. The prevalence of gastric and duodenal ulcer is increased two-fold in smokers compared with non-smokers[87,88]. Smoking delays ulcer healing and favours ulcer relapse[89-91], and mortality from peptic ulcer is higher in smokers than non-smokers[92,93]. In clinical trials, non-smoking proved as effective in healing acute duodenal ulcer and preventing ulcer relapse as intake of H_2-receptor antagonists[90,91]. While both ulcer types are unfavourably affected by smoking, duodenal ulcer is more sensitive to nicotine consumption than gastric ulcer[94-96].

For a cohort analysis of cigarette smoking, the United Kingdom showed to have the best statistics dealing with cigarette consumption covering the whole period since the beginning of cigarette consumption about 100 years ago[97]. Estimates of male and female cigarette consumption for each five-year age group in each year during the period 1890–1975 and 1972–1982 were taken

21

from the Tobacco Research Council in England and the British Office of Population Censuses and Surveys (OPCS). An index of the average deliveries of tar and nicotine of cigarettes manufactured in the United Kingdom since 1934 had been studied by Wald and coworkers[98]. A table of the age-specific annual numbers of cigarettes consumed per adult male and female during each year of the period 1890–1979 was then used to accumulate consumption per lifetime for the various birth-cohorts. Using the average deliveries of tar and nicotine per cigarette for each year since 1934, cumulative cigarette consumption was also converted to consumption of constant tar and constant nicotine cigarettes. Cumulative cigarette consumption increased in all male cohorts born between 1845 and 1915 and remained constant for all subsequent birth-cohorts. Cumulative cigarette consumption based on constant tar or constant nicotine cigarettes showed a peak for men born around 1915 (Figure 1.13). In women, cumulative cigarette consumption in terms of total cigarettes, constant tar cigarettes, or constant nicotine cigarettes increased for all cohorts born between 1835 and 1955. In both men and women from the United Kingdom, mortality from gastric and duodenal ulcer was highest in the cohorts born around 1885. Thus, from the lack of coincidence of the peaks of peptic ulcer mortality and cumulative cigarette consumption, it must be concluded that cigarette consumption is not responsible for the birth-cohort patterns of the death rates from gastric and duodenal ulcer.

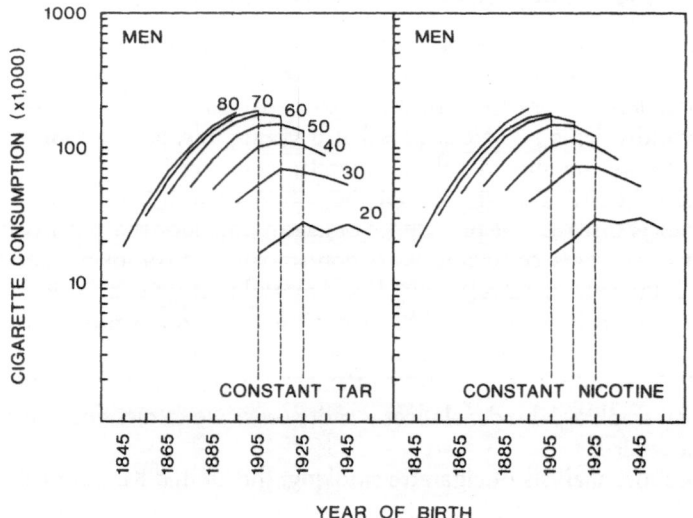

Figure 1.13 Cohort-age contours of cumulative cigarette consumption in terms of constant tar cigarettes and constant nicotine cigarettes in men from the United Kingdom. Calculation was based on tar and nicotine deliveries published by Wald et al.[98]

ASPIRIN AND OTHER NON-STEROIDAL ANTI-INFLAMMATORY DRUGS (NSAIDs)

Chronic consumption of aspirin increases the risk of contracting gastric ulcer five- to ten-fold compared to controls[99–104]. In 17 per cent of patients under long-term treatment with aspirin for rheumatic disease, upper gastrointestinal endoscopy revealed gastric ulceration[104]. The risk for duodenal ulcer is only slightly increased by chronic aspirin intake[88]. There is evidence that NSAIDs other than aspirin increase the risk for gastric ulcer by a factor of two. Older patients seem particularly susceptible to gastric perforation during chronic ingestion of NSAIDs[105,106]. The reason for the increased risk at higher ages is unknown but it might be owing to the age-related increase in gastritis[107] and the underlying cohort phenomenon. Aspirin, however, cannot be held responsible for the birth-cohort pattern. The first bottle of aspirin was purchased in Germany only in 1899. The decline in gastric ulcer and its geographic distribution are not matched by parallel changes in aspirin consumption.

ALCOHOL CONSUMPTION AND DIETARY FIBRE

Acute exposure of the stomach to concentrated solutions of alcohol disrupts mucosal defences and induces haemorrhagic erosions. Such findings in the experimental animal, however, do not necessarily apply to repeated ingestion of alcoholic beverages in man. Repeated exposures to mild irritants increase the resistance of the gastric mucosa to subsequent exposures to strong irritants[108]. In evaluating the effect of alcohol consumption, moderate drinking must be differentiated from heavy drinking leading to liver cirrhosis. Liver cirrhosis itself, irrespective of its etiology, appears to predispose to both ulcer types[109–111]. Westlund[112] and Bonnevie[113] found a higher prevalence of liver cirrhosis in ulcer patients than in the general population. Other studies which ascribed an unfavourable effect to alcohol consumption used subjects who consumed more than 60 g alcohol per day[114]. On the other hand, if the effect of moderate consumption was assessed separately, no effect or even beneficial effects on ulcer prevalence and healing were observed[90,91,103,115].

Dietary fibre has been claimed to promote ulcer healing and to prevent ulcer recurrences[17,18,116]. The results of clinical trials have not been convincingly supportive of this hypothesis[117,118]. The evolution of industrial food processing has led to a decrease in dietary intake of fibre. Since the decrease occurred simultaneously with the decline in ulcer prevalence, dietary fibre cannot play an important role in the epidemiology of peptic ulcer disease.

A UNIFIED THEORY OF PEPTIC ULCER DISEASE

The interaction of the two risk factors, workload and salt, in the pathogenesis of peptic ulcer is summarized in Figure 1.14. In order to maintain thermodynamic equilibrium, increased workload must be met with increased food intake. In some occupations, such as in coal miners and foundry workers, increased workload is also related to high rates of sweating and salt losses being replaced by salty food. Salty food may also result from dietary habits, such as in fish-eating countries, where salt is frequently used for food preservation. Physical stress alone or structural changes associated with chronically high food intake increase gastric acid secretion and further the development of duodenal ulcer. This may occur in all persons or only in those responsive to this kind of stimulus. Dietary consumption of salt independently of, or in conjunction

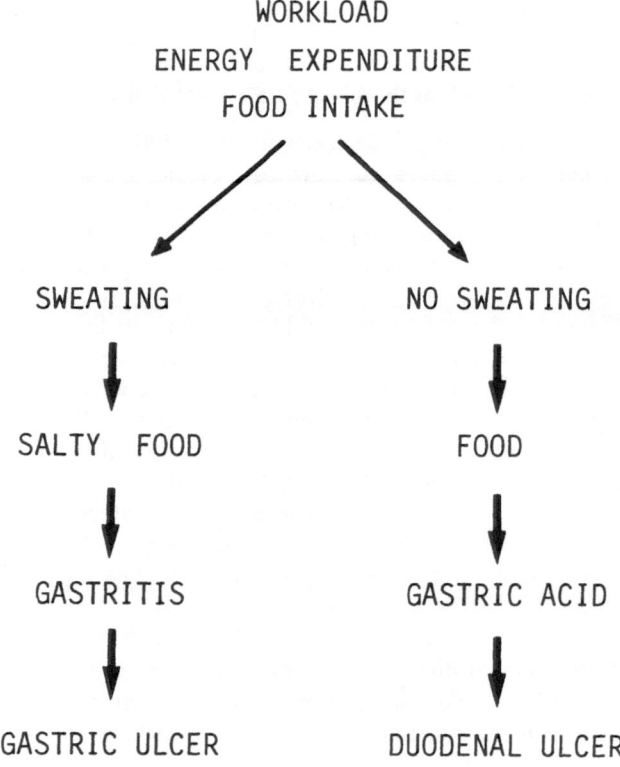

Figure 1.14 Model for the interaction of workload and dietary salt as risk factors for gastric and duodenal ulcer

with, high occupational workload and sweating leads to gastritis and gastric ulceration.

The onset of environmental influence before the age of 15 years in gastric and duodenal ulcer fits into this model. Dietary habits like adding salt are adopted at a rather young age. The picture is completed when one realises that from the late 19th century until the First World War, children entered the workforce at the age of 10–14 years and even until the 1950s, a large fraction of the population started gainful work at the age of 14–15 years.

This model helps to explain several characteristic features of ulcer epidemiology. Duodenal ulcer used to occur more frequently in urban than in rural communities[55], since factories and heavy industry were located in the townships. The amount of acid output being proportional to body weight, men secrete more acid than women. The higher portion of men than women being involved in occupations demanding physical stress probably adds to the high male incidence of duodenal ulcer. During the past decades the male/female ratio of duodenal ulcer dropped from 4/1 to 2/1[119], reflecting the evening-out in the lifestyles and types of occupations of the two sexes. The 'ulcer facies' described by former clinicians to be typical of duodenal ulcer patients probably relates to the lean lineaments of hard-working people. The beneficial effect of hospitalization on ulcer healing is based on abstinence from physical work and energy expenditure[120–122]. The seasonal fluctuations in ulcer relapse which became less obvious in present times followed similar fluctuations in workload. Some industries, such as building, pause in winter. In former times, workload started to increase as daylight grew longer during spring. In other industries, such as agriculture, maximum workload occurs in autumn. The dip of ulcer incidence reported nowadays during summer relates to the time of vacation[123–125].

In gastric ulcer the male/female ratio has dropped from 2/1 to 1/1[119,121]. The mean age of patients with gastric ulcer is 60 years, that is 10–20 years older than in duodenal ulcer. This difference is probably owing to the time it takes for gastritis to develop. The reduction in dietary intake of salt resulted in a general decline of ulcer prevalence and in longer time-spans for the development of gastritis. In conjunction with the cohort phenomenon, the age of those affected by gastric ulceration became shifted towards older age groups. In addition to the decline of gastric ulcer, the decline in salt consumption also led to a decline in gastric cancer. Although it has been unequivocally shown that benign gastric ulcers do not turn into gastric cancer, gastritis forms a common basis for both diseases, hence the higher chances of developing cancer of the gastric remnant after partial gastrectomy for gastric than for duodenal ulcer[127–131].

SUMMARY

Thus far, epidemiology of peptic ulcer disease has been able to unravel four distinct environmental risk factors for peptic ulcer disease. While aspirin and salt challenge the gastric mucosa, smoking and workload mainly promote ulceration of the duodenal mucosa. The distinction between gastric and duodenal risk factors, however, does not represent an absolute distinction, since each of the four risk factors affects both mucosae. Circumstantial evidence suggests that workload exerts its effect by increasing acid secretion and that salt acts by favouring the development of gastritis. The mechanism of aspirin and smoking is still an enigma. Although both factors have been shown to reduce mucosal prostaglandin synthesis, this may be neither the only nor the decisive link to the pathophysiology of ulcer disease. Both factors also reduce mucosal blood flow and alter bicarbonate secretion. Changes in exposure to these environmental risk factors explain many of the epidemiologic and clinical features of peptic ulcer disease. It still remains to be shown how these environmental factors interact with the pathophysiology of peptic ulcer disease at the mucosal, cellular and subcellular levels.

ACKNOWLEDGEMENT

This work was supported by grant # So 172/1-1 from the Deutsche Forschungsgemeinschaft.

REFERENCES

1. Sonnenberg, A. (1985). Geographic and temporal variations in the occurrence of peptic ulcer disease. *Scand. J. Gastroenterol.*, **20**, (Suppl. 110), 11–24
2. Elashoff, J.D. and Grossman, M.I. (1975). Trends in hospital admissions and death rates for peptic ulcer in the United States from 1970 to 1978. *Gastroenterology*, **68**, 280–5
3. Hoogendoorn, D. (1984). Interesting changes of the epidemiological pattern of peptic ulcer. *Ned. Tijschr. Geneeskd.*, **128**, 484–91
4. Kurata, J.H. and Haile, B.M. (1982). Racial differences in peptic ulcer disease: fact or myth? *Gastroenterology*, **83**, 162–72
5. Fineberg, H.V. and Pearlman, L.A. (1981). Surgical treatment of peptic ulcer in the United States. Trends before and after the introduction of cimetidine. *Lancet*, **i**, 1305–7
6. Smith, M.P. (1977). Decline in duodenal ulcer surgery. *J. Am. Med. Assoc.*, **237**, 987–8
7. Vogt, T.M. and Johnson, R.E. (1980). Recent changes in the incidence of duodenal and gastric ulcer. *Am. J. Epidemiol.*, **111**, 713–20
8. Sonnenberg, A. (1987). Changes in physician visits for gastric and duodenal ulcer in the United States during 1958–1984 as shown by the National Disease and Therapeutic Index (NDTI). *Dig. Dis. Sci.*, **32**, 1–7
9. Coggon, D., Lambert, P. and Langman, M.J.S. (1981). 20 years of hospital admissions for peptic ulcer in England and Wales. *Lancet*, **i**, 1302–4
10. Wylie, C.M. (1981). The complex wane of peptic ulcer. I. Recent national trends in deaths and hospital care in the United States. *J. Clin. Gastroenterol.*, **3**, 327–32
11. Kurata, J.H., Elashoff, J.D., Haile, B.M. and Honda, G.D. (1983). A reappraisal of time trends in ulcer disease: Factors related to changes in ulcer hospitalization and mortality rates. *Am. J. Publ. Health*, **79**, 1066–72
12. Ishimori, A. and Kawamura, T. (1979). Epidemiology of peptic ulcer disease in Japan. In

26

Fisher, RS (ed.) *Peptic Ulcer Disease: An Update*, pp. 153–64. (New York: Biomedical Information Corporation Publications)

13. Kurata, J.H., Honda, G.D. and Frankl, H. (1985). The incidence of duodenal and gastric ulcers in a large health maintenance organization. *Am. J. Publ. Health*, **75**, 625–9
14. Litton, A. and Murdoch, W.R. (1963). Peptic ulcer in south-west Scotland. *Gut*, **4**, 360–6
15. Dunlop, J.M. (1968). Peptic ulcer in central Scotland. *Scott. Med. J.*, **13**, 192–201
16. Sonnenberg, A., Arnold, R. and Fritsch, A. (1982). Epidemiologie und Genetik der Ulcuskrankheit. In Blum, A.L. and Siewert, J.R. (eds) *Ulcus-Therapie*, pp. 3–22. (Berlin, Heidelberg, New York: Springer)
17. Tovey, F. (1975). Duodenal ulcer in Black populations in Africa south of the Sahara. *Gut*, **16**, 564–76
18. Tovey, F. (1979). Peptic ulcer in India and Bangladesh. *Gut*, **20**, 239–47
19. Sonnenberg, A. (1987). Causative factors in the etiology of peptic ulcer disease become effective before the age of 15 years. *J. Chronic Dis.*, **40**, 193–202
20. Langman, M.J.S. (1979). *The Epidemiology of Chronic Digestive Disease*. (London: Edward Arnold Publishers)
21. Kahn, H.A. (1983). *An Introduction to Epidemiologic Methods*, pp. 63–78. (New York: Oxford University Press)
22. Jennings, D. (1940). Perforated peptic ulcer. Changes in age-incidence and sex-distribution during the last 150 years (parts 1 and 2). *Lancet*, **i**, 395–8 and 444–7
23. Susser, M. and Stein, Z. (1962). Civilization and peptic ulcer. *Lancet*, **i**, 115–19
24. Susser, M. (1982). Period effects, generation effects and age effects in peptic ulcer mortality. *J. Chronic Dis.*, **35**, 29–40
25. Sonnenberg, A. (1984). The occurrence of a cohort phenomenon in peptic ulcer mortality from Switzerland. *Gastroenterology*, **86**, 398–401
26. Sonnenberg, A., Müller, H. and Pace, F. (1985). Birth-cohort analysis of peptic ulcer mortality in Europe. *J. Chronic Dis.*, **38**, 309–17
27. Sonnenberg, A. and Müller, H. (1984). Cohort and period effects in peptic ulcer mortality from Japan. *J. Chronic Dis.*, **37**, 699–704
28. Monson, R.R. and MacMahon, B. (1969). Peptic ulcer in Massachusetts physicians. *N. Engl. J. Med.*, **281**, 11–15
29. Sonnenberg, A. and Fritsch, A. (1983). Changing mortality of peptic ulcer disease in Germany. *Gastroenterology*, **84**, 1553–7
30. Bonnevie, O. (1975). The incidence of gastric ulcer in Copenhagen County. *Scand. J. Gastroenterol.*, **10**, 231–9
31. Bonnevie, O. (1975). The incidence of gastric ulcer in Copenhagen County. *Scand. J. Gastroenterol.*, **10**, 385–93
32. Sonnenberg, A. (1985). Disability pensions due to peptic ulcer in Germany between 1953 and 1983. *Am. J. Epidemiol.*, **122**, 106–11
33. Richardson, T.C. (1985). Pathogenetic factors in peptic ulcer disease. *Am. J. Med.*, **75**, Suppl. 2C, 1–7
34. MacMahon, B. and Pugh, T.F. (1970). *Epidemiology – Principles and Methods*, pp. 184–98. (Boston: Little, Brown & Co.)
35. Passmore, R. and Draper, M.H. (1965). Energy metabolism. In Albanese, AA (ed.) *Newer Methods of Nutritional Biochemistry*, pp. 41–83. (New York: Academic Press)
36. Kuczynski, J. (1961–1971). *Die Geschichte der Lage der Arbeiter unter dem Kapitalismus. Teil I. Die Geschichte der Lage der Arbeiter in Deutschland von 1789 bis zur Gegenwart*, Vols. 1–4. (Berlin, East Germany: Akademie Verlag)
37. Thomson, D. (1983). *England in the Nineteenth Century 1815–1914*. (Harmondsworth, England: Penguin Books Ltd.)
38. Sonnenberg, A., Sonnenberg, G.S. and Wirths, W. (1987). Historic changes of occupational workload and mortality from peptic ulcer in Germany. *J. Occup. Med.*, **28**, 756–61
39. Wirths, W. (1965). Veränderungen der Arbeitsbedingungen aus arbeits- und ernährungsphysiologischer Sicht. *Ernährungs-Umschau*, **12**, 29–35
40. Wirths, W., Keller, W. and Kraut, H. (1966). Work and food. *Nutr. Dieta.*, **8**, 168–78

41. Kraut, H., Kofranyi, E., Mohr, E. and Wirths, W. (1981). *Der Nahrungsbedarf des Menschen*. Vol. 1. pp. 68–117. (Darmstadt, West Germany: Dr Dietrich Steinkopf Verlag)
42. Nasiry, R. and Piper, D.W. (1983). Social aspects of chronic duodenal ulcer. A case control study. *Digestion*, **27**, 196–202
43. Würsch, T.G., Hess, H., Walser, R., *et al.* (1978). Die Epidemiologie des Ulcus duodeni. Untersuchungen an 1105 Patienten in Zürich. *Dtsch. Med. Wschr.*, **103**, 613–19
44. Horn, J. and Herfarth, C. (1978). Das Gastarbeiterulkus. *Med. Klin.*, **173**, 1417–21
45. Quaquish, I., Burkhardt, H.U. and Heilmann, K.L. (1979). Magenerkrankungen bei ausländischen Arbeitnehmern in der Bundesrepublick Deutschland. *Münch. Med. Wschr.*, **121**, 1563–5
46. Schmid, E., Vollmer, K., Allmendinger, G., Blaich, E. and Hofgärtner, F. (1984). Epidemiologische Resultate der endoskopischen Untersuchungen beim Ulcus ventriculi und duodeni. *Med. Welt*, **35**, 281–5
47. Lewis, J.H. (1942). *The Biology of the Negro*, p. 307. (Chicago: University of Chicago Press)
48. Jennison, J. (1938). Observations made on a group of employees with duodenal ulcer. *Am. J. Med. Sci.*, **196**, 654–62
49. Duesberg, R. (1938). Ulcus ad pylorum und Arbeitspause – Statistische Erhebungen. *Med. Welt*, **12**, 595–7
50. Schellong, I. (1937). Die Häufigkeit der Magengeschwürserkrankung bei den (ostpr.) Bauarbeitern und ihre soziale Bedeutung. *Z. Ärztl. Fortb.*, **34**, 245–51
51. Sallström, T. (1945). Regarding occupational factors in gastric ulcer and duodenal ulcer. *Acta Med. Scand.*, **120**, 340–8
52. Rietschel, E. (1978). Magen-Zwölffingerdarmgeschwüre und Arbeitswelt (Felduntersuchung in einem Großbetrieb). *Arbeitsmed. Präventivmed. Sozialmed.*, **13**, 197–201
53. Ihre, J.E. and Müller, R. (1943). Gastric and duodenal ulcer. Study of 1193 cases collected during 1930 to 1940 in Stockholm. *Acta Med. Scand.*, **116**, 33–57
54. Doll, R., Avery Jones, F. and Buckatzsch, M.M. (1951). *Occupational Factors in the Etiology of Gastric and Duodenal Ulcers with an Estimate of their Incidence in the General Population*, pp. 1–96. (London: HMSO)
55. Pulvertaft, C.N. (1968). Comments on the incidence and natural history of gastric and duodenal ulcers. *Postgrad. Med. J.*, **44**, 597–602
56. Emery, Jr, E.S. and Monroe, R.T. (1935). Peptic ulcer. Nature and treatment based on a study of one thousand, four hundred and thirty-five cases. *Arch. Int. Med.*, **55**, 271–92
57. Sonnenberg, A. and Sonnenberg, G.S. (1986). Occupational factors in disability pensions for gastric and duodenal ulcer. *J. Occup. Med.*, **28**, 87–90
58. Sonnenberg, A. and Sonnenberg, G.S. (1986). Occupational mortality from gastric and duodenal ulcer. *Br. J. Ind. Med.*, **43**, 50–5
59. Sonnenberg, A. and Haas, J. (1986). The joint effect of occupation and nationality on the prevalence of peptic ulcer in German workers. *Br. J. Ind. Med.*, **43**, 490–3
60. Markiewicz, K., Cholewa, M. and Lukin, M. (1979). Gastric basal secretion during exercise and restitution in patients with chronic duodenal ulcer. *Hepato-Gastroenterol.*, **26**, 160–5
61. Markiewicz, K., Cholewa, M., Gorski, L. and Chmura, J. (1977). Effect of physical exercise on gastric basal secretion in healthy men. *Hepato-Gastroenterol.*, **24**, 377–80
62. Øktedalen, O., Guldvog, I., Opstad, P.K., Berstad, A., Gedde-Dahl, E. and Jorde, R. (1984). The effect of physical stress on gastric secretion and pancreatic polypeptide levels in man. *Scand. J. Gastroenterol.*, **19**, 770–8
63. Seidel, H. and Woller, R. (1980). *Das Geschenk der Erde. Vom Salz zur modernen Chemie*, pp. 71–6. (Düsseldorf, West Germany: Econ Verlag)
64. Denton, D. (1982). *The Hunger for Salt*, pp. 76–90. (New York: Springer-Verlag)
65. Stemmermann, G., Haenszel, W. and Locke, F. (1977). Epidemiologic pathology of gastric ulcer and gastric carcinoma among Japanese in Hawaii. *J. Natl. Cancer Inst.*, **58**, 13–19
66. Sato, T., Fukuyama, T., Suzuki, T., Takayanagi, J., Murakami, T., Shiotsuki, N., Tanaka, R. and Tsuji, R. (1959). Studies of the causation of gastric cancer. 2. The relation between gastric cancer mortality rate and salted food intake in several places in Japan. *Bull. Inst. Publ. Health*, **8**, 187–98
67. Joossens, J.V. (1980). Stroke, stomach cancer and salt. In Kesteloot, H. and Joossens, J.V.

(eds) *Epidemiology of Arterial Blood Pressure*, pp. 489–508. (The Hague: Martinus Nijhoff Publishers)
68. Whelton, P.K. and Goldblatt, P. (1982). An investigation of the relationship between stomach cancer and cerebrovascular disease. *Am. J. Epidemiol.*, **115**, 418–27
69. Joossens, J.V. and Geboers, J. (1981). Nutrition and gastric cancer. *Nutr. Cancer*, **2**, 250–61
70. Joossens, J.V. (1980). Dietary salt restriction – The case in favour. In Robertson, J.I.S., Pickering, G.W. and Caldwell, A.D.S. (eds) *The Therapeutics of Hypertension*, Royal Society of Medicine Series No. 26. pp. 243–50. (London: Academic Press)
71. Tuomilehto, J., Geboers, J., Joossens, J.V., Salonen, J.T. and Tanskanen, T. (1984). Trends in stomach cancer and stroke in Finland. Comparison to northwest Europe and USA. *Stroke*, **15**, 823–8
72. Segi, M., Fujisaku, S. and Kurihara, M. (1959). Mortality for gastric and duodenal ulcer in countries and its geographical correlation to mortality for gastric and intestinal cancer. *Schweiz. Z. Path. Bakt.*, **22**, 777–84
73. Sonnenberg, A. (1986). Dietary salt and gastric ulcer. *Gut*, **27**, 1138–42
74. Sonnenberg, A. (1987). Gastric cancer, gastric ulcer, and hypertensive diseases – A common epidemiologic risk factor? (Abstr.) *Gastroenterology*, **92**, 1649
75. Kang, J.Y., Canalese, J., Ellard, K., Ng, J. and Piper, D.W. (1980). Urinary salt excretion in peptic ulcer patients. *Aust. N.Z. J. Med.*, **10**, 682
76. Svanes, K., Ito, S., Takeushi, K. and Silen, W. (1982). Restitution of the surface epithelium of the *in vitro* frog gastric mucosa after damage with hyperosmolar sodium chloride. *Gastroenterology*, **82**, 1409–26
77. Haenszel, W., Kurihara, M., Segi, M. and Lee, R.K.C (1972). Stomach cancer among Japanese in Hawaii. *J. Natl. Cancer Inst.*, **49**, 969–88
78. Du Plessis, D.J. (1965). Pathogenesis of gastric ulceration. *Lancet*, **i**, 974–8
79. Oi, M., Ito, Y., Kumagai, F., Yoshida, K., Tanaka, Y., Yoshikawa, K., Miho, O. and Kijima, M. (1969). A possible dual control mechanism in the origin of peptic ulcer. A study on ulcer location as affected by mucosa and musculature. *Gastroenterology*, **57**, 280–3
80. Gear, M.W.L., Truelove, S.C. and Whitehead, R. (1971). Gastric ulcer and gastritis. *Gut*, **12**, 639–45
81. Stadelmann, O., Elster, K., Stolte, M., Miederer, S.E., Deyhle, P., Demling, L. and Siegenthaler, W. (1971). The peptic gastric ulcer – histotopography and functional investigations. *Scand. J. Gastroenterol.*, **4**, 613–21
82. Tatsuta, M. and Okuda, S. (1975). Location, healing, and recurrence of gastric ulcers in relation to fundal gastritis. *Gastroenterology*, **69**, 897–902
83. Tatsuta, M., Iishi, H. and Okuda, S. (1986). Location of peptic ulcers in relation to antral and fundic gastritis by chromoendoscopic follow-up examinations. *Dig. Dis. Sci.*, **31**, 7–11
84. Marshall, B.J. and Warren, J.R. (1984). Unidentified curved bacilli in the stomach of patients with gastritis and peptic ulceration. *Lancet*, **i**, 1311–14
85. Editorial (1984). Campylobacters in Ottawa. *Lancet*, **ii**, 135
86. Rudell, W.S.J., Bone, E.S., Hill, M.J. and Walters, C.L. (1978). Pathogenesis of gastric cancer in pernicious anemia. *Lancet*, **i**, 521–3
87. Friedman, G.D., Siegelaub, A.B. and Seltzer, C.C. (1974). Cigarettes, alcohol, coffee and peptic ulcer. *N. Engl. J. Med.*, **290**, 469–73
88. Piper, D.W., Nasiry, R., McIntosh, J., Shy, C.M., Pierce, J. and Byth, K. (1984). Smoking, alcohol, analgesics, and chronic duodenal ulcer. *Scand. J. Gastroenterol.*, **19**, 1015–21
89. Korman, M.G., Shaw, R.G., Hansky, J., Schmidt, G.T. and Stern, A.I. (1981). Influence of smoking on healing rate of duodenal ulcer in response to cimetidine or high-dose antacid. *Gastroenterology*, **80**, 1451–3
90. Sonnenberg, A., Müller-Lissner, S.A., Vogel, E., Schmid, E., Gonvers, J.J., Peter, P., Strohmeyer, G. and Blum, A.L. (1981). Predictors of duodenal ulcer healing and relapse. *Gastroenterology*, **81**, 1061–7
91. Sontag, S., Graham, D.Y., Belsito, A., *et al.* (1984). Cimetidine, cigarette smoking, and recurrence of duodenal ulcer. *N. Engl. J. Med.*, **311**, 689–93

29

92. Heuman, R., Larsson, J. and Norrby, S. (1983). Perforated duodenal ulcer – long-term results of following simple closure. *Acta Chir. Scand.*, **149**, 77–81
93. McLean Ross, A.G., Smith, M.A., Anderson, J.R. and Small, W.P. (1982). Late mortality after surgery for peptic ulcer. *N. Engl. J. Med.*, **307**, 519–22
94. Doll, R., Jones, F.A. and Pygott, F. (1958). Effect of smoking on the production and maintenance of gastric and duodenal ulcers. *Lancet*, **i**, 657–62
95. Piper, D.W., Hunt, J. and Heap, T.R. (1980). The healing rate of chronic gastric ulcer in patients admitted to hospital. *Scand. J. Gastroenterol.*, **15**, 113–17
96. Okada, M., Yao, T., Fuchigami, T., Imamura, K. and Omae, T. (1984). Factors influencing the healing rate of gastric ulcer in hospitalised subjects. *Gut*, **25**, 881–5
97. Sonnenberg, A. (1986). Smoking and mortality from peptic ulcer in the United Kingdom. *Gut*, **27**, 1369–72
98. Wald, N., Doll, R. and Copeland, G. (1981). Trends in tar, nicotine, and carbon monoxide yields of UK cigarettes manufactured since 1934. *Br. Med. J.*, **282**, 763–5
99. Gillies, M.A. and Skyring, A. (1969). Gastric and duodenal ulcer – The association between aspirin ingestion, smoking and family history of ulcer. *Med. J. Aust.*, **2**, 280–5
100. Levy, M. (1974). Aspirin use in patients with major upper gastrointestinal bleeding and peptic-ulcer disease. *N. Engl. J. Med.*, **290**, 1158–62
101. McIntosh, J.H., Byth, K. and Piper, D.W. (1985). Environmental factors in aetiology of chronic gastric ulcer: a case control study of exposure variables before the first symptoms. *Gut*, **26**, 789–98
102. Piper, D.W., McIntosh, J.H., Ariotti, D.E., Fenton, B.H. and MacLennan, R. (1981). Analgesic ingestion and chronic peptic ulcer. *Gastroenterology*, **80**, 427–32
103. Piper, D.W., McIntosh, J.H., Greig, M. and Shy, C.M. (1982). Environmental factors and chronic gastric ulcer. A case control study of the association of smoking, alcohol, and heavy analgesic ingestion with the exacerbation of chronic gastric ulcer. *Scand. J. Gastroenterol.*, **17**, 721–9
104. Silvoso, G.R., Ivey, K.J., Butt, J.H., Lockard, O.O., Holt, S.D., Sisk, C., Baskin, W.N., Mackercher, P.A. and Hewett, J. (1979). Incidence of gastric lesions in patients with rheumatic disease on chronic aspirin therapy. *Ann. Int. Med.*, **91**, 517–20
105. Collier, D.S.J. and Pain, J.A. (1985). Non-steroidal anti-inflammatory drugs and peptic ulcer perforation. *Gut*, **26**, 359–63
106. Sommerville, K., Faulkner, G. and Langman, M.J.S. (1986). Non-steroidal anti-inflammatory drugs and bleeding peptic ulcer. *Lancet*, **i**, 462–4
107. Steinheber, F.C. (1985). Aging and the stomach. *Clin. Gastroenterol.*, **14**, 657–88
108. Robert, A. (1979). Cytoprotection by prostaglandins. *Gastroenterology*, **77**, 761–7
109. Swisher, W.P., Baker, L.A. and Bennett, H.D. (1955). Peptic ulcer in Laennec's cirrhosis. *Am. J. Dig. Dis.*, **22**, 291–4
110. Tabaqchali, S. and Dawson, A.M. (1964). Peptic ulcer and gastric secretion in patients with liver disease. *Gut*, **5**, 417–21
111. Kirk, A.P., Dooley, J.S. and Hunt, R.H. (1980). Peptic ulceration in patients with chronic liver disease. *Dig. Dis. Sci.*, **25**, 756–60
112. Westlund, K. (1963). Mortality of peptic ulcer patients. *Acta Med. Scand.*, **174**, (Suppl. 402), 1–110
113. Bonnevie, O. (1977). Causes of death in duodenal and gastric ulcer. *Gastroenterology*, **73**, 1000–4
114. Hagnell, O. and Wretmark, G. (1957). Peptic ulcer and alcoholism. A statistical study in frequency, behaviour, personality traits, and family occurrence. *J. Psychosomatic Res.*, **2**, 35–44
115. Piper, D.W., McIntosh, J. and Hudson, H.M. (1985). Factors relevant to the prognosis of chronic duodenal ulcer. *Digestion*, **31**, 9–16
116. Malhotra, S.L. (1978). A comparison of unrefined wheat and rice diets in the management of duodenal ulcer. *Postgrad. Med. J.*, **54**, 6–9
117. Rydning, A., Berstad, A., Aadland, E. and Odegaard, B. (1982). Prophylactic effect of dietary fibre in duodenal ulcer disease. *Lancet*, **ii**, 736–9
118. Rydning, A. and Berstad, A. (1985). Fibre diet and antacids in the short-term treatment of duodenal ulcer. *Scand. J. Gastroenterol.*, **20**, 1078–82

119. Kurata, J.H., Haile, B.M. and Elashoff, J.D. (1985). Sex differences in peptic ulcer disease. *Gastroenterology*, **88**, 96–100
120. Doll, R. and Pygott, F. (1952). Factors influencing the rate of healing of gastric ulcers. Admission to hospital, phenobarbitone, and ascorbic acid. *Lancet*, **i**, 171–5
121. Binder, H.J., Cocco, A., Crossley, R.J., *et al.* (1978). Cimetidine in the treatment of duodenal ulcer. A multicentre double blind study. *Gastroenterology*, **74**, 380–8
122. Malchow, H., Sewing, K.F., Albinus, M., Horn, H., Schomerus, H. and Dölle, W. (1979). Cimetidin in der stationären Behandlung des peptischen Ulkus. *Dtsch. Med. Wschr.*, **103**, 149–52
123. Hall, W.H., Read, R.C., Wesard, L., Lee, L.E. and Robinette, C.D. (1972). The calendar and duodenal ulcer. *Gastroenterology*, **62**, 1120–4
124. Gibinski, K., Rybicka, J., Nowak, A. and Czarnecka, K. (1982). Seasonal occurrence of abdominal pain and endoscopic findings in patients with gastric and duodenal ulcer disease. *Scand. J. Gastroenterol.*, **17**, 481–5
125. Palmas, F., Andriulli, A., Canepa, G., Gardino, L., Boero, M., Rocca, G. and Verme, G. (1984). Monthly fluctuations of active duodenal ulcers. *Dig. Dis. Sci.*, **29**, 983–7
126. Glynn, M.J. and Kane, S.P. (1985). Benign gastric ulceration in a health district: incidence and presentation. *Postgrad. Med. J.*, **61**, 695–700
127. Kühlmayer, R. and Rokitansky, P. (1954). Das Magenstumpfkarzinom als Spätproblem der Ulkustherapie. *Langenbeck's Arch. Chir.*, **278**, 361–75
128. Griesser, G. and Schmidt, H. (1964). Statistische Erhebungen über die Häufigkeit des Karzinoms nach Magenoperation wegen eines Geschwürsleidens. *Med. Welt*, **15**, 1836–40
129. Kootz, F. (1967). Das Stumpfkarzinom nach Operation eines benignen Magenleidens. *Brun's Beitr. Klin. Chir.*, **215**, 275–94
130. Hilbe, G., Salzer, G.M., Hussl, H. and Kutschera, H. (1968). Die Carcinomgefährdung des Resektionsmagens. *Langenbeck's Arch. Chir.*, **323**, 142–53
131. Caygill, C.P., Hill, M.J., Kirkham, J.S. and Northfield, T.C. (1986). Mortality from gastric cancer following gastric surgery for peptic ulcer. *Lancet*, **i**, 929–30

31

2
Human gastric acid secretion and intragastric acidity

R. E. POUNDER

Since the mid-1970s, there has been a move away from the assessment of gastric secretion of acid by man in response to a single pharmacological stimulus to either the measurement of 'natural' gastric acid secretion in response to a whole meal or the measurement of intragastric acidity (which is the end-result of not only gastric acid secretion, but also food and liquid taken by mouth and also gastric emptying).

The purpose of this chapter is to review what is known about naturally-stimulated gastric acid secretion, and also 24-hour intragastric acidity in man.

FOOD STIMULATED GASTRIC ACID SECRETION

In 1973 Fordtran and Walsh described a novel technique for measuring the rate of gastric acid secretion in human subjects in response to eating a 'normal meal'[1]. A double lumen nasogastric tube was passed into the stomach of a fasting patient. The meal consisted of a hamburger eaten with a drink of 360 ml of water. The pH of intragastric contents was adjusted to 5.5 and, as the stomach secreted acid in response to the meal, sodium bicarbonate was infused to maintain gastric luminal pH at either 5 or 5.5. Hence, the amount of sodium bicarbonate required per hour to keep the pH constant was equal to the rate of acid secretion (expressed as mmol of hydrochloric acid per hour). Thus the technique allowed intragastric titration of gastric acid as it was secreted.

A subsequent paper from the same group used a mixture of protein hydrolysate and carbohydrate to stimulate gastric acid secretion[2]. In this study they measured the gastric secretory response to the meal by intragastric titration at four different pH values – 5.5, 4.0, 3.0 and 2.5. The rate of acid secretion in response to the meal was highest at pH 5.5 but it was only 60% of that produced by a steak meal at the same pH. As the pH of the amino acid meal was decreased, there was a step-wise decrease of acid secretion, so that at pH 2.5 the rate of secretion was only half as great as that at pH 5.5.

In a recent study, the authors have compared peak acid output, in response to either pentagastrin or histamine, and food-stimulated gastric acid secretion in duodenal ulcer patients and normal subjects[3]. Mean peak acid output was significantly higher in the duodenal group than controls (36.3 versus 15.8 mmol/h, $p < 0.001$). However, gastric acid secretion was similar in the two groups when food was used as stimulant (Figure 2.1), mean acid secretion for the entire two-hour experiment being only 3.4 mmol/h higher in the duodenal ulcer group (24.3 versus 20.9 mmol/h). Thus, although duodenal ulcer patients had a much higher maximal secretory capacity (peak acid output) than healthy subjects, they had a similar acid secretory response to food. Serum gastrin concentrations in response to the same meal increased by similar amounts in the two groups (Figure 2.1). This study is considerably larger than

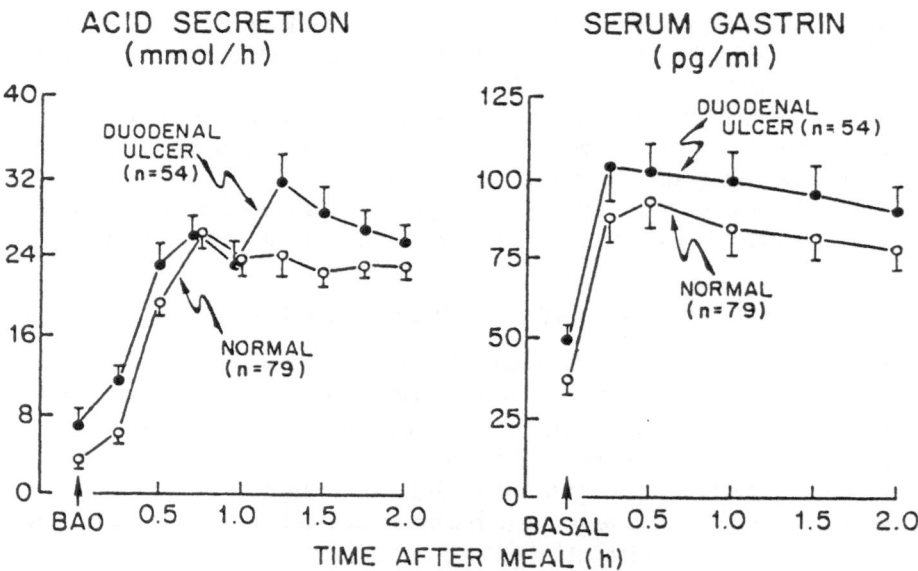

Figure 2.1 The mean (±SEM) acid secretion (left) and serum gastrin concentration (right) in response to intragastric meal infusion in normal subjects and duodenal ulcer patients. Basal acid output is also shown. Reproduced from *J. Clin. Invest.*[3], with permission

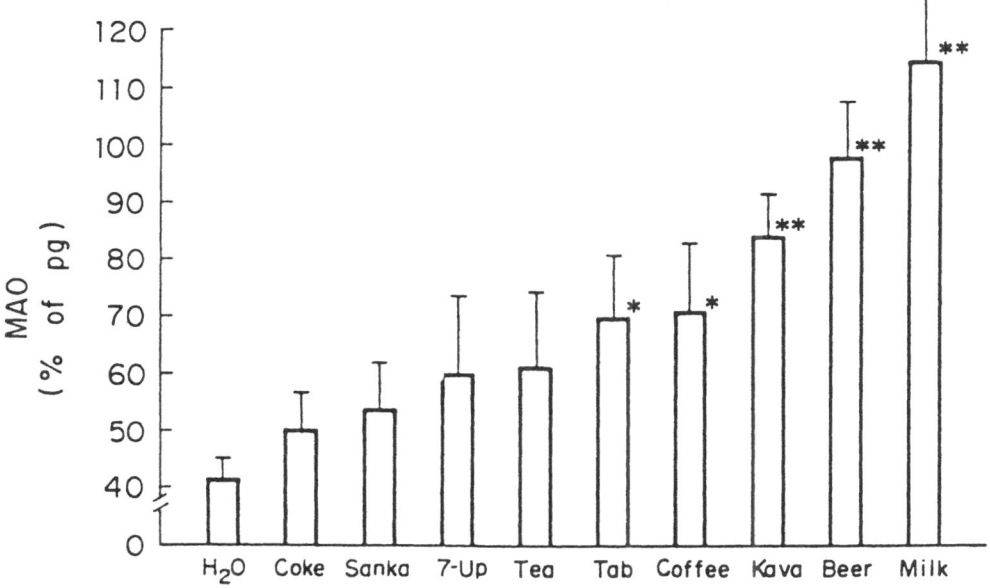

Figure 2.2 Mean maximum acid output to nine beverages, and water control, expressed as percent of maximum acid response to pentagastrin. Vertical bars indicate ± 1 SEM. The mean response to pentagastrin in these healthy subjects was 27 mmol/h. Reproduced from *Gastroenterology*[9], with permission

earlier studies, three of which had suggested that food-stimulated gastric acid secretion was higher in duodenal ulcer patients than normal subjects[4–6], and two of which found no difference in the secretory responses[7,8]. Overall, it would now appear that the acid-secretory response, measured under conditions of intragastric titration with alkali, is similar in duodenal ulcer patients and healthy subjects.

Although the original technique for the measurement of intragastric acidity depended upon the response to a whole hamburger, later studies all homogenized the hamburger with water, so that particles of food would not block the nasogastric tube. There have been a number of studies looking at the secretory response to various test meals. In India the type of meal did not influence the acid secretory response[5] while an American study showed very considerable variation in the secretory response to different beverages[9]. Jalan and colleagues[5] could not detect any difference in the gastric secretory response to a rice-based meal, consisting of rice, fish, vegetables, yoghurt and spices (similar to one commonly consumed by the population of eastern India) and a wheat-based meal where the rice was substituted by whole wheat flour made into chapatties, and the fish was replaced by goat meat (similar to food consumed in the north-west of India)[5]. McArthur and colleagues looked at the effect of nine commonly ingested beverages on gastric acid secretion in humans – each beverage was swallowed at its usually consumed temperature and gastric acid secretion was measured by intragastric titration[9]. The results are shown in Figure 2.2 – where it can be seen that the greatest responses were to either milk or beer, and the smallest response was to Coke!

24-HOUR GASTRIC ACID SECRETION

The technique of intragastric titration has now been developed to measure 24-hour gastric acid secretion rates in duodenal ulcer patients and healthy controls[10]. The technique involves intragastric titration of acid secretion in response to breakfast, lunch and dinner, together with continuous aspiration between each of the three meals for the remaining parts of the 24-hour study. Intragastric titrations were performed for three 120-minute periods after the same 600 ml meal (homogenized sirloin steak, toast, butter and water adjusted to a pH of 5) at 0900, 1400 and 1900 hours. The subjects received intravenous saline throughout the study, to stop them becoming dehydrated.

Figure 2.3 shows that throughout the 24-hour study, mean acid secretion was higher in non-operated duodenal ulcer patients than in normal controls;

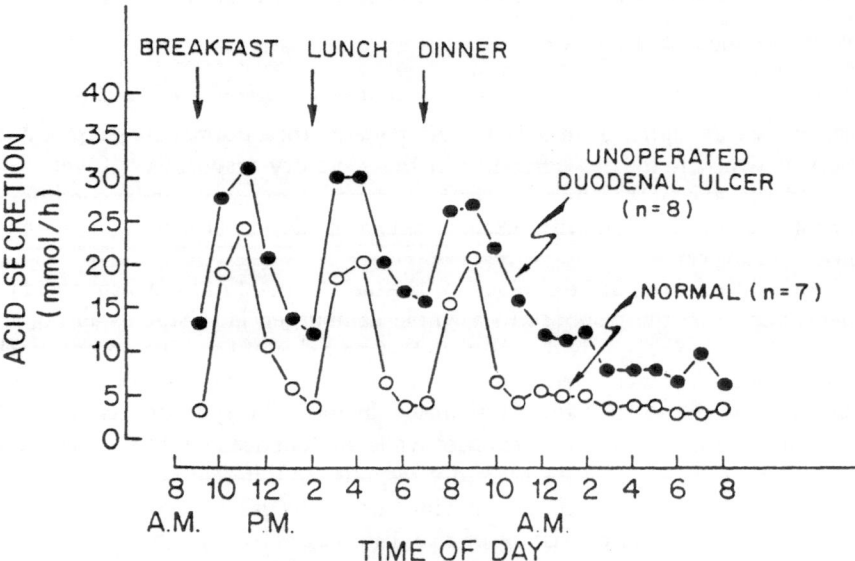

Figure 2.3 Mean hourly gastric acid secretion during a 24-hour period in eight non-operated duodenal ulcer patients and in seven normal men. Reproduced from *Gastroenterology*[10], with permission

36

the 24-hour acid secretion being 408.3 versus 208.3 mmol/24 h. The greater gastric acid secretion in the ulcer patients was owing to a higher rate of secretion in the interprandial periods and during the night. The response of the ulcer patients and healthy subjects to the three standard meals was similar, the incremental rise of gastric acid secretion being the same in both groups. In the same study, vagotomy produced a profound decrease of interprandial and nocturnal gastric acid secretion without abolishing the post-prandial release of gastric acid (Figure 2.4).

The measurement of 24-hour gastric acid secretion is a formidable task and, although it has been repeated once by the same group[11], it is unlikely to become a standard technique for measuring gastric secretory responses in clinical practice. The other disadvantage of measuring 24-hour gastric acid secretion is that the technique only approximates to what happens in everyday life – the experiment being, to a degree, rather artificial. There are three principal reasons for this: firstly, the meal is a homogenized hamburger – which, despite the hamburger's popularity, is not a normal balanced meal; secondly, the intragastric environment is abnormal – as alkali is infused into the stomach to hold pH at approximately 5.0; and thirdly, between the meals

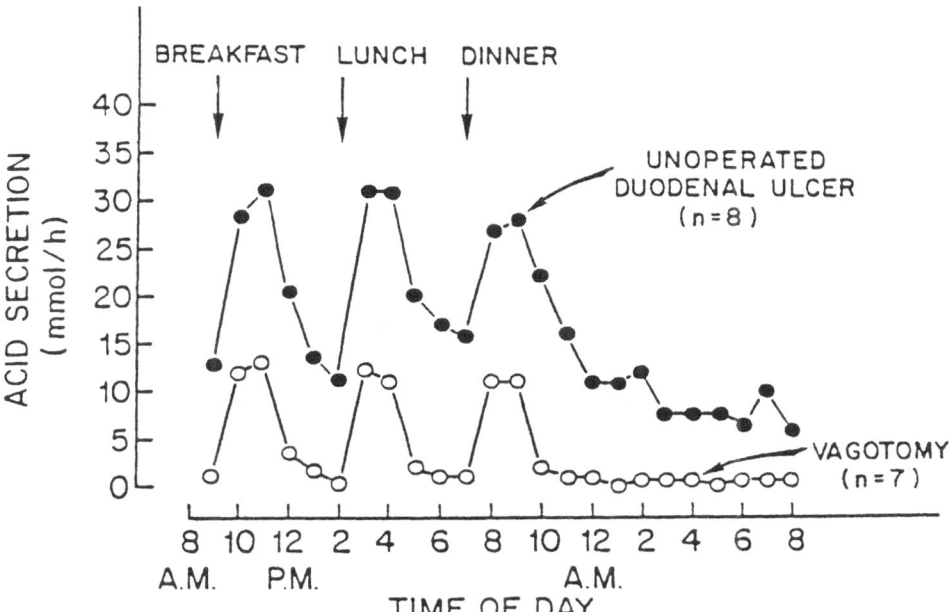

Figure 2.4 Mean hourly gastric acid secretion during a 24-hour period in eight non-operated duodenal ulcer patients and in seven duodenal ulcer patients treated by a parietal cell vagotomy. Reproduced from *Gastroenterology*[10], with permission

there is continuous gastric aspiration – which means that the stomach is kept empty and no gastric contents are passing into the small intestine.

24-HOUR INTRAGASTRIC ACIDITY

The measurement of 24-hour intragastric acidity allows the investigator to observe exactly what happens in the stomach, whilst the subjects eat normal meals, and are fully ambulant. The technique was originally used to observe different patterns of acidity in patients with a variety of peptic disorders[12-14], and was later used to assess the effects of different therapeutic diets[15-17]. In the early 1970s, the technique was rediscovered and applied to the evaluation of new antisecretory drugs that were being developed[18,19]. The new experiments were performed under much more controlled conditions than hitherto, usually involving the simultaneous investigation by medical investigators of large numbers of subjects or patients[20-24].

The technique involves fasting subjects attending an investigation ward and the swallowing of a fine bore nasogastric tube[25]. The subjects are allowed full mobility during the study, and consume six normally-prepared standard meals at fixed times throughout a 24-hour period. Every hour, on the hour, a small sample of gastric juice is aspirated from the stomach and its acidity measured using a glass electrode. Figure 2.5 shows a typical profile of 24-hour

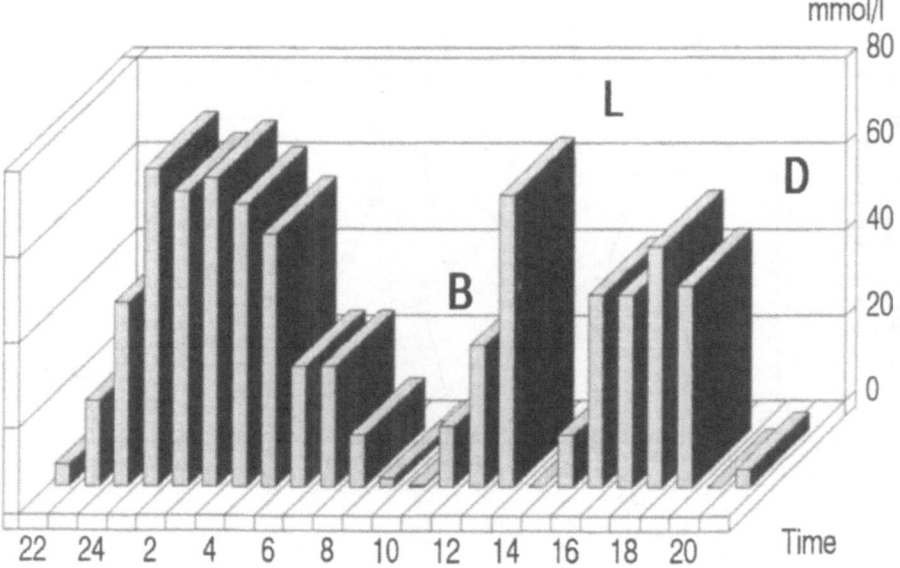

Figure 2.5 Median hourly intragastric acidity in ten healthy subjects who received a placebo tablet at 2100 hours. B = breakfast; L = lunch; D = dinner

38

intragastric acidity in a group of ten healthy subjects. The study lasted from 2200 to 2100 hours the following evening. Breakfast, taken at 0915 hours, neutralises intragastric acidity, but is followed by a rapid build-up of acidity during the morning. Lunch, taken at 1315 hours, again neutralises acidity and is followed by a build-up of acidity during the afternoon and early evening. Dinner, taken at 1915 hours causes a more prolonged decrease of intragastric acidity, with a build-up of acidity in the late evening. Acidity peaks in the early hours of the morning, and then falls away to reach a low level by 0800 hours. It is interesting to compare this profile of intragastric acidity with the profile of 24-hour gastric acid secretion seen in Figure 2.3. The response to a meal is completely different in the two studies – measurement of intragastric acidity demonstrating a decrease of acidity following a meal, and quantitation of acid secretion showing stimulation of acid output by a meal. So what is really happening when a human being eats a meal? The answer is that eating a meal stimulates gastric acid secretion, but any meal entering the stomach at a pH between 5 and 7 has a considerable buffering capacity. The stomach secretes acid in response to the meal, and gradually the buffering capacity of the meal is exhausted. At the same time, the stomach is emptying the meal and several hours after ingestion either its buffering capacity has been

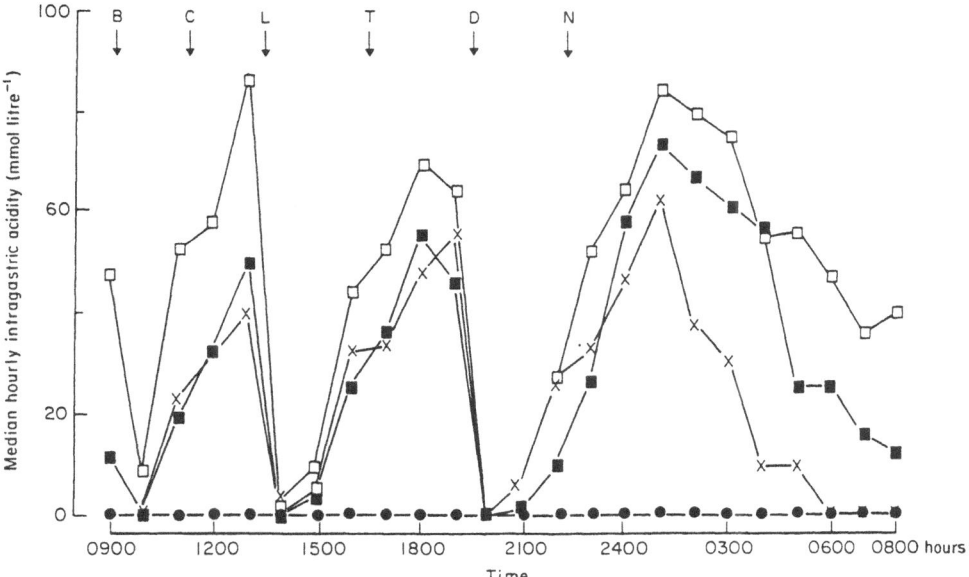

Figure 2.6 Twenty-four hour median intragastric acidity in healthy subjects (■, $n = 16$), patients with a history of duodenal ulcer (□, $n = 12$) or gastric ulceration (×, $n = 10$), or pernicious anaemia patients (●, $n = 8$). B = breakfast; C = coffee; L = lunch; T = tea; D = dinner; N = night snack. Reproduced from *Aliment. Pharmacol. Therapeut.*[25], with permission

completely exhausted or the meal has disappeared into the small intestine. Either way, intragastric acidity begins to rise to a peak as interprandial gastric acid is secreted into an empty stomach.

Intragastric acidity has been measured in four groups of subjects, each studied under identical environmental conditions and with the same meals[25]. The study involved the investigation of 12 duodenal ulcer patients, 16 healthy subjects, 10 gastric ulcer patients, and 8 patients with a history of pernicious anaemia. Figure 2.6 shows the profile of 24-hour median intragastric acidity in all these subjects, and Figure 2.7 shows integrated 24-hour intragastric acidity in the same subjects. It can be seen that duodenal ulcer patients have a significantly higher 24-hour intragastric acidity than all other groups. There is no difference of acidity between healthy subjects and gastric ulcer patients, and patients with pernicious anaemia have virtually no acid in their stomach.

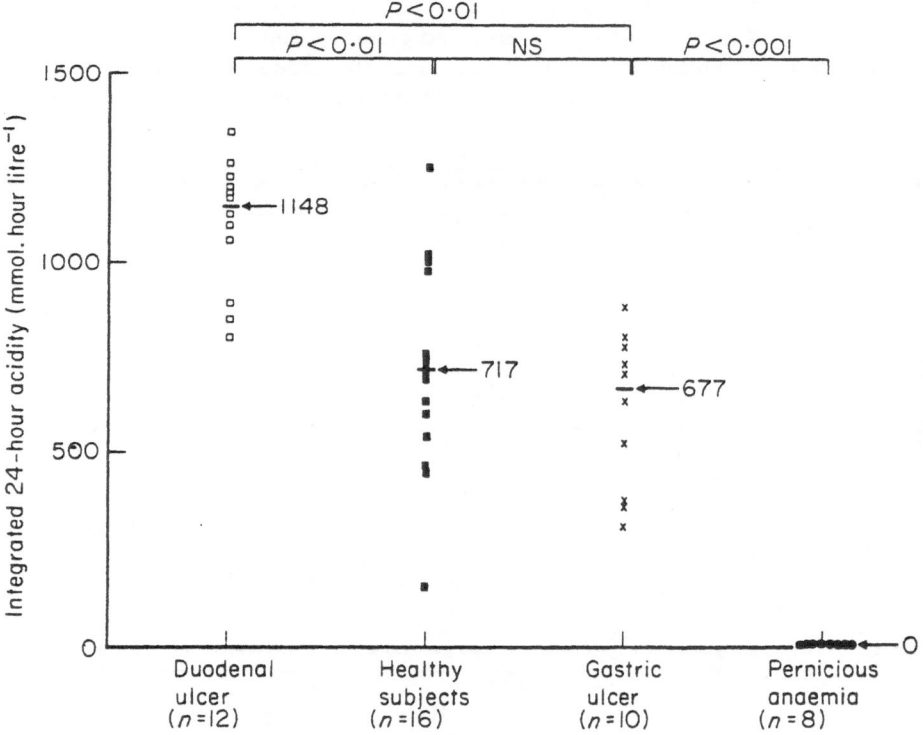

Figure 2.7 Integrated 24-hour intragastric acidity in healthy subjects, and patients with a history of duodenal or gastric ulceration, or pernicious anaemia. Arrows indicate the median value for each group. Reproduced from *Aliment. Pharmacol. Therapeut.*[25], with permission

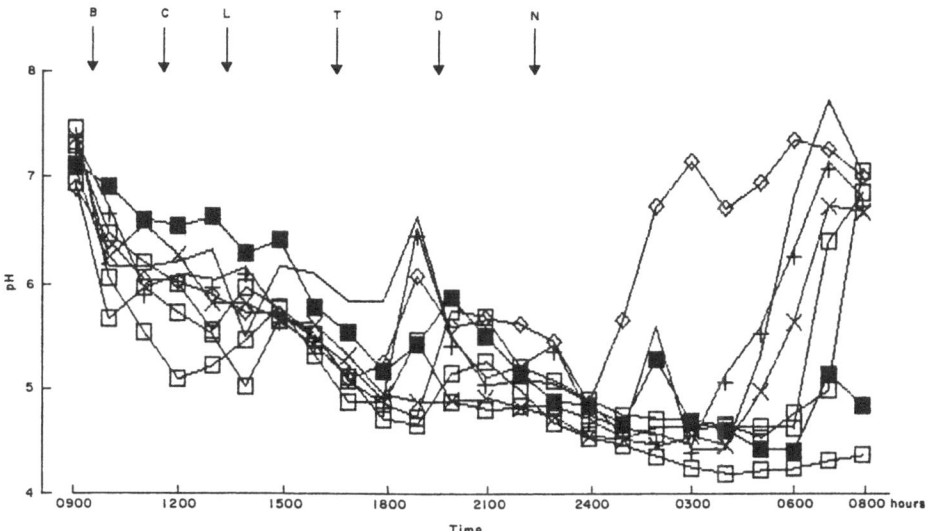

Figure 2.8 Hourly intragastric pH in eight patients with pernicious anaemia. Reproduced from *Aliment. Pharmacol. Therapeut.*[25], with permission

Pernicious anaemia patients do have a degree of gastric acidity in that their intragastric pH ranges between 7.6 and 4.2 (Figure 2.8). This intragastric 'acidity' is partly owing to the ingestion of meals which have a pH ranging between 5.1 and 6.4, but it may be partly due to either a very small amount of residual gastric acid secretion, or the production of organic acids by intragastric bacteria.

Recently, a number of electronic systems have been developed for the measurement of intragastric acidity using pH probes that are kept within the stomach for 24 hours[27]. The theoretical advantage of such techniques is the acquisition of very much larger amounts of data concerning intragastric acidity – for example, intragastric acidity can be measured every 10 seconds, which should improve the precision of the observations. However, the electrode is out of sight, and it may become contaminated by the intragastric environment which contains proteins and fats, or mispositioned in the mucus gel layer or duodenal cap. The technology for electronic measurement of intragastric acidity is also relatively expensive, particularly as most studies involve the simultaneous investigation of a number of subjects. However, the considerable advantage of the *simultaneous* investigation of subjects is that it allows very close control of the environmental conditions, when a team of investigators can measure not only intragastric acidity but also concentrations of drugs and polypeptide hormones in the blood.

41

Circadian rhythm of gastric acid secretion

Fasting humans have a circadian rhythm of their gastric acid secretion. In a series of reports from 1970 to 1986, Moore has reported patterns of 24-hour fasting gastric acid secretion[28-31]. A peak of acid secretion occurs in the late evening and early hours of the night, with low secretion rates during the morning (Figure 2.9). Duodenal ulcer patients have a consistently higher rate of secretion than healthy subjects[31]. It is not known what happens when night-workers go on holiday!

24-hour plasma gastrin concentration

The technique for the measurement of 24-hour intragastric acidity has recently been used to correlate plasma polypeptide hormone levels with intragastric acidity[24-26]. Obviously, such a correlation would be useless in any study that involves intragastric titration with alkali. In the study[25] involving healthy subjects, and patients with duodenal ulcer, gastric ulcer or pernicious anaemia, 24-hour plasma gastrin concentration was measured (Figure 2.10). All groups, except the pernicious anaemia patients, showed a prompt rise of plasma gastrin concentration in response to each of the three main meals. The pernicious anaemia patients, neither as a group nor as individuals, showed any gastrin response to the three main meals and throughout the 24 hours plasma gastrin concentration was constantly elevated.

ASSESSMENT OF ANTISECRETORY DRUGS USING 24-HOUR INTRAGASTRIC ACIDITY

The present technique of measurement of 24-hour intragastric acidity was developed for the assessment of the antisecretory effects of cimetidine[18,19]. The idea behind these experiments was to develop the most economic dose of cimetidine that would cause a 24-hour decrease of intragastric acidity. Figure 2.11 shows the profiles of three subjects that were treated with cimetidine 200 mg q.d.s., and three subjects who receive cimetidine 400 mg q.d.s. It is amusing to note that the final dosage of cimetidine (200 mg t.d.s. with 400 mg at bed-time) never had its 24-hour profile of acidity measured until some years after the drug was introduced!

In the last 15 years, many hundreds of 24-hour intragastric acidity profiles have been recorded, and recently these profiles have been compared with the duodenal ulcer healing action of a range of therapeutic regimens (Figure 2.12)[32]. It seems that the night-time period of intragastric acidity is exceptionally important and the benefits of existing therapeutic regimens using H_2-receptor blockers with a short half-life are related to their ability to control nocturnal intragastric acidity. However, if the regression line is extended so that there

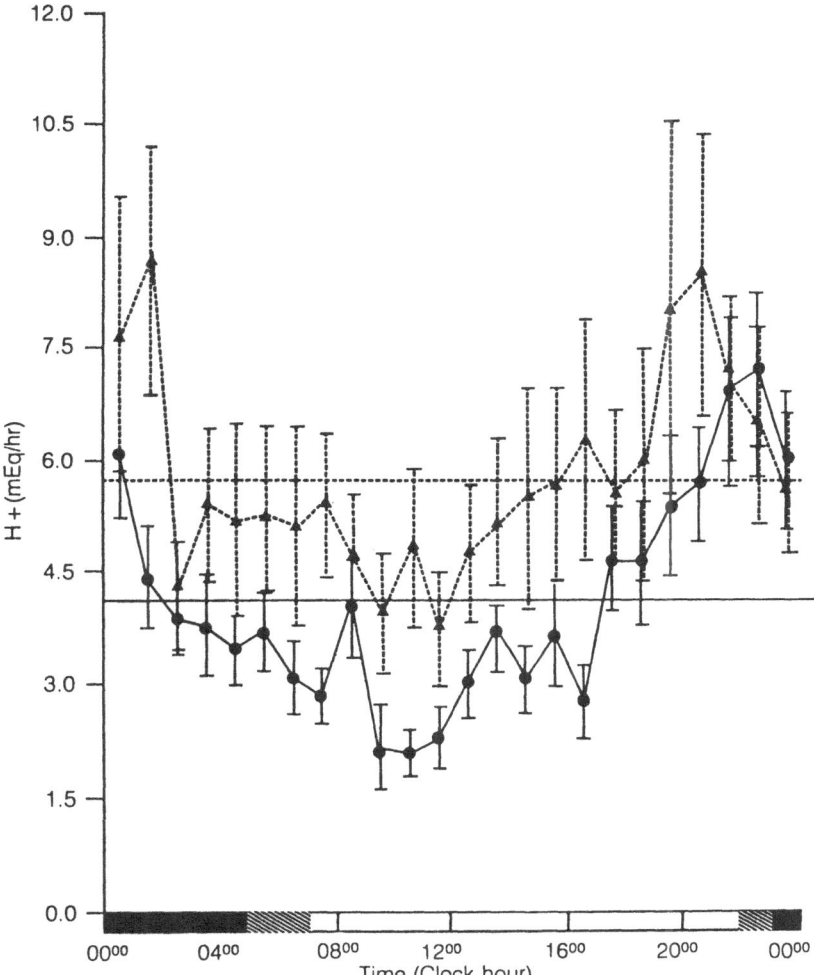

Figure 2.9 Mean hourly gastric acid secretion in 14 healthy volunteers (●) and 21 patients with an active duodenal (▲). Each point represents the mean ± SEM. Both groups show a low morning, and high evening, rate of acid secretion. The broken horizontal line represents the mean 24-hour secretory rate for ulcer patients (5.8 mmol/h) and the straight horizontal line represents the mean rate for the healthy volunteers (4 mmol/h,. Reproduced from *Dig. Dis. Sci.*[31], with permission

is a 100% decrease of nocturnal acidity, it can be predicted that only about 85% of ulcers will heal after four weeks of treatment. It is therefore likely that day-time acidity is also important and the extra benefits of omeprazole in terms of duodenal ulcer healing[33–35] are probably related to the ability of omeprazole to control both day-time and nocturnal acidity (Figure 2.13)[24].

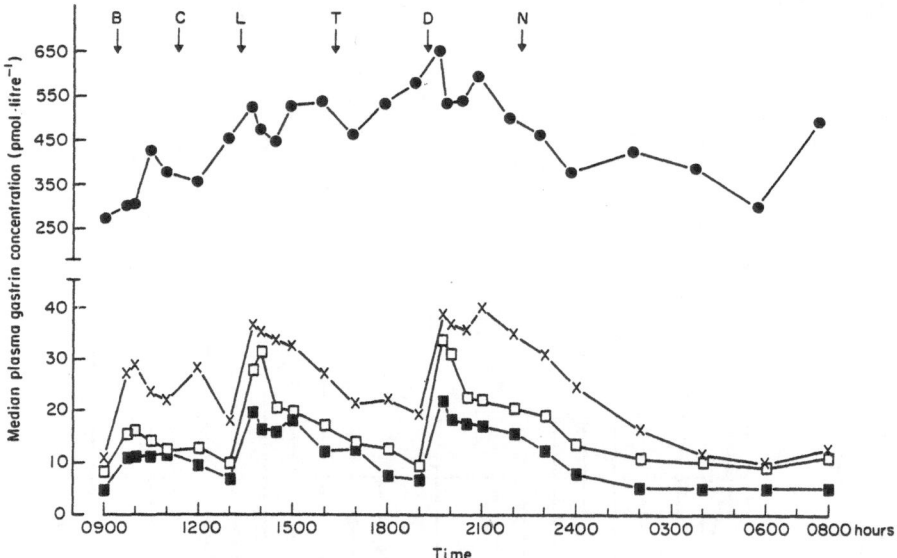

Figure 2.10 Twenty-four hour plasma gastrin concentration in healthy subjects (■, $n = 16$) and patients with a history of duodenal (□, $n = 12$) or gastric ulceration (×, $n = 10$), or pernicious anaemia (●, $n = 8$). Reproduced from *Aliment. Pharmacol. Therapeut.*[25], with permission

The analysis of data from studies of 24-hour intragastric acidity

The analysis of data from 24-hour studies arouses considerable controversy and a degree of excitement whenever there is a meeting of investigators that use this technique. Data collected from these studies should be handled as follows. The individual pH values should be immediately transformed to hydrogen ion activity expressed as mmol/litre; acidity values, usually collected at hourly intervals, should be expressed as a median value for each interval (Figure 2.13); 24-hour intragastric acidity should be expressed as the integrated value for 24 hours – that is the area under the curve (Figure 2.14); and finally, the data should also be analysed as 'meal-related intervals'. The three main meals (breakfast, lunch and dinner) all cause a prompt decrease of acidity so that the data can be divided into morning, afternoon, evening, and night-time (representing the period after the subjects go to bed).

Thus, the data shown in Figures 2.13 and 2.14 can also be expressed in terms of 'meal-related intervals' as in Figure 2.15. In untreated duodenal ulcer patients, the 'meal-related intervals' occur naturally with each major meal causing a sudden decrease of intragastric acidity (Figure 2.5). Such an analysis not only allows one to see the 24-hour effect of a drug, but it also allows the duration of activity of any dose to be assessed in terms of the four 'meal-

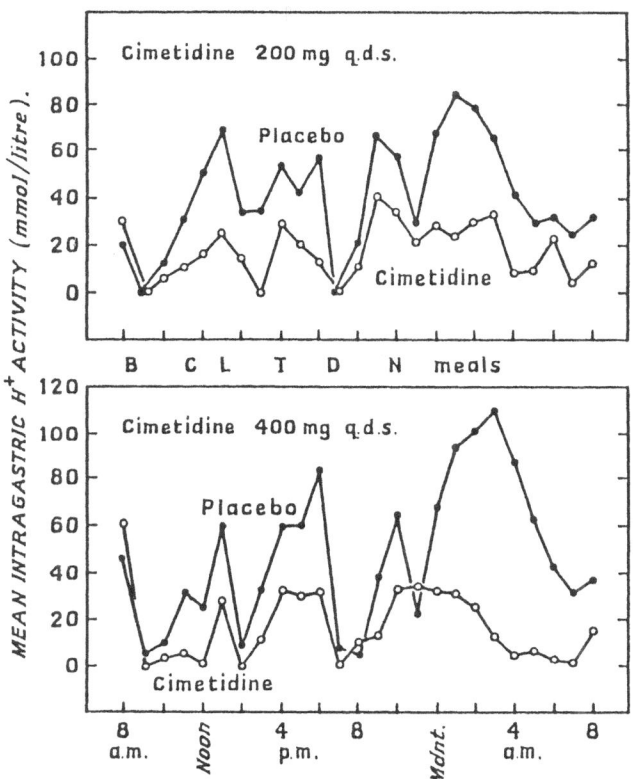

Figure 2.11 Mean hourly intragastric acidity in two groups of three duodenal ulcer patients, given cimetidine (200 mg q.d.s. or 400 mg q.d.s.) or placebo. Reproduced from *Lancet*[18], with permission

related intervals'. For example, Figure 2.14 shows that ranitidine 150 mg b.d. has little effect on intragastric acidity in the afternoon, and no effect on acidity in the evening.

WHY HAVE INTRAGASTRIC ACID?

What is the role of acid in the human stomach? It seems unlikely that it is really important in terms of digestion, as most patients with pernicious anaemia have no problem with malabsorption of food. It seems more likely that intragastric acid is present as an 'antiseptic seal' to the alimentary tract, essentially sterilizing food before it passes into the small and large intestines[36,37]. A range of alimentary infections have been associated with decreased intragastric acidity: typhoid and non-typhoid salmonellosis[38-41], bacillary dys-

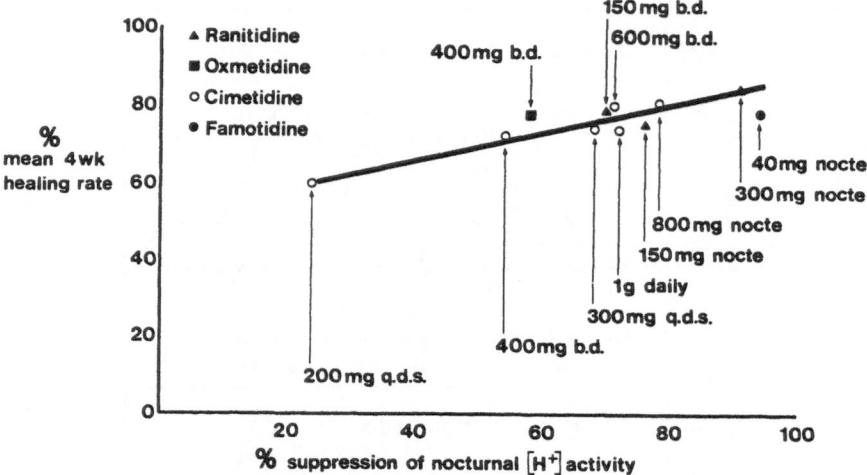

Figure 2.12   Correlation between the four-week duodenal ulcer healing rate and suppression of nocturnal acidity with different H_2 receptor antagonist regimens. Reproduced from *Scand. J. Gastroenterol.* [32], with permission

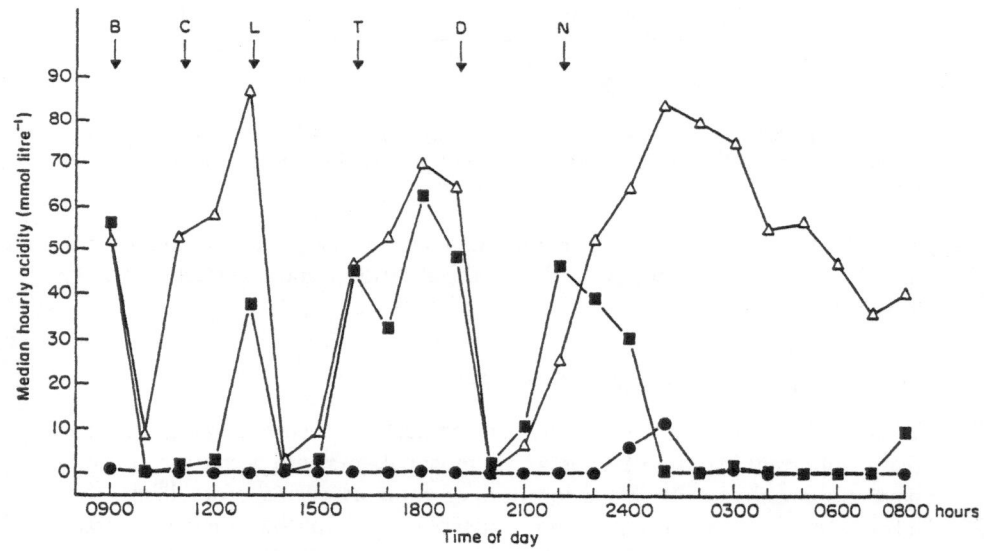

Figure 2.13   Twenty-four hour median intragastric acidity before treatment ($\triangle$) and on the 28th day of treatment with either ranitidine 150 mg b.d. ($\blacksquare$) or omeprazole 20 mg o.m. ($\bullet$) in 12 duodenal ulcer patients. Reproduced from *Aliment. Pharmacol. Therapeut.* [24], with permission

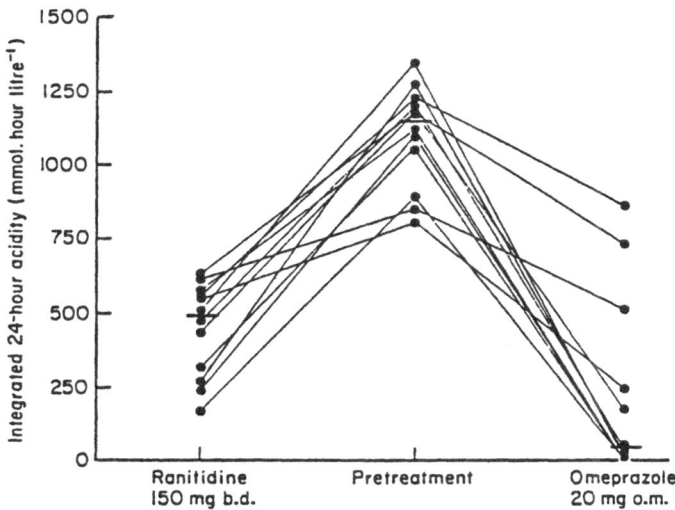

Figure 2.14 Integrated 24-hour intragastric acidity pre-treatment, and on the 28th day of treatment with either ranitidine 150 mg b.d. or omeprazole 20 mg o.m., in 12 duodenal ulcer patients. Horizontal bar indicates the median value for each group. Reproduced from *Aliment. Pharmacol. Therapeut.*[24], with permission

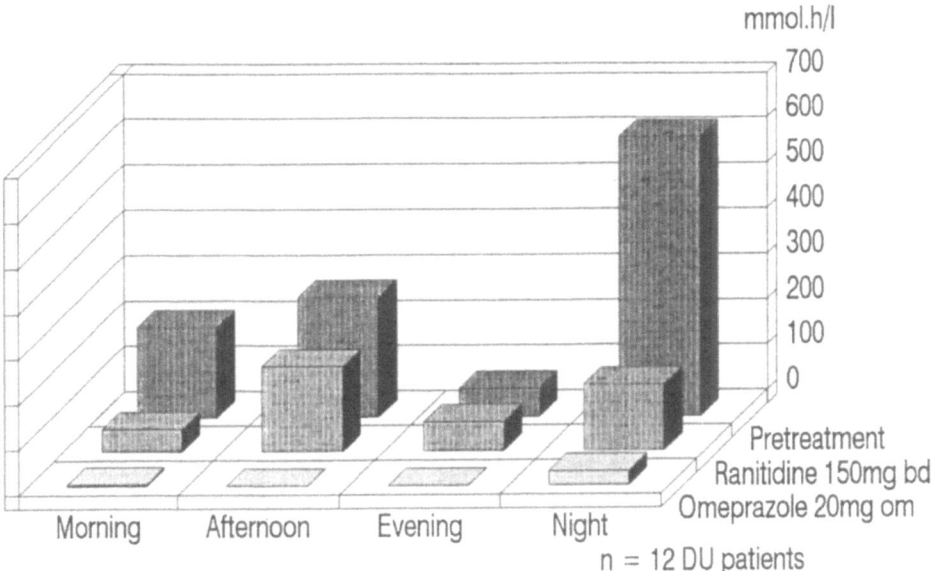

Figure 2.15 Median integrated intragastric acidity in 12 duodenal ulcer patients, analysed according to 'meal-related intervals'. Calculated from data in *Aliment. Pharmacol. Therapeut.*[24], with permission

entery[42], cholera[43-44], brucellosis[45], giardiasis[46], pseudomembranous colitis[47], and even infestation with *Strongyloidis stercoralis* or *Diphyllobothrium latum*[39].

Modern treatment with histamine H_2-receptor antagonists normally involves the use of medication at bed-time – with a pulse of inhibition of acid secretion during the night, and unchanged acid secretion during the following day. Such regimens should minimize the risk of patients developing food-borne intestinal infections.

ACKNOWLEDGEMENTS

The figures have been reproduced with the kind permission of the relevant authors and journals. The manuscript was prepared by Mrs Julie Young.

REFERENCES

1. Fordtran, J.S. and Walsh, J.H. (1973). Gastric acid secretion rate and buffer content of the stomach after eating. Results in normal subjects and in patients with duodenal ulcer. *J. Clin. Invest.*, **52**, 645–57
2. Walsh, J.H., Richardson, C.T. and Fordtran, J.S. (1975). pH dependence of acid secretion and gastrin release in normal and ulcer subjects. *J. Clin. Invest.*, **55**, 462–8
3. Blair, A.J., Feldman, M., Barnett, C., Walsh, J.H. and Richardson, C.T. (1987). Detailed comparison of basal and food-stimulated gastric acid secretion rates and serum gastrin concentrations in duodenal ulcer patients and normal subjects. *J. Clin. Invest.*, **79**, 582–7
4. Fordtran, J.S. and Walsh, J.H. (1973). Gastric acid secretion rate and buffer content of the stomach after eating: results in normal subjects and in patients with duodenal ulcer. *J. Clin. Invest.*, **52**, 654–7
5. Jalan, K.N., Mahalanabis, D., Maitra, T.K. and Agarwal, S.K. (1979). Gastric acid secretion rate and buffer content of the stomach after a rice- and a wheat-based meal in normal subjects and patients with duodenal ulcer. *Gut*, **20**, 389–93
6. Bodemar, G., Walan, A. and Lundquist, G. (1978). Food-stimulated acid secretion measured by intragastric titration with bicarbonate in patients with duodenal and gastric ulcer disease and in controls. *Scand. J. Gastroenterol.*, **13**, 911–18
7. Malagelada, J.-R., Longstreth, G.F., Deering, T.B., Summerskill, W.H.J. and Go, V.L.W. (1977). Gastric secretion and emptying after ordinary meals in duodenal ulcer. *Gastroenterology*, **73**, 989–94
8. Gross, R.A., Isenberg, J.I., Hogan, D. and Samloff, I.M. (1978). Effect of fat on meal-stimulated duodenal acid load, duodenal pepsin load, and serum gastrin in duodenal ulcer and normal subjects. *Gastroenterology*, **75**, 357–62
9. McArthur, K., Hogan, D. and Isenberg, J.I. (1982). Relative stimulatory effects of commonly ingested beverages on gastric acid secretion in humans. *Gastroenterology*, **83**, 199–203
10. Feldman, M. and Richardson, C.T. (1986). Total 24-hour gastric acid secretion in patients with duodenal ulcer. *Gastroenterology*, **90**, 540–4
11. Richardson, C.T. and Feldman, M. (1986). Effects of transdermal scopolamine, alone or in combination with cimetidine on total 24 hour gastric acid secretion in patients with duodenal ulcer. *Gut*, **27**, 1493–7
12. James, A.H. and Pickering, G.W. (1949). The role of gastric acidity in the pathogenesis of peptic ulcer. *Clin. Sci.*, **8**, 181–210
13. Watkinson, G. (1951). A study of the changes of pH of gastric contents in peptic ulcer using the twenty-four hour test meal. *Gastroenterology*, **18**, 377–90
14. Watkinson, G. and James, A.H. (1951). Twenty-four hour gastric analysis in patients with histamine achlorhydria. *Clin. Sci.*, **10**, 255–66

15. Lennard-Jones, J.E. (1961). Experimental and clinical observations on poldine in the treatment of duodenal ulcer. *Brit. Med. J.*, **1**, 1071–6
16. Lennard-Jones, J.E. and Babouris, N. (1965). Effect of different foods on the acidity of the gastric contents in patients with duodenal ulcer. I. A comparison between two 'therapeutic' diets and freely-chosen meals. *Gut*, **6**, 113–17
17. Babouris, N., Fletcher, J. and Lennard-Jones, J.E. (1965). Effect of different foods on the acidity of the gastric contents in patients with duodenal ulcer. II. Effect of varying the size and frequency of the meals. *Gut*, **6**, 118–20
18. Pounder, R.E., Williams, J.G., Milton-Thompson, G.J. and Misiewicz, J.J. (1975). Twenty-four hour control of intragastric acidity by cimetidine in duodenal ulcer patients. *Lancet*, **ii**, 1069–70
19. Pounder, R.E., Williams, J.G., Milton-Thompson, G.J. and Misiewicz, J.J. (1976). Effect of cimetidine on 24-hour intragastric acidity in normal subjects. *Gut*, **17**, 133–8
20. Walt, R.P., Male, P.J., Rawlings, J., Hunt, R.N., Milton-Thompson, G.J. and Misiewicz, J.J. (1981). Comparison of the effects of ranitidine, cimetidine and placebo on the 24-hour intragastric acidity and nocturnal acid secretion in patients with duodenal ulcer. *Gut*, **22**, 49–54
21. Gledhill, T., Howard, O.M., Buck, M., Paul, A. and Hunt, R.H. (1983). Single nocturnal dose of an H_2-receptor antagonist for the treatment of duodenal ulcer. *Gut*, **24**, 904–8
22. Sharma, B.K., Walt, R.P., Pounder, R.E., Gomes M. de F.A., Wood, E.C. and Logan, L.H. (1984). Optimal dose of oral omeprazole for maximal 24 hour decrease of intragastric acidity. *Gut*, **25**, 957–64
23. Pritchard, P.J., Yeomans, N.D., Mihaly, G.W., *et al.* (1983). Effect of daily oral omeprazole on 24-hour intragastric acidity. *Gastroenterology*, **287**, 1378–9
24. Lanzon-Miller, S., Pounder, R. E., Hamilton, M.R., *et al.* (1987). 24-hour intragastric acidity and plasma gastrin concentration before and during treatment with either ranitidine or omeprazole. *Aliment. Pharmacol. Therapeut.*, **1**, 239–52
25. Lanzon-Miller, S., Pounder, R.E., Hamilton, M.R., Ball, S., Chronos, N.A.F., Olausson, M. and Cederberg, C. (1987). 24-hour intragastric acidity and plasma gastrin concentration in healthy subjects and patients with duodenal or gastric ulcer, or pernicious anaemia. *Aliment. Pharmacol. Therapeut.*, **1**, 228–38
26. Mahachai, V., Walker, K. and Thomson, A.B.R. (1985). Comparison of cimetidine and ranitidine on 24-hour intragastric acidity and serum gastrin profile in patients with esophagitis. *Dig. Dis. Sci.*, **30**, 321–8
27. Fimmel, C. J ., Etienne, A. and Cilluffo, T., *et al.* (1985). Long-term ambulatory gastric pH monitoring: validation of a new method of effect of H_2-antagonists. *Gastroenterology*, **88**, 1842–57
28. Moore, J.G. and Englert, E. (1970). Circadian rhythm of gastric acid secretion in man. *Nature (London)*, **226**, 1261–2
29. Moore, J.G. and Wolfe, M. (1973). The relation of plasma gastrin to the circadian rhythm of gastric acid secretion in man. *Digestion*, **9**, 97–107
30. Moore, J.G. and Wolfe, M. (1974). Circadian plasma gastrin patterns in feeding and fasting man. *Digestion*, **11**, 226–31
31. Moore, J.G. and Halberg, F. (1986). Circadian rhythm of gastric acid secretion in men with active duodenal ulcer. *Dig. Dis. Sci.*, **31**, 1185–91
32. Hunt, R.H., Howden, C.W., Jones, D.B., Burget, D.W. and Kerr, G.D. (1986). The correlation between acid suppression and duodenal ulcer healing. *Scand. J. Gastroenterol.*, **21** (Suppl. 125), 22–8
33. Classen, M., Dammann, H.G. and Domschke, W., *et al.* (1985). Omeprazole heals duodenal, but not gastric ulcers more rapidly than ranitidine. Results of two German multicentre trials. *Hepatogastroenterology*, **32**, 243–5
34. Lauritsen, K., Rune, S.J. and Bytzer, P., *et al.* (1985). Effect of omeprazole and cimetidine on duodenal ulcer, a double-blind comparative trial. *N. Engl. J. Med.*, **312**, 958–61
35. Bardhan, D.K., Bianchi Porro, G. and Bosel, K., *et al.* (1986). A comparison of two different doses of omeprazole versus ranitidine in treatment of duodenal ulcers. *J. Clin. Gastroenterol.*, **8**, 408–13

36. Cook, G.C. (1985). Infective gastroenteritis and its relationship to reduced gastric acidity. *Scand. J. Gastroenterol.*, **20**, 17–22
37. Howden, C.W. and Hunt, R.H. (1987). Relationship between gastric secretion and infection. *Gut*, **28**, 96–107
38. Giannella, R.A., Broitman, S.A. and Zamchek, N. (1971). *Salmonella* enteritis. I. Role of reduced gastric secretion in pathogenesis. *Am. J. Dig. Dis.*, **16**, 1000–6
39. Giannella, R.A., Broitman, S.A. and Zamchek, N. (1973). Influence of gastric acidity on bacterial and parasitic infections. A perspective. *Ann. Intern. Med.*, **78**, 271–6
40. Waddell, W.R. and Kunz, L.J. (1956). Association of *Salmonella* enteritis with operations on the stomach. *N. Engl. J. Med.*, **255**, 555–9
41. Gray, J.A. and Trueman, A.M. (1971). Severe *Salmonella* gastroenteritis associated with hypochlorhydria. *Scott. Med. J.*, **16**, 255–8
42. Dupont, H.L., Hornick, R.B., Snyder, M.J., Libonati, J.P., Formal, S.B. and Gangarosa, E.J. (1972). Immunity in shigellosis. I. Response of man to attenuated strains of *Shigella*. *J. Infect. Dis.*, **125**, 5–11
43. Cash, R.A., Music, S.I., Libonati, J.P., Snyder, M.J., Wenzel, R.P. and Hornick, R.B. (1974). Response of man to infection with *Vibrio cholerae*. I. Clinical, serologic and bacteriologic responses to a known inoculum. *J. Infect. Dis.*, **129**, 45–52
44. Nalin, D.R., Levine, R.J. and Levine, M.M., *et al.* (1978). Cholera, non-*Vibrio* cholera and stomach acid. *Lancet*, **ii**, 856–9
45. Steefan, R. (1977). Antacids – a risk factor in travellers' brucellosis. *Scand. J. Infect. Dis.*, **9**, 311–12
46. Anon. (1982). Battles against *Giardia* in gut mucosa. (Leading article.) *Lancet*, **ii**, 527–8
47. Gurian, L., Ward, T.T. and Katon, R.M. (1982). Possible foodborne transmission in a case of pseudomembranous colitis due to *Clostridium difficile*. Influence of gastrointestinal secretions on *Clostridium difficile* infection. *Gastroenterology*, **83**, 465–9

3
Duodenogastric reflux and other motility disorders in gastric ulcer disease

I. A. EYRE-BROOK and A. G. JOHNSON

The significance of duodenogastric reflux (DGR) in the pathogenesis of gastric ulcer disease is still uncertain. Much of this uncertainty arises because the complex process of reflux has been studied in many different ways and usually only one aspect or marker has been measured at a time. This limits the value of comparisons between DGR measurements by different workers. Although various duodenal constituents, particularly bile acids, have been shown to damage gastric mucosa in experimental studies, great caution is required before results of such animal experiments are used to implicate DGR in the aetiology of human gastric ulcer disease (GU). In this chapter the evidence from human and animal studies which suggest that DGR can cause gastric ulceration will be reviewed. The motor abnormalities in gastric ulcer disease which could predispose to reflux will then be considered.

METHODS OF ASSESSMENT

Reflux is not an 'all or none' phenomenon and to assess its significance in various conditions it is necessary to define its character fully (Table 3.1). Every method of reflux measurement fails to answer all these questions. Techniques of DGR measurement fall into three categories.

Table 3.1   Characterization of reflux

---

1. The process of reflux:
   How much refluxes?
   When does it reflux?
   How often does it reflux?
   How long does it remain in the stomach?

2. The nature of the refluxed material:
   What is its chemical composition?

3. The state of the stomach:
   How good is the mucosal protection?
   What is the gastric acid secretory status?
   Is gastritis already present?
   Is there food in the stomach?

---

(1) Assessment of reflux of marker substances

Capper's radiological 'pyloric regurgitation test' was first reported in 1966[1] and has been used extensively since; it is a qualitative assessment of reflux. An oroduodenal tube is passed and a 30-ml bolus of barium sulphate is injected to fill the proximal duodenum. Reflux is assessed radiologically by screening for three minutes. This test is no longer considered safe because of the prolonged x-ray screening required. Capper's original observation that the introduction of barium led to an increased frequency of duodenal retro-peristaltic contractions suggests that the barium bolus disrupts normal fasting motor activity. The technique offers an assessment of reflux over a very short period under non-physiological conditions. Barium is a very heavy hyperosmolar material with no calorific value and the test simulates neither the fasting nor the postprandial state.

To avoid the use of a transpyloric tube others have injected an intravenous marker such as bromsulphthalein[2], indocyanine green[3] or the radio-pharmaceutical [99m]technetium iminodiacetic acid (HIDA)[4] and assessed recovery of the marker from gastric aspirates. These agents are excreted in the bile but excretion is neither uniform nor predictable[5]. Reflux values quoted as a proportion of the injected dose may well reflect variations in the biliary excretion of the marker rather than genuine reflux. Similar objections apply to labelling the bile salt pool with ^{14}C chenodeoxycholic acid[6] since distribution may not be uniform. Muller-Lissner has overcome some of these problems by using the gamma-camera to calculate the duodenal content of ^{99m}Tc HIDA after an intravenous injection and expressing the amount of HIDA in gastric aspirates as a proportion of the duodenal activity[7].

52

(2) Measurement of intragastric concentrations of bile acids and other duodenal secretions

These techniques again involve the passage of a gastric tube but leave the pylorus undisturbed. Both the gastric tube itself and the aspiration of gastric contents disturb the normal gastroduodenal physiology. These tests do not simply measure the movement of duodenal contents into the stomach but instead reflect the complicated balance between secretion into the duodenum and stomach and the movement of these contents orally and aborally. However, despite their limitations, these tests provide the most important parameters of reflux since they measure the concentrations of bile acids and other duodenal constituents in the stomach.

(3) Non-invasive measurements

Intravenous HIDA is rapidly taken up by hepatocytes and excreted in the bile ducts. Bile discharge into the duodenum can then be observed on the gamma-camera and reflux assessed as the movement of activity into the gastric region[8]. This is certainly the most physiological technique. The major technical problem is that the duodenojejunal flexure frequently lies behind the body of the stomach and it is often difficult to distinguish genuine reflux from activity in the duodenojejunal flexure.

Our knowledge of reflux in health and disease comes from observations using these three techniques, none of which provides all the information shown in Table 3.1. Since each technique provides a different 'glimpse' of the process of reflux, it is difficult to compare results.

REFLUX IN HEALTH

William Beaumont, who published his results in 1833, is usually cited as the first man to study DGR. His subject, Alexis St Martin, had a traumatic gastric fistula through which Beaumont observed the passage of bile across the pylorus. He concluded that 'bile is seldom found in the stomach except under peculiar circumstances'[9] and later studies using Capper's pyloric regurgitation test seemed to confirm this conclusion. Capper reported no reflux of barium from duodenum to stomach in 21 healthy subjects[10] and others have confirmed this finding. Barium reflux has been noted in only one of 112 healthy subjects studied in the literature[11-14]. However, the value of these studies is limited by their non-physiological nature.

Muller Lissner, who studied the proportion of duodenal HIDA which was aspirated from the stomach during two hours of fasting, reported that DGR did occur in his six healthy volunteers. Duodenal HIDA refluxed into the stomach at a mean rate of 0.42% of the intraduodenal HIDA per minute (range 0.06–0.97% per minute)[7].

While Capper's technique does not allow post-prandial observation, Muller Lissner's studies suggest that reflux rates in the fasting and post-prandial states are similar. He found mean reflux after a meal of (20%) Intralipid to be 0.3% per minute[7]. Non-invasive HIDA studies confirm that post-prandial reflux can occur in health although reflux is undetectable in the majority of healthy subjects[8,15].

More prolonged measurement of bile acid concentration in gastric aspirates indicates that bile acids may be present in the gastric aspirate of healthy subjects[15-19]. Although it has been argued that intubation of the stomach, necessary in these tests, may itself induce abnormal reflux, this has not been confirmed during HIDA studies of the intubated subject[20]. Concentrations of bile acid in the fasting state are usually low or unrecordable. Reported post-prandial values range from 11–88 μmol/litre but individual values as high as 550 μmol/litre have been observed. Concentrations of bile acids after a variety of liquid fat-containing test meals are also low but individual levels as high as 690 μmol/litre have been observed. All these values have been obtained in studies lasting 1 to 4 h but marked variations in bile acid reflux may occur over more prolonged periods[21]. The only prolonged study of bile acid reflux reported marked fluctuations over 24 h in a small group of eight subjects. Mean intragastric bile acid concentrations rose as high as 700 μmol/litre in the early hours of the morning[22].

THE IMPORTANCE OF TECHNIQUE

Aspiration

Two important aspects of technique must be stressed. The first is the method of aspiration. If this is continuous, the refluxed juice has no chance to empty back into the duodenum and the suction itself could encourage reflux. If aspiration is intermittent, emptying the stomach completely each time has its disadvantages, whereas a small sample may be unrepresentative. Probably the best method is intermittent complete aspiration with reintroduction of all but the small sample required for analysis.

Stimuli

Of even greater significance is the variety of different stimuli used during reflux studies. Cholecystokinin (CCK) for example, produces a sudden secretion of bile and inhibition of antral contractions. It is only one of many hormones released by a meal and reflux certainly cannot be considered normal if it is produced in healthy subjects by this stimulus alone. Intralipid also has the disadvantage that it is an artificial meal, but is more physiological than CCK. The most physiological meal is the balanced Lundh meal but its contents and consistency make bile salt analysis difficult. The most physiological study is a 24-h study with normal meals, but this also presents technical problems.

REFLUX IN GASTRIC ULCER DISEASE

Early studies using Capper's radiological pyloric regurgitation test demonstrated a clear difference between gastric ulcer patients and controls[10–12]. Reflux of barium has been observed in nearly all gastric ulcer patients studied, but in none of the control patients (Table 3.2). These results indicate that the antroduodenal region of GU patients is abnormal. The constancy of the results leaves little doubt that the response of the antroduodenal region to the instillation of barium is different in GU patients than in controls. However, the pyloric regurgitation test is not a physiological test and there may be no difference in the response of the antroduodenal region to more physiological stimuli. Unfortunately there are no more prolonged studies of fasting marker reflux available although Muller Lissner's studies of post-prandial HIDA reflux across the pylorus have failed to substantiate increased reflux rates in GU patients. High reflux rates (> 0.2% of duodenal HIDA per minute) occurred

Table 3.2 Radiological studies of reflux using Capper's pyloric regurgitation test

Disease studied	Authors of study (Reference no.)	Number studied	Number of reflux negative	Number of reflux positive*	Subjects reflux negative (%)	Subjects reflux positive (%)
Normal controls	Capper[10]	21	21	0	100	0
Normal controls	Flint and Grech[11]	12	11	1	92	8
Normal controls	Cocking and Grech[12]	10	10	0	100	0
Normal controls	Johnson[13]	4	4	0	100	0
Normal controls	Giacosa et al.[14]	65	65	0	100	0
Gastric ulcer	Capper[10]	20	0	20	0	100
Gastric ulcer	Flint and Grech[11]	21	2	19	9	91
Gastric ulcer	Cocking and Grech[12]	10	0	10	0	100
Duodenal ulcer	Capper et al.[30]	41	18	23	44	56
Duodenal and pre-pyloric ulcer	Flint and Grech[11]	16	2	14	13	87
Gallstones	Johnson[13]	18	6	12	33	67
Hiatus hernia	Gillison et al.[31]	80	24	56	30	70
Hiatus hernia	Giacosa et al.[14]	35	14	21	40	60

* Reflux-positive patients have reflux of barium solution into the stomach observed radiologically after instillation of barium into the duodenum.

more frequently in his 17 GU patients than in the 10 control subjects, but there was no statistical differences between the two groups[7]. However Niemela, using an entirely non-invasive HIDA technique, has found a difference between post-prandial reflux rates in 33 GU patients and 33 non-ulcer controls[23]. Nevertheless, many of Niemela's GU patients still had low reflux values which were well within the control range.

Most studies of bile acid concentration in the stomach have confirmed a difference between gastric ulcer patients and controls both in the fasting and post-prandial states (Tables 3.3 and 3.4)[6,16,19,24,25]. Mean bile acid concentrations in GU patients are significantly higher than in controls but there is an enormous scatter of bile acid values in gastric ulcer patients. This is quite unlike the consistent results seen in the pyloric regurgitation test. Many GU patients have bile acid concentrations well within the control range and in some GU patients bile acids are not detectable in the stomach.

The results summarized in Table 3.3 come from studies lasting only a few hours. Many of the results were obtained before gastroenterologists were aware that fasting gastroduodenal motility was cyclical. Since Szurszewski first described the migrating myoelectrical complex in dogs[26], similar electrical and motility patterns have been demonstrated in man[21]. Reflux of duodenal markers

Table 3.3 Fasting studies of intragastric bile acid concentrations (μmol/litre)*

Disease studied	Authors of study (Reference no.)	Number studied	Mean values during study**	Range of values	Statistical difference from control group†
Normal controls	DuPlessis[16]	13	88 ± 40		
Normal controls	Rhodes et al.[6]	10	80 ± 30	10–330	
Normal controls	Black et al.[25]	13		0–120	
Normal controls	Stol et al.[17]	13	80 ± 70	0–200	
Normal controls	Dewar et al.[19]	9	11 ± 11	0–200	
Normal controls	Eyre-Brook et al.[25]	6	24 ± 4	10–33	
Gastric ulcer	DuPlessis[16]	14	490 ± 350		
Gastric ulcer	Rhodes et al.[6]	10	660 ± 340	30–3170	$p = 0.05$
Gastric ulcer	Black et al.[24]	32		0–3200	$p < 0.001$
Gastric ulcer	Dewar et al.[19]	11	885 ± 700		
Gastric ulcer	Eyre-Brook et al.[25]	11	277 ± 120	10–1270	$p < 0.01$
Duodenal ulcer	DuPlessis[16]	22	200 ± 150		$p < 0.01$
Duodenal ulcer	Dewar et al.[19]	16	381 ± 150		$p < 0.001$
Non-functioning gallbladder	Eyre-Brook et al.[25]	11	613 ± 329		$p < 0.01$
Hiatus hernia	Stol et al.[17]	22	320 ± 320	0–1030	

* All quoted concentrations have been converted to μmol/litre using mean molecular weight of bile acids = 450.

** Mean values are the mean of concentrations during all sampling periods (± SEM).

† Probabilities are those quoted in each publication and represent the statistical difference from the control group in the same study.

Table 3.4 Post-prandial studies of intragastric bile acid concentrations (μmol/litre)*

Disease studied	Authors of study	Number studied	Mean values during study**	Peak values during study	Range of values	Statistical difference from control group†
Normal controls	Rhodes et al.[6]	10	60 ± 10		10–690	
Normal controls	Black et al.[24]	13			0–480	
Normal controls	Dewar et al.[18]	9	51 ± 20			
Normal controls	Eyre-Brook et al.[25]	6		46 ± 8	23–74	
Gastric ulcer	Rhodes et al.[6]	10	780 ± 330	1100 ± 330	90–29 000	$p < 0.01$
Gastric ulcer	Black et al.[24]	32			0–7400	$p < 0.01$
Gastric ulcer	Dewar et al.[19]	9	671 ± 400			$p < 0.001$
Gastric ulcer	Eyre-Brook et al.[25]	11		812 ± 383	33–4375	$p < 0.01$
Duodenal ulcer	Dewar et al.[18]	16	516 ± 200	906 ± 250		$p < 0.001$
Non-functioning gallbladder	Eyre-Brook et al.[25]	11		435 ± 228	29–2000	$p < 0.01$

*All quoted concentrations have been converted to μmol/litre using mean molecular weight of bile acids = 450.

** Mean values are the mean of concentrations during all post-prandial sampling periods ($\pm$ SEM) in all patients.

† Probabilities are those quoted in each publication and represent the statistical difference from the control.

into the duodenum can be shown to vary with the migrating motor complex (MMC) and peak reflux occurs at the end of phase II[27]. Only one prolonged study of intragastric bile acid concentration in GU patients has been reported. In this study, gastric contents were sampled hourly for 24 h in seven GU patients and eight controls[22]. Individual results were not given but mean results showed great variations over the 24 h with no obvious difference between GU patients and controls. Unfortunately no prolonged studies are available comparing reflux at different phases of the MMC in GU and control subjects. Results from bile acid studies currently available suggest that GU patients comprise a heterogeneous group with some patients having bile acid concentrations much greater than those seen in controls.

REFLUX IN OTHER DISEASES

Increased DGR has also been reported in other diseases not associated with gastric mucosal ulceration.

(1) Duodenal ulcer

Abnormal reflux has been reported in duodenal ulcer disease but the degree of reflux seems less than in gastric ulcer patients (Tables 3.2 to 3.4). The simultaneous occurrence of gastric ulcer and duodenal ulcer suggests common variables in their pathogenesis. Capper, using his radiological pyloric regurgitation test, noted reflux of barium in all 20 active GU patients and in 18 of 41 duodenal ulcer patients, but in no controls[10]. Fiddian-Green *et al.* used the sodium content of gastric aspirates to infer reflux[28] and reported greater reflux in 59 duodenal ulcer patients than in 50 controls after histamine stimulation. Dewar *et al.* have confirmed earlier reports of intragastric bile acid concentrations. Fasting and post-prandial bile acid concentrations in 16 duodenal ulcer patients (mean 38 and 516 μmol/litre) were significantly greater than in nine controls (mean 11 and 52 μmol/litre) but lower than results in gastric ulcer disease (mean 885 and 671 μmol/litre)[18,19]. In studies of gastric lysolecithin concentration at night[29], DU patients appear to comprise two populations, one with very little reflux, similar to normals, and one with significant reflux but less than GU patients. There is a type-II GU which is associated, and probably preceded by duodenal ulcer disease, and so this reflux in some duodenal ulcer patients may be significant.

(2) Gallbladder disease

Capper reported reflux of barium from duodenum to stomach in 16 of 18 patients with gallstones and implicated reflux as the cause of symptoms of flatulent dyspepsia associated with gallstones[30].

We have corroborated the relationship between barium reflux and the symptoms of flatulent dyspepsia[13] but have been unable to demonstrate this relationship with studies of intragastric bile acid concentrations[25]. Non-invasive HIDA studies suggest that reflux in gallbladder disease is more closely related to the loss of normal gallbladder motility owing to cholelithiasis, than to the symptoms of flatulent dyspepsia (Figure 3.1)[15].

Both studies of intragastric bile acids and non-invasive HIDA studies have confirmed that DGR is more common in patients with gallstones than in controls[15,25]. We have compared bile acid reflux in 11 patients with gastric ulcer and 11 patients with gallstones in a non-functioning gallbladder on oral cholecystogram. Both fasting and post-prandial reflux were similar in the two diseases and results in each group were different from control subjects (Figures 3.2 and 3.3)[25].

(3) Oesophagitis

Gillison and Airth, working with Capper, reported barium reflux from duo-

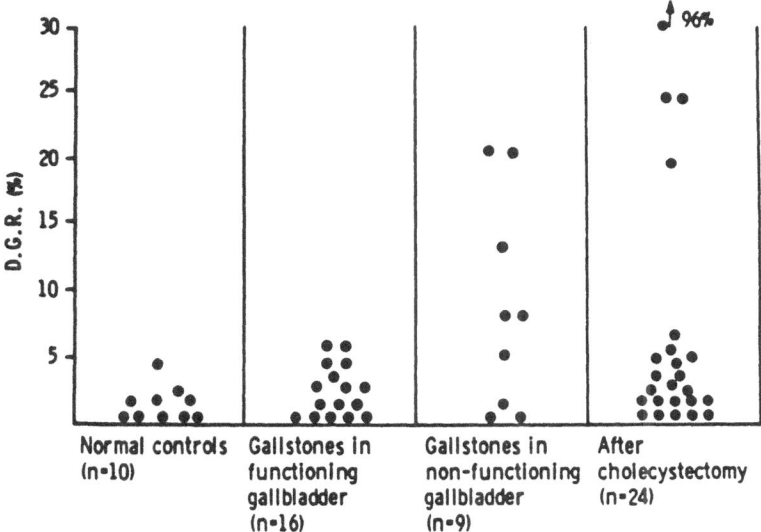

Figure 3.1 HIDA reflux in patients with and without radiological gallbladder function. DGR (%) is the percentage of HIDA secreted by the liver which refluxes into the stomach

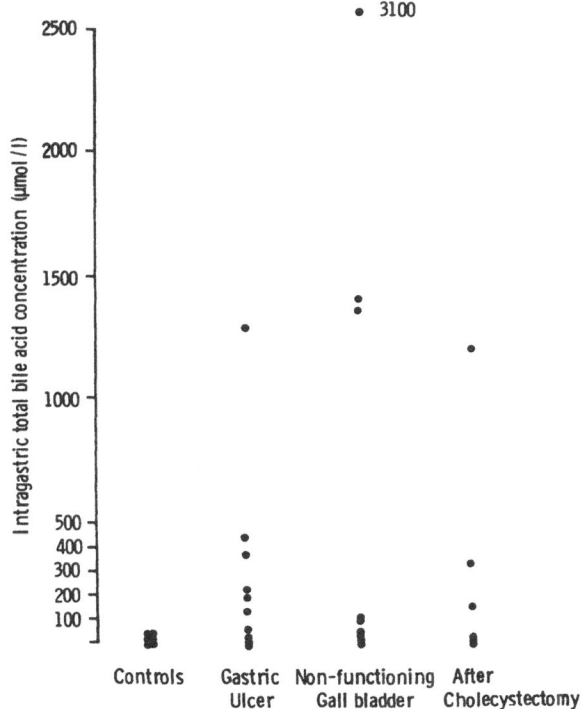

Figure 3.2 Bile acid reflux in the fasted state

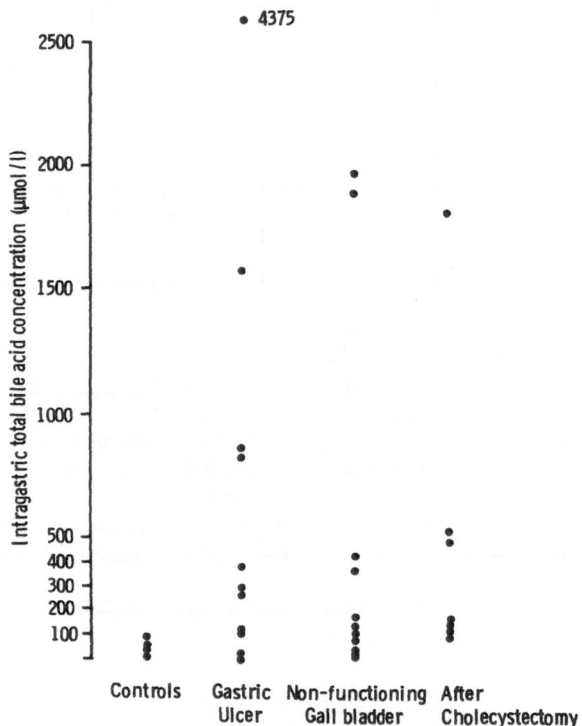

Figure 3.3 Bile acid reflux after an intralipid meal

denum to stomach in 56 of 80 patients with hiatus hernia[31]. Symptoms of heartburn were present in 52 of 56 with DGR but in only seven of 24 who did not have DGR on screening. Giacosa *et al.*, using Capper's technique, suggested a relationship between oesophagitis and DGR[14]. Although Stol *et al.* found intragastric bile acid concentrations to be significantly higher in 22 patients with symptomatic hiatus hernia (mean 330 μmol/litre) than in 13 controls (mean 80 μmol/litre)[17], this finding has not been supported by Collins *et al.*[32].

EXPERIMENTAL STUDIES

If DGR is significant in the aetiology of gastric ulcer disease, we must seek to explain why reflux can occur in other diseases without causing mucosal ulceration. Experiments on the development of gastric mucosal injury in animals after exposure to duodenal contents, provide valuable insight into the possible effects of duodenal contents on the gastric mucosa.

(1) Acute changes on exposure to pancreatic and biliary secretions

Gastric stress ulceration induced in animals by a variety of physiological stresses is intimately associated with the presence of duodenal contents in the stomach and can be prevented by avoiding duodenogastric reflux. Smith first demonstrated this in dogs and cats in 1914[33]. Roux-en-Y diversion can prevent the induction of stress ulceration both in the dog[34] and in the piglet[35], while intragastric administration of 5 mmol/litre taurocholic acid reverses this protective action[34]. Ligation of the pylorus similarly prevents the ulcerogenic effects of haemorrhagic shock in dogs and rats but ulcers return with intragastric administration of 15 mmol/litre taurocholate[36-38]. Similar results have been found in rats using water immersion stress[39] and restraint stress[40].

Intragastric bile acids alone, however, even in concentrations far in excess of those seen clinically, do not produce gastric ulceration in the dog[39,41]. A series of elegant experiments using vascularised full thickness wedges of canine gastric wall mounted in lucite chambers has defined more clearly the environmental conditions in which 'physiological' concentrations of bile acids can induce gastric mucosal ulceration[41]. Significant ulcer formation occurs only with the simultaneous topical administration of hydrochloric acid and bile acids to mucosa rendered ischaemic with intra-arterial vasopressin. The incidence of ulcers in the presence of luminal acid and mucosal ischaemia is linearly dependent upon the concentration of bile acids (taurocholic 1 to 5 mmol/litre) while in the presence of 'physiological' concentrations of taurocholic acid (1 and 2 mmol/litre) ulceration in ischaemic mucosa varies linearly with hydrogen ion concentration. Sub-ulcerogenic mucosal damage has been assessed by monitoring hydrogen (H^+) and sodium (Na^+) ion fluxes and potential difference changes across the mucosa. Although the value of these changes as indicators of mucosal damage has been questioned[41,42], most workers accept their value. The gastric mucosal barrier normally restricts movement of H^+ down its concentration gradient from lumen to blood (back diffusion), and the movement of Na^+ in the reverse direction down its concentration gradient (forward diffusion). In non-ischaemic mucosa, 'physiological' concentrations of bile salts in an acid medium produce a significant concentration-dependent increase in H^+ back diffusion and Na^+ forward diffusion, together with a fall in potential difference across the mucosa. These changes are generally greater in ischaemic mucosa preceding ulcer formation[41]. Progressive changes in these parameters have also been demonstrated with increasing acid concentrations in bile salt-exposed mucosa[41]. Davenport[43], and Duane and Wiegand[44] claimed that taurocholate (10, 20 and 40 mmol/litre) in neutral solution also produced these fluxes. However, in these Heidenhain pouch experiments the test solutions which commenced at neutral pH were often acid (pH 3) when removed from the pouch. Davenport[43] has also shown that both bile salts and natural bile can break the mucosal barrier when administered at a concentration of 40 mmol/litre with a liquid, mixed fat-containing meal.

(2) The mechanism of bile salt injury

Bile salts appear to disrupt the gastric mucosal barrier thereby permitting H^+ to enter and disrupt mucosal cells. Bile salts and synthetic detergents applied topically to gastric mucosa undoubtedly increase the rate at which H^+ passes from the lumen of the canine Heidenhain pouch[43,45]. Ulcer formation is associated with a profound fall in intramucosal pH[46] and gastric venous acidosis[41], while induced alkalosis of the gastric vasculature will prevent mucosal damage[47].

Cholestyramine, which binds bile salts, virtually abolishes H^+ back diffusion and prevents ulceration[36]. However, certain inconsistencies exist. Hamza and Den Beston[36] demonstrated that topical bile salts led to ulcers in dogs subjected to haemorrhagic shock, without increasing the magnitude of H^+ back diffusion. Ritchie's findings[41] that ulceration was not linearly related to H^+ back diffusion but was enhanced by mucosal ischaemia, led him to propose that ulcerogenesis was less dependent on the absolute magnitude of the H^+ back diffusion than on the mucosa's capacity to respond to the insult. This mucosal capacity was felt to depend on mucosal blood flow acting as an 'alkaline tide' to neutralize H^+. Blood flow findings, however, have been confusing. O'Brien and Silen[48] reported that high concentrations of luminal bile acid reduced mucosal blood flow as assessed by aminopyrine clearance, while others have found a lower concentration of bile acid (10 mmol/litre) to increase mucosal blood flow[49]. Experiments performed with intravenous vasopressin demonstrate that it prevents the bile acid-induced increase in mucosal flow and leads to ulceration[41]. This synergism between mucosal flow and H^+ back diffusion is illustrated by Ritchie's work[41]. Ulcerogenesis could be prevented either by improving mucosal flow despite continued back diffusion of H^+ or by preventing H^+ back diffusion with cholestyramine despite continued impairment of mucosal flow.

OTHER COMPONENTS OF REFLUX

Duodenal contents other than bile acids have also been shown to damage gastric mucosa. Stress ulceration in the dog, prevented by Roux-en-Y diversion, can be induced again by intragastric administration of lysolecithin (0.2 mmol-/litre)[34]. Lysolecithin in concentrations similar to those seen in gastric ulcer patients (100 mg%) can produce gastric ulceration in the guinea-pig stomach, these changes being preceded by a transmucosal potential difference shift[50]. H^+ back diffusion and Na^+ forward diffusion has been demonstrated with lysolecithin in the canine Heidenhain pouch[51]. Phospholipase A_2, which can damage the phospholipid-containing membranes of the erythrocyte, may also damage the gastric mucosal barrier, although results are far from conclusive[51].

Several studies have examined concentrations of lysolecithin and phospholipase A_2 in the human stomach[18,19,25,29]. The distribution of results both in gastric ulcer and controls resembles the pattern of bile acid results. Thus, although lysolecithin and phospholipase A_2 are statistically greater in GU patients there is a considerable scatter of results. Many GU patients have very low concentrations which are well within the range of values seen in controls[18,19]. It is interesting that Dewar, who found a difference between lysolecithin concentrations in gastric ulcer patients and controls, found no difference between DU patients and controls. This might suggest that duodenal ulcer patients reflux less lysolecithin than gastric ulcer patients and thereby avoid gastric mucosal damage. However, differences in lysolecithin reflux would not seem to explain the absence of mucosal ulceration in patients with gallstones. We have measured phospholipase A_2 concentrations in the stomach of controls, gastric ulcer patients and those with gallstones[25]. Patterns of fasting and post-prandial phospholipase A_2 reflux were similar in gastric ulcer patients and in those with gallstones in a non-functioning gallbladder, and both groups had greater concentrations than in controls. However, the low phospholipase A_2 results seen after cholecystectomy might help explain why patients with bile reflux after cholecystectomy avoid gastric ulcer.

SIGNIFICANCE OF DGR IN GU

Some of the results from studies of DGR in health and disease appear contradictory but certain conclusions can be drawn from the available data. Although reflux of barium in the radiological pyloric regurgitation test appears a consistent finding in gastric ulcer disease, all other techniques of reflux measurement indicate that gastric ulcer patients are a heterogeneous group. Some GU patients have markedly greater reflux than healthy controls but many other GU patients have negligible reflux detected and reflux varies considerably over a period of 12 h during day or night. Clearly reflux is not the cause of all gastric ulcer disease. If reflux is to be considered a significant factor in some GU patients, we must explain why patients who reflux with duodenal ulcer disease, hiatus hernia and cholelithiasis do not develop gastric ulcers. Although gastritis is a common feature in all these diseases, an increased predisposition to gastric ulceration has only been noted in duodenal ulcer disease. GU is probably multifactorial and other abnormalities need to be considered:

(a) *Slow gastric emptying.* This has been proposed as an additional factor in gastric ulceration[52,53]. It is tempting to propose that delayed emptying of refluxed duodenal contents prolongs the 'contact time' between noxious chemicals and the gastric mucosa. Miller *et al.* have demonstrated delayed emptying of solids as well as increased reflux of bile in GU patients[52].

(b) *Mucosal factors.* Experiments in the isolated animal stomach implicate three principal factors in the aetiology of acute gastric ulceration[54]. These are intragastric bile acid concentrations, intragastric pH and mucosal ischaemia, but these parameters may not be as relevant in the intact animal. Bile and pancreatic juice alone, or in combination, have been diverted into the canine stomach without mucosal changes even after a year[55]. Yet under other experimental conditions, diversion of duodenal contents initiates marked gastritis[56]. Menguy and Max[57] noted severe inflammatory and proliferative changes in the gastric mucosa after pancreatico-biliary diversion which were similar to those seen in gastric ulceration in man. Lawson[56] has demonstrated that gastritis is most severe with diversion of both bile and pancreatic fluid together while gastritis is minimal when only pancreatic juice is diverted. Roux-en-Y diversion of duodenal contents reverses these changes[58]. Hydrogen-ion back diffusion has been demonstrated in five healthy human volunteers subjected to intragastric infusions of 5 mmol/litre taurocholate[59] and a fall in intramucosal potential difference has been observed following instillation of pancreatico-biliary secretions in nine volunteers[60].

The capacity of the postoperative stomach to tolerate large quantities of intragastric bile, frequently without symptoms, gastritis or ulceration, suggests that high intragastric pH may protect against bile acid damage. Despite rather low acid secretion in GU patients, ulceration could still be related to a decreased capacity of the mucosal 'alkaline tide' to neutralize normal H^+ back diffusion. Certainly both vagotomy[61] and H_2-receptor blockade[62] promote ulcer healing. However, if a low pH is central to bile acid-induced mucosal damage it is difficult to explain why duodenal ulcer patients who reflux do not get gastric ulcers. Thomas has suggested *local* hypersecretion of acid adjacent to gastric ulcers[63] but this has not been demonstrated. Bile-induced H^+ back diffusion, however, is postulated to release histamine locally[64] and this could induce local hypersecretion of acid. If differences in lysolecithin reflux in gastric ulcer and DU could be demonstrated, this might provide a further possible explanation.

The role of mucosal ischaemia in gastric ulcer disease is unknown. It has not been demonstrated in gastric ulcer disease and we have no knowledge of the comparative vascularity of mucosa in GU, DU, hiatus hernia and cholelithiasis.

Individual bile acids differ in their capacity to damage gastric mucosa and differences in bile acid composition could help explain why patients with gallstones who reflux do not get ulcers. Unfortunately, changes in individual bile acids seen after cholecystectomy would be expected to make the reflux more damaging to the gastric mucosa[65]!

Only limited studies of the reflux of phospholipase A_2 and lysolecithin have been performed but these have failed to identify a difference between reflux of phospholipase A_2 in gallbladder disease and cholelithiasis but the lack of phospholipase A_2 reflux after cholecystectomy could explain why these patients avoid ulcers[25].

An interesting observation by Ritchie and Delaney[66] that mucosa rendered previously atrophic is more susceptible to chemical injury than is normal mucosa, suggests that mucosal atrophy in gastric ulcer disease might be a primary defect rendering gastric mucosa more susceptible to H^+ back diffusion. However, mucosal atrophy has been reported in cholelithiasis[30] as well as in GU disease although the extent and severity of the atrophic changes in the two conditions has not been compared.

The more detailed aspects of mucosal protection will be discussed in Chapters 6 to 10.

CONCLUSION

The evidence we have reviewed points to duodenogastric reflux playing some part in the aetiology of GU and gastritis. Only a few studies have been done during the night and it is quite likely that this is the time when the stomach is empty and reflux is most damaging. However, one person's gastric mucosa may be sensitive to the effects of duodenal juice whereas another's may not.

A simple analogy will help to illustrate this principle: If a fair-skinned person sits in the sun with a dark-skinned friend, he will be sunburnt the next day, whereas his friend will not, even though they have both received the same 'dose' of ultraviolet rays. The degree of sunburn will depend on the sun's intensity and the length of the exposure. The dark-skinned person, however, is relatively 'resistant' to sunburn. The fair-skinned person can produce a degree of protection by sunbathing a little at a time so that his skin becomes trained ('adaptive cytoprotection'). He can also prevent the sunburn by putting a 'barrier' between his skin and the sun in the form of sunscreen cream, or he can stop the sun reaching the skin at all by sitting under a sun-shade! The parallels for the treatment of gastric ulcer are obvious, but mucosal resistance and sensitivity to a variety of damaging agents is just as important as the particular concentration of these agents in the stomach.

MOTILITY PATTERNS IN REFLUX

An understanding of the physiological mechanisms by which reflux is pre-vented in health but permitted in some patients with gastric ulceration would allow a logical approach to reflux prevention.

The pylorus

The extent to which the pylorus itself is an anti-reflux mechanism is a matter of debate. Surgical procedures which disrupt the anatomy of the antropyloroduodenal segment (Figure 3.4) are usually associated with increased reflux but these procedures do not only distort the pylorus. Thus most studies of DGR after vagotomy and pyloroplasty have identified increased reflux while antropyloric resections are associated with marked and consistent increased reflux[19].

The pylorus certainly differs from the adjacent antrum and duodenum anatomically, both in its muscle physiology and histochemistry, and this implies a separate function for the pylorus. The pylorus comprises two distinct loops of circular muscle[67]. Physiological studies in the length–tension relation-ship of isolated pyloric muscle from various species have identified muscle physiology distinct from surrounding antral and duodenal muscle[68]. Histo-chemical studies have identified a dense network of nerve fibres with ence-

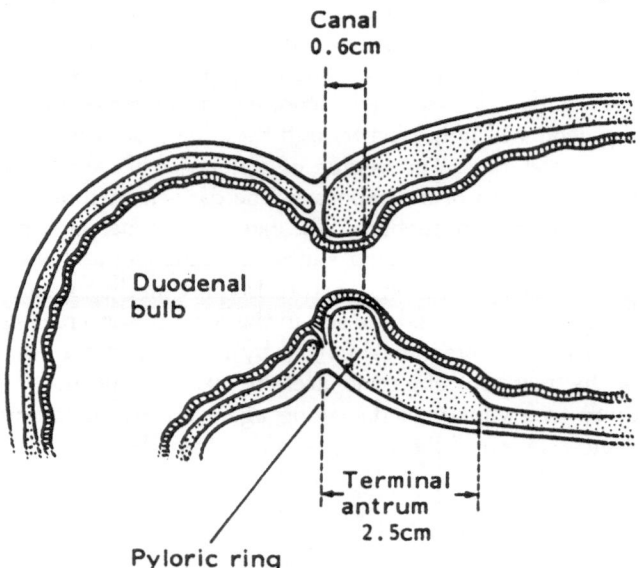

Figure 3.4   Diagram of the pylorus

phalin-like immunoreactivity lying parallel to the muscle fibres of the pylorus[69]. Studies in the intact cat have confirmed a separate non-cholinergic, non-adrenergic neural control of the pylorus in which encephalinergic neuro-transmission plays a central role. Studies in the cat also show the pylorus to be richly endowed with VIP nerve fibres which are usually a hallmark of muscle with a physiological sphincter function[70].

Early radiological studies in the cat suggested that the pylorus did work as a sphincter which controlled gastric emptying, being closed except when peristaltic antral contractions approached[71]. However, the majority of sub-sequent research has failed to corroborate these findings. Carlson *et al.*, studying canine gastric emptying, radiologically observed that the pylorus was open much of the time[72]. The terminal antrum and pyloric ring contracted almost simultaneously, propelling a small amount of barium into the duodenum and 'retropelling' the remainder back into the stomach as it came up against the pylorus. Duodenal contraction occurred just as the pyloric ring closed and reflux was prevented by the closed pylorus (Figure 3.5). Only 11% of duodenal contractions occurred with the pylorus open. Further confirmation of the anti-reflux role of the pylorus in dogs comes from studies in which the pylorus is kept open with a metal tube[73]. Gastric emptying rates are not altered by this procedure but bile reflux into the stomach is much increased.

Studies of pressure within the human pyloric canal have produced conflicting results but most of the evidence suggests that the human pyloric canal is *not* a high-pressure zone like the gastro-oesophageal junction or the anal canal. Early pull-through studies in man using balloons and non-perfused catheters failed to detect a zone of increased pressure at the pylorus[74] but later work

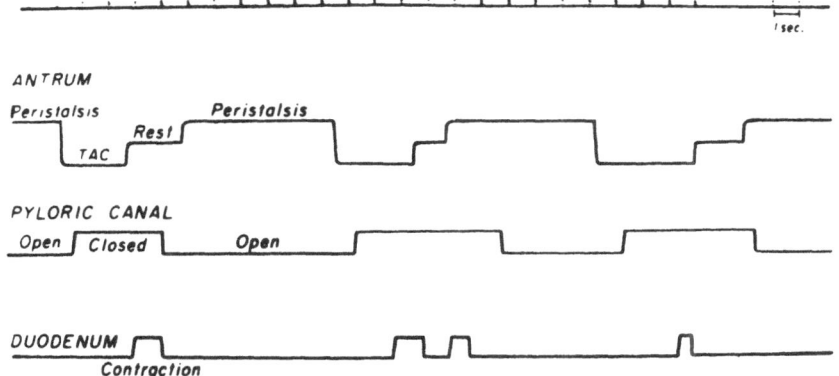

Figure 3.5 Detection of motor activity from projected cineradiograph of an unanaesthetized dog using three observers to record: progression of antral peristaltic wave and its transformation into terminal antral contraction (TAC); opening (visualization) and closure of pyloric canal; contractions in proximal duodenum. (After Carlsson *et al.*[72])

by Fisher and Cohen[75] and by Valenzuela et al.[76] recorded a high-pressure zone at the pylorus. Pressure within this zone increased following duodenal stimulation with fat or acid. However, these findings, which suggest that the pylorus acts as a sphincter, have not been confirmed using circumferentially-sensitive miniature transducers[77] or using a pull-through technique with a 2-mm balloon at endoscopy[78]. The cause of this discrepancy is probably technical. Fisher's recordings show the gastroduodenal mucosal junction (denoted by the change in mucosal potential difference) to be positioned in the middle of a 2.5-cm long high-pressure zone. This is incompatible with our knowledge of the pylorus which is only 6-mm long and lies entirely beneath gastric-type mucosa. The subjects were in the right lateral position. Recorded elevations of pressure at the pylorus may be because the catheter at this point is tightly opposed to mucosa as it moves from the posteriorly-orientated proximal duodenum into the transversely-orientated antrum. Occlusion of the orifice of a side-opening catheter by mucosa at this point may thus cause a rise in pressure resembling a contraction (Figure 3.6). Kaye et al. repeated Fisher's pull-through studies using three catheters with side-openings arranged circumferentially at the same level. They detected a tonic elevation of pyloric pressure in all three leads simultaneously in only one of 10 subjects and concluded that the pylorus was open most of the time in healthy individuals[77].

Although the resting state of the pylorus is debated, one thing is clear: if

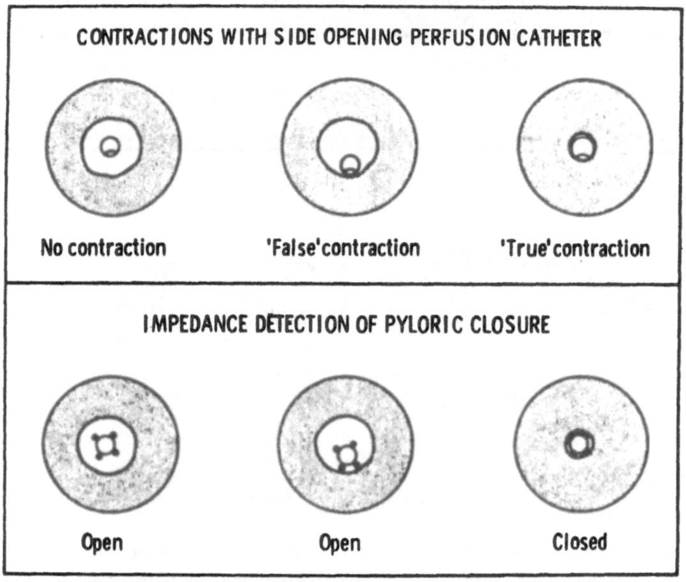

Figure 3.6 Detection of pyloric 'contractions' using manometric and impedance techniques (see text)

the pylorus is to act as a competent barrier to reflux, it must either remain closed or, if open, be capable of closing in response to isolated duodenal contractions which would otherwise induce reflux. White *et al.* have attempted to locate the orifice of a side-opening perfused catheter at the pylorus during dynamic studies by mounting it between two potential difference electrodes positioned to straddle the gastroduodenal junction[79]. Since the side-opening of their catheter was mounted between electrodes 2-cm apart, it could easily miss contractions of the pyloric ring which is only 6-mm long. This limits the reliability of their observation that the pylorus does not respond consistently to isolated duodenal contractions.

We have used an impedance technique to study closure of the pylorus at endoscopy. Antral and duodenal pressure profiles were measured using air-filled Fogarty balloon catheters. Pyloric closure was registered by monitoring the impedance across two pairs of electrodes arranged, equally spaced, around the circumference of the duodenal catheter, 5-cm proximal to the balloon. The duodenal catheter was positioned endoscopically with the balloon in the proximal duodenum and the four electrodes lying in the pyloric ring (Figure 3.7). Pyloric closure brings mucosa into contact with the electrodes lying within the pyloric canal. This contact induces a fall in the impedance and a fall in impedance between both pairs of electrodes was recorded only when the

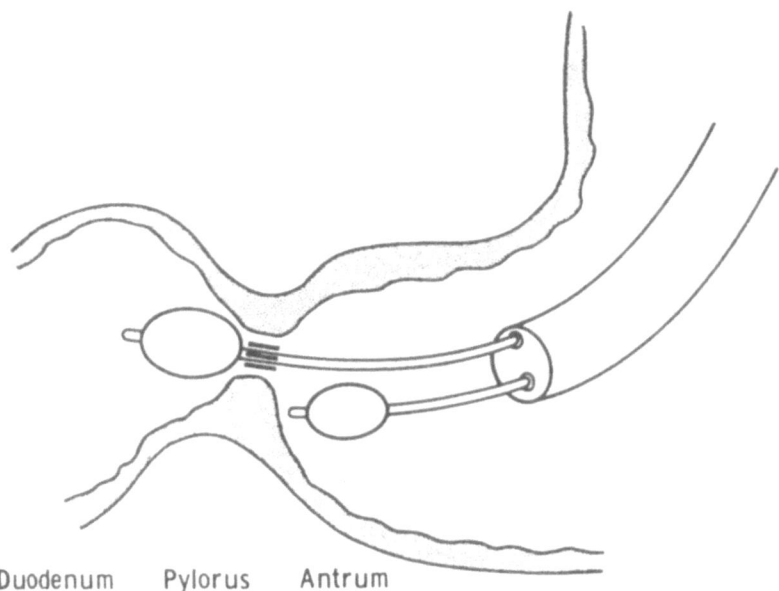

Duodenum   Pylorus   Antrum

Figure 3.7 Arrangement of antral and duodenal balloon catheters during impedance studies at endoscopy. The four impedance electrodes are sited in the pyloric canal

pylorus was closed tightly around the catheter. This avoids the problem of the 'false contraction' observed when a perfused manometric system lies eccentrically within the lumen of a viscus with the side orifice occluded by mucosa (Figure 3.6). The electrodes in this system are 6-mm long and can be accurately positioned to lie within the pyloric canal. Using this technique, we have been able to record coordinated antropyloroduodenal activity during phase III of the MMC (Figure 3.8) which closely resembles the coordination

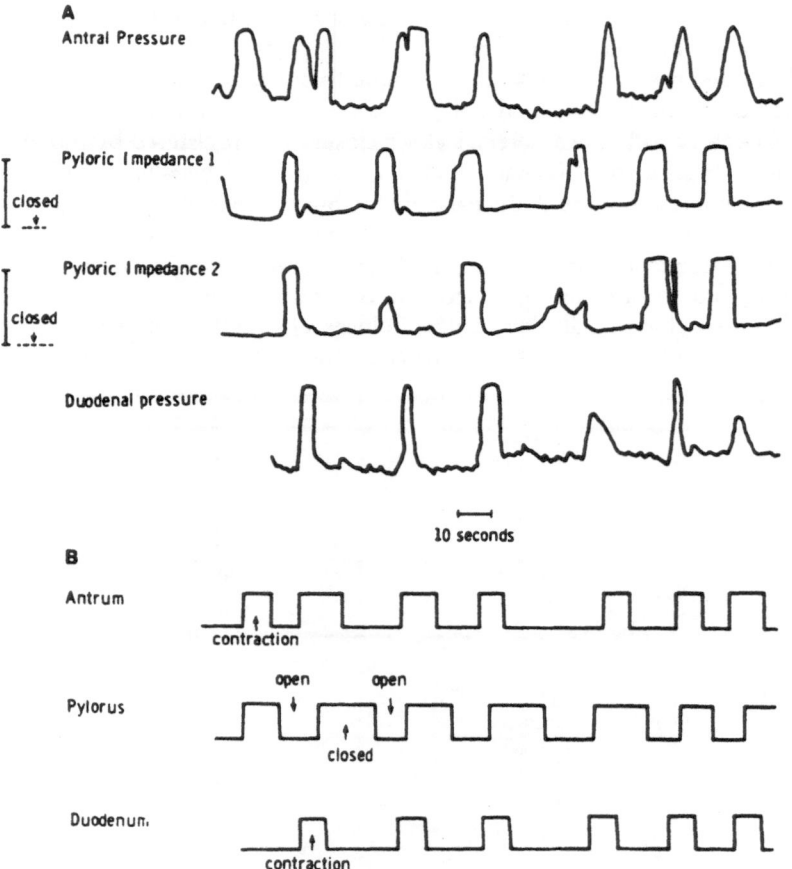

Figure 3.8 Pyloric behaviour recorded with impedance technique during antral phase-III activity. **A.** Actual traces – antral and duodenal pressure profiles are shown at the top and bottom respectively with the impedance traces in the two pairs of pyloric electrodes in the centre. The pylorus is closed only when both impedance traces are near the baseline. **B.** Schematic representation of the same result. Note that pyloric closure here is indicated in the same way as an antral or duodenal contraction with an upward deflection (the opposite of the actual trace)

observed in radiological studies in dogs (Figure 3.5) and in man. When an isolated duodenal contraction occurred with the pylorus open, we usually observed a brisk pyloric closure (Figure 3.9). Thus, in a study of 20 subjects, we observed 137 isolated duodenal contractions but the pylorus remained open after such a contraction in only 12.5% of cases—similar to Carlson and Code's original observations[72].

A. Contractions with pylorus open at onset   = 54
   (i) pyloric closure within 2 seconds   = 44
   (ii) pylorus remains open   = 10
B. Contractions with pylorus closed at onset   = 83
   (i) pyloric opening within 2 seconds   = 7
   (ii) pylorus remains closed   = 76

It is difficult to compare these results with those of manometric studies as the impedance technique measures mucosal contact around the catheter and cannot necessarily be equated with pressure recordings. However, when the pylorus was open the pyloric response to the isolated duodenal contraction was remarkably constant, four of every five such contractions being associated with pyloric closure. Such a relationship strongly suggests that the isolated duodenal contraction triggers pyloric closure. Such a pattern of activity would be appropriate if the pylorus was indeed a barrier to duodenogastric reflux.

If the pylorus is a barrier to reflux, it is pertinent to look for a defect in gastric ulcer disease. Fisher and Cohen[81] and Valenzuela and Defillipi[82] have implicated abnormal pyloric function in gastric ulcer disease but the interpretation of their work is difficult since the very existence of a pyloric high-pressure zone is debated. Valenzuela and Defillipi found the high-pressure zone on pull-through manometry to be significantly reduced in 11 patients with type-I gastric ulcer compared with 13 controls. Intraduodenal hydrochloric acid increased 'pyloric' pressure in controls but not in GU patients. Eight duodenal ulcer patients had 'pyloric' pressures similar to controls with a normal response to acid. Fisher and Cohen, on the other hand, found different basal pyloric pressures between 10 gastric ulcer patients and 10 controls but the raised pressure zone in gastric ulcer patients failed to respond normally to intraduodenal acid, olive oil, amino acid or to exogenous cholecystokinin and secretin. The reduction in Phenol Red reflux from the duodenum seen on acidification in controls was also absent. Unfortunately only four of Fisher and Cohen's 10 gastric ulcer patients had a type-I GU and the presence of a prepyloric ulcer in the remainder may have influenced their pyloric pressures and could account for discrepancies between their and Valenzuela and Defillipi's results.

71

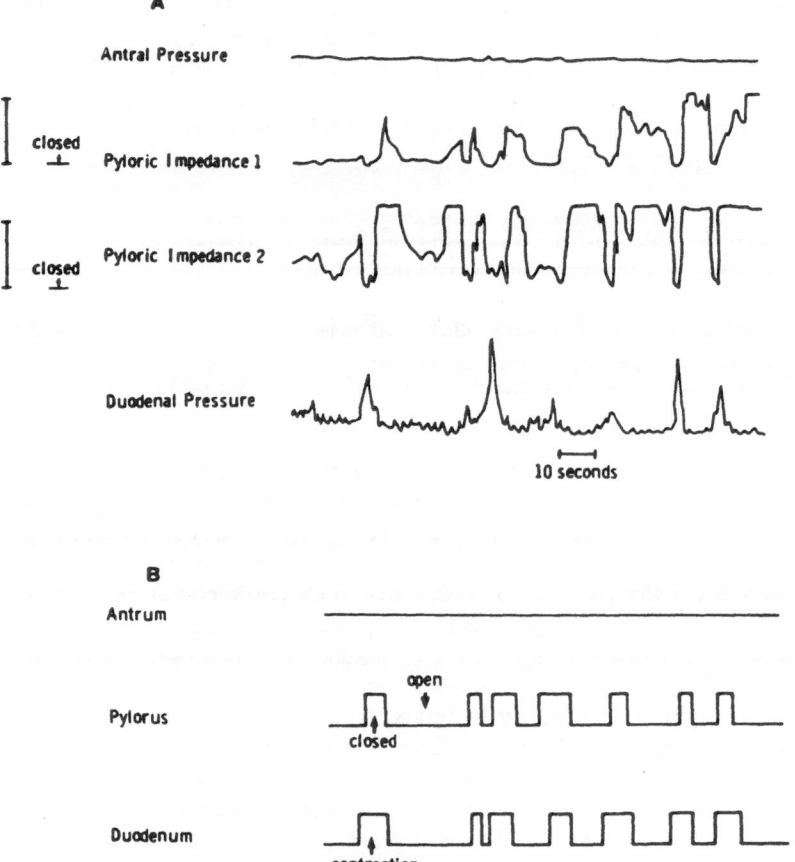

Figure 3.9 Isolated duodenal contractions with pylorus open at onset. A. Actual trace. B. Schematic representation (see Figure 3.8 for explanation)

We have noted the 'resting' diameter of the pylorus at endoscopy (the maximum relaxation diameter between contractions) to be wider in type-I GU than in controls and over twice as wide as in the patients with duodenal ulcer.

We also noted a significantly greater contractile response of the pyloric canal to CCK in GU patients than in controls[83] but it is difficult to see the pathophysiological significance of this finding which is at variance with Fisher and Cohen's observations[81]. If the pylorus is a barrier to reflux it is difficult to see how this pyloric abnormality could render GU patients more liable to reflux.

We have so far not been able to identify a pyloric malfunction in gastric

72

ulcer patients using our impedance technique. We have only studied a small number of patients but results suggest a normal pyloric closure mechanism but increased numbers of isolated duodenal contractions (contractions without preceding antral contraction).

The antrum and duodenum

The capacity of the duodenum to produce reflux through an incompetent pylorus will depend upon two factors:

(1) coordination of antral and duodenal contractions; and
(2) the frequency and the direction of propagation of isolated duodenal contractions.

In the post-prandial state both in dogs and man, duodenal contractions are usually associated with preceding antral activity, though not always on a one-to-one basis. The mechanism by which the rather poor antroduodenal coordination seen in the fasting state is improved after feeding is not known. The pylorus was initially believed to act as an electrical insulator[84] but studies in dogs[85] and man[86] have shown that the antral slow-wave activity spreads across the pylorus. Although antral electrical activity can augment the duodenal slow wave, thereby increasing the probability of duodenal contractions, the occurrence of duodenal contractions in the fasting state cannot be shown to depend primarily on antral contraction strength or frequency[87].

We have observed movements of barium across the pylorus in man during simultaneous manometric and radiological studies[88]. We observed that antral contractions can prevent retropulsive duodenal waves from inducing reflux across the pylorus (Figure 3.10). Thus the antral hypomotility noted in gastric ulcer disease would favour duodenogastric reflux. In a well-designed study, Miller et al. found that in gastric ulcer disease there is delayed emptying of solids but normal emptying of liquids as well as increased reflux[52]. Since solid emptying is primarily dependent on antral contractions, these findings implicate a defect in antral motility. Antral hypomotility in gastric ulcer disease has been reported during motility studies[54].

However, several observations suggest that antroduodenal coordination is not the major extrapyloric mechanism for reflux prevention. In the first place, most studies find reflux to be greater after meals than in the fasting state despite improved antroduodenal coordination seen in the post-prandial state[6,18,19,25]. Secondly, reflux is minimal in health despite frequent isolated duodenal contractions and a 'pyloric closure mechanism' which is not fully competent.

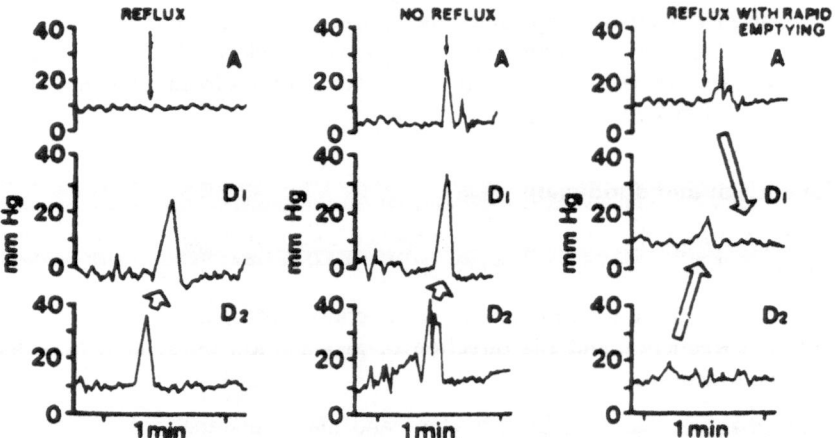

Figure 3.10 Three tracings of antral (A), proximal duodenal (D1) and distal duodenal (D2) contractions in one individual during combined manometric and radiological study. Large arrows indicate movement of intraduodenal barium

Direction of propagation of duodenal contraction

Experimental evidence that the nature and direction of propagation of duodenal contractions are important in the genesis of reflux comes from two sources: the study of electrical pacing of the duodenum and the study of motility patterns in nausea and vomiting. Kelly and Code placed electrodes in the proximal and distal duodenal wall in dogs and were able to pace the duodenum by stimulating at frequencies greater than the intrinsic pacemaker[89]. Stimulation of the proximal electrode which produced aborally-propagated contractions resulted in no increased reflux of a duodenally-infused marker, while distal stimulation, resulting in retroperistaltic contractions, markedly increased reflux from duodenum to stomach. Similar results have been reported in the cat[90].

Further evidence suggests that retroperistaltic duodenal contractions also induce reflux in the absence of electrical pacing. Alvarez first reported this in 1925 whilst studying the vomiting reflex in the cat[91] and this association with nausea has been confirmed both in animals and man[92,93]. Ehrlein, however, has observed reflux in dogs to be more commonly associated with atypical duodenal bulb contractions than with mass peristalsis[94].

Unfortunately duodenal motility studies in man are more difficult to perform and as yet we have few duodenal motility studies in gastric ulcer disease. Reflux certainly varies with the migrating motor complex in man and seems to peak at the end of phase-II activity[27]. We do not know what factors control duodenal motility and it is interesting that bile acids themselves can alter duodenal motility and thus could predispose to reflux by stimulating contractions in the second part of the duodenum[95].

CONCLUSIONS AND IMPLICATIONS FOR TREATMENT

If reflux of duodenal juice is an important factor in gastric mucosal damage, albeit not the only one, then correction of abnormal motility is a possible approach to treatment: either the prevention of reflux or speeding the emptying of refluxed juice would help. There are three 'prokinetic' drugs—metoclopramide, domperidone and cisapride—which speed gastric emptying and increase the coordination at the antroduodenal junction. This motility change would tend to prevent reflux but it is difficult to demonstrate that it does so because the reflux is often so intermittent. Research workers are just beginning to realize the importance of motility changes in the aetiology and treatment of peptic ulcer and this is a fruitful line of future research.

REFERENCES

1. Capper, W.M., Airth, G.R. and Kilby, J.O. (1966). A test for pyloric regurgitation. *Lancet*, **ii**, 621–3
2. Faber, R.G., Russell, R.C.G. and Royston, C.M. (1974). Duodenal reflux during insulin-stimulated secretion. *Gut*, **15**, 880–4
3. Fiddian-Green, R.G., Whitfield, P., Russell, R.C.G. and Hobsley, M. (1974). Indocyanine green as a marker of duodenal reflux in aspirated gastric juice. *Br. J. Surg.*, **61**, 323–4
4. Schmidt, G.F., Schneider, J.A., Bauer, H., Frey, K.W. and Holle, F. (1982). Measurement of duodenogastric reflux with ^{99m}Tc HIDA in duodenal ulcer patients. *World J. Surg.*, **6**, 98–102
5. Van Berg Henegouwen, G.P. and Hofmann, A.F. (1978). Nocturnal gallbladder storage and emptying in gallstone patients and healthy subjects. *Gastroenterology*, **75**, 879–85
6. Rhodes, J., Barnado, D.E. and Phillips, S.F. (1969). Increased reflux of bile into the stomach in patients with gastric ulcer. *Gastroenterology*, **57**, 241–52
7. Muller-Lissner, S.A., Fimmel, C.J., Sonnenberg, A., Will, N., Muller-Duysing, W., Heinzel, F., Muller, R. and Blum, A.L. (1983). Novel approach to quantifying duodenogastric reflux in healthy volunteers and in patients with type I gastric ulcer. *Gut*, **24**, 510–18
8. Tolin, R.D., Malmud, L.S., Stelzer, F., Menin, R., Todd Makler, P., Applegate, G. and Fisher, R.S. (1979). Enterogastric reflux in normal subjects and patients with Billroth II gastroenterostomy. *Gastroenterology*, **77**, 1027–33
9. Beaumont, W. (1833). *Experiments and Observations on Gastric Juice and the Physiology of Digestion.* (Plattsburgh: F.P. Allen)
10. Capper, W.M. (1967). Factors in the pathogenesis of gastric ulcer. *Ann. Roy. Coll. Surg. Engl.*, **40**, 21–35
11. Flint, F.J. and Grech, P. (1970). Pyloric regurgitation and gastric ulcer. *Gut*, **2**, 735–7
12. Cocking, J.B. and Grech, P. (1973). Pyloric reflux and the healing of gastric ulcer. *Gut*, **14**, 555–7
13. Johnson, A.G. (1975). Cholecystectomy and gallstone dyspepsia. *Ann. R. Coll. Surg. Engl.*, **56**, 69–80
14. Giacosa, A., Bocchini, R. and Molinari, F. (1981). Reflux esophagitis and duodenogastric reflux. *Scand. J. Gastroenterol.*, **16**, (Suppl. 67), 125–8

15. Eyre-Brook, I.A., Holroyd, A.M. and Johnson, A.G. (1983). A single isotope method of postprandial duodenogastric reflux assessment using ^{99m}Tc labelled IDA in patients with gallstones. *Clin. Phys. Physiol. Meas.*, **4**, 299–307

16. DuPlessis, D.J. (1965). Pathogenesis of gastric ulceration. *Lancet*, **i**, 974–8

17. Stol, D.W., Murphy, G.M. and Leigh-Collis, J. (1974). Duodenogastric reflux and acid secretion in patients with symptomatic hiatus hernia. *Scand. J. Gastroenterol*, **9**, 91–101

18. Dewar, P., King, R. and Johnston, D. (1982). Bile acid and lysolecithin concentrations in the stomach in patients with duodenal ulcer before operation and after treatment by highly selective vagotomy, partial gastrectomy, or truncal vagotomy and drainage. *Gut*, **23**, 569–77

19. Dewar, P., King, R. and Johnston, D. (1983). Bile acid and lysolecithin concentrations in the stomach of patients with gastric ulcer: before and after treatment by highly selective vagotomy, Billroth I partial gastrectomy and truncal vagotomy and pyloroplasty. *Br. J. Surg.*, **70**, 401–5

20. Wolverson, R.L., Sorgi, M., Mosimann, F., Donovan, I.A., Harding, L.K. and Alexander-Williams, J. (1983). Does gastric intubation cause enterogastric reflux? *Scand. J. Gastroenterol.*, **19**, (Suppl. 92), 36–40

21. Rees, W.D.W. Go, V.L.W. and Malagelada, J.R. (1979). Simultaneous measurement of antroduodenal motility, gastric emptying and duodenogastric reflux in man. *Gut*, **20**, 963–70

22. Poxon, V., Hogg, B., Youngs, D., Morris, D.L. and Keighley, M.R.B. (1986). Incidence of bile reflux in gastric ulcer and after partial gastrectomy. *Br. J. Surg.*, **73**, 295–7

23. Niemela, S. (1985). Duodenogastric reflux in patients with upper abdominal complaints or gastric ulcer. *Scand. J. Gastroenterol*, **20**, (Suppl. 115), 1–56

24. Black, R.B., Roberts, G. and Rhodes, J. (1971). The effect of healing on bile reflux in gastric ulcer. *Gut*, **12**, 552–8

25. Eyre-Brook, I.A., Smythe, A., Bird, N.C., Mangall, Y.F. and Johnson, A.G. (1987). Total bile acid and pancreatic phospholipase A_2 in the stomach in patients with gastric ulcer and gallstone disease. *Br. J. Surg.*, **74**, 721–5

26. Szurszewski, J.H. (1969). A migrating electric complex of the canine small intestine. *Am. J. Physiol.*, **217**, 1757–63

27. Keane, F.B., DiMagno, E.P. and Malagelada, J.R. (1981). Duodenogastric reflux in humans: its relationship to fasting antroduodenal motility and gastric, pancreatic and biliary secretions. *Gastroenterology*, **81**, 726–31

28. Fiddian-Green, R., Russell, R.C.G. and Hobsley, M. (1973). Pyloric reflux in duodenal ulceration and its relationship to smoking. *Br. J. Surg.*, **60**, 321 (Abstract)

29. Johnson, A.G. and McDermot, S.J. (1974). Lysolecithin: A factor in the pathogenesis of gastric ulceration. *Gut*, **15**, 710–713

30. Capper, W.M., Butler, T.J., Kilby, J.O. and Gibson, M.J. (1967). Gallstones, gastric secretion and flatulent dyspepsia. *Lancet*, **i**, 413–15

31. Gillison, E.W., Capper, W.M. and Airth, G.R. (1969). Hiatus hernia and heartburn. *Gut*, **10**, 609–13

32. Collins, B.J., Crothers, G., McFarland, R.J. and Love, A.H.G. (1985). Bile acid concentrations in the gastric juice of patients with erosive gastritis. *Gut*, **26**, 495–9

33. Smith, G.M. (1914). An experimental study of the relation of bile to ulceration of the mucous membrane of the stomach. *J. Med. Res.*, **30**, 147–83

34. Clemencon, G.H., Finger, J. and Fehr, H.F. (1981). The role of taurocholic acid, glycocholic acid and lysolecithin in experimental stress ulcer in the rat. *Scand. J. Gastroenterol.*, **16**, (Suppl. 67), 137–40

35. Kivilaakso, E., Ehnholm, C., Kalima, T. and Lempinen, M. (1976). Duodenogastric reflux of lysolecithin in the pathogenesis of experimental porcine stress ulcer. *Eur. Surg. Res.*, **8**, (Suppl. 2), 55–6

36. Hamza, K.N. and Den Beston, L. (1972). Bile salts producing stress during experimental shock. *Surgery*, **71**, 161–7

37. Mersereau, W.A. and Hinchey, E.J. (1973). Effect of gastric acidity on gastric ulceration

induced by hemorrhage in the rat utilising a gastric chamber technique. *Gastroenterology*, **64**, 1130–5

38. Ischihara, Y. and Okabe, S. (1981). Effects of cholestyramine and synthetic hydrotalcite on acute gastric or intestinal lesion formation in rats and dogs. *Dig. Dis. Sci.*, **26**, 553–60

39. Okale, S., Hung, C.R., Takeuchi, K. and Takago, K. (1976). Effects of L-glutamine and acetylsalicylic acid on taurocholic acid-induced gastric lesions and secretory changes in pylorus ligated rats under normal and stress conditions. *Jpn. J. Pharmacol.*, **26**, 455–60

40. Hemmati, M., Abtahi, F., Farroksiar, M. and Djahanguiri, B. (1974). Prevention of restraint and indomethacin induced gastric ulceration by bile duct or pylorus ligation in rats. *Digestion*, **10**, 108–12

41. Ritchie, W.P. (1981). Role of bile acid reflux in acute hemorrhagic gastritis. *World J. Surg.*, **5**, 189–98

42. Moody, F.G. and Aldrete, J.S. (1971). Hydrogen permeability of canine gastric secretory epithelium during formation of acute superficial erosions. *Surgery*, **70**, 154–60

43. Davenport, H.W. (1968). Destruction of the gastric mucosal barrier by detergents and urea. *Gastroenterology*, **54**, 175–81

44. Duane, W. and Wiegand, D.M. (1980). Mechanisms by which bile salt disrupts the gastric mucosal barrier in the dog. *J. Clin. Invest.*, **66**, 1044–9

45. Black, R.B., Hole, D. and Rhodes, J. (1971). Bile damage to the gastric mucosal barrier; the influence of pH and bile acid concentration. *Gastroenterology*, **61**, 178–84

46. Kivilaakso, E., Fromm, M.D. and Silen, W. (1978). Relationship between ulceration and intramural pH of gastric mucosa during hemorrhagic shock. *Surgery*, **85**, 70–8

47. Cheung, L.Y. and Porterfield, G. (1979). Protection of gastric mucosa against acute ulceration by intravenous infusion of sodium bicarbonate. *Am. J. Surg.*, **137**, 106–10

48. O'Brien, P.E. and Silen, W. (1973). Effect of bile salts and aspirin on the gastric mucosal blood flow. *Gastroenterology*, **64**, 246–53

49. Davenport, W.H. and Munro, D. (1973). Aminopyrine clearance in the damaged gastric mucosa: reconciliation of conflicting data. *Gastroenterology*, **65**, 512–14

50. Orchard, R., Reynolds, K., Fox, B., Andrews, R., Parkin, R.A., and Johnson, A.G. (1977). Effect of lysolecithin on gastric mucosal structure and potential difference. *Gut*, **18**, 457–61

51. Davenport, H.W. (1970). Effect of lysolecithin, digitoxin and phospholipase A upon the dog gastric mucosal barrier. *Gastroenterology*, **59**, 505–9

52. Miller, L.J., Malagelada, J.R., Longstreth, G.F. and Go, V.L.W. (1980). Dysfunction of the stomach with gastric ulceration. *Dig. Dis. Sci.*, **25**, 857–64

53. Moore, S.C., Malagalada, J.R., Shorter, R.G. and Zinmeister, A.R. (1986). Interrelationships among gastric mucosal morphology, secretion and motility in peptic ulcer disease. *Dig. Dis. Sci.*, **31**, 673–84

54. Ritchie, W.P. (1975). Acute gastric mucosal damage induced by bile salts, acid and ischaemia. *Gastroenterology*, **68**, 699–707

55. Byers, F. and Jordon, P. (1962). Effect of bile upon gastric mucosa. *Proc. Soc. Exp. Biol. Med.*, **110**, 864–66

56. Lawson, H.H. (1981). The postoperative stomach as seen clinically and experimentally. *Scand. J. Gastroenterol.*, **16**, (Suppl. 67) 157–60

57. Menguy, R. and Max, M.H. (1970). Influence of bile on the canine gastric antral mucosa. *Am. J. Surg.*, **119**, 177–82

58. Lawson, H.H. (1981). The production of chronic gastritis under experimental conditions. *Scand. J. Gastroenterol.*, **16**, (Suppl. 67) 91–8

59. Ivey, K.J., Den Beston, L. and Clifton, J.A. (1970). Effect of bile salts on ionic movement across the human gastric mucosa. *Gastroenterology*, **59**, 683–90

60. Geale, M.G., Phillips, S.F. and Summerskill, W.H.J. (1970). Profile of gastric potential difference in man. Effects of aspirin, alcohol, bile and endogenous acid. *Gastroenterology*, **58**, 437–43

61. Duthie, H.L., Moore, K.T.H., Bardsley, D. and Clark, R.G. (1970). Surgical treatment of gastric ulcers. Controlled comparison of Billroth I and vagotomy and pyloroplasty. *Br. J. Surg.*, **57**, 784–7

62. Ashton, M.G., Holdsworth, C.D., Ryan, F.P. and Moore, M. (1982). Healing of gastric ulcers after one, two and three months of ranitidine. *Br. Med. J.*, ii, 795–7
63. Thomas, W.E.G. (1980). Duodenogastric reflux–a common factor in the pathogenesis of gastric and duodenal ulcer. *Lancet*, ii, 1166–8
64. Davenport, H.W., Warner, H.A. and Code, C.F. (1964). Functional significance of gastric mucosal barrier to sodium. *Gastroenterology*, 47, 142–52
65. Malagelada, J.R., Go, V.L.W., Summerskill, W.H.J. and Gamble, W.S. (1973). Bile acid secretion and biliary bile acid composition altered by cholecystectomy. *Am. J. Dig. Dis.*, 18, 455–9
66. Ritchie, W.P. and Delaney, J.P. (1971). Susceptibility of experimental atrophic gastritis to ulceration. *Gastroenterology*, 60, 554–9
67. Torgersen, J. (1942). The muscular build and movements of the stomach and duodenal bulb especially with regard to the problem of the segmental divisions of the stomach in the light of comparative anatomy and embryology. *Acta Radiol. (Stockholm)*, Suppl. 45, 1–187
68. Anuras, S., Cooke, A.R. and Christensen, J. (1974). An inhibitory innervation of gastro-duodenal junction. *J. Clin. Invest.*, 54, 529–35
69. Edin, R., Lundberg, J., Terenius, L., Dahlstrom, A., Hokfelt, T., Kewenter, J. and Ahlman, H. (1980). Evidence for vagal enkephalinergic neural control of the feline pylorus and stomach. *Gastroenterology*, 78, 492–7
70. Alumets, J., Fahrenkrug, J., Hakanson, R., Schaffalitzky, de Muckadell, O., Sundler, F. and Uddman, R. (1979). A rich VIP nerve supply is characteristic of sphincters. *Nature (London)*, 208, 155–6
71. Cannon, W.B. (1898). The movements of the stomach by means of roentgen rays. *Am. J. Physiol.*, 1, 359–82
72. Carlson, H.C., Code, C.F. and Nelson, R.A. (1966). Motor action of the canine gastroduodenal junction: a cineradiographic, pressure and electric study. *Am. J. Dig. Dis.*, 11, 155–72
73. Crider, J.D. and Thomas, J.E. (1937). A study of gastric emptying with the pylorus open. *Am. J. Dig. Dis. Nutr.*, 4, 295
74. Atkinson, M., Edwards, D.A.W., Honour, A.J. and Rowlands, E.N. (1951). Comparison of cardiac and pyloric sphincters. *Lancet*, ii, 918–22
75. Fisher, R.S. and Cohen, S. (1973). Physiological characteristics of human pyloric sphincter. *Gastroenterology*, 64, 67–75
76. Valenzuela, J.E., Defilippi, C. and Csendes, A. (1976). Manometric studies on the human pyloric sphincter. Effect of cigarette smoking, metoclopramide and atropine. *Gastroenterology*, 70, 481–3
77. Kaye, M.D., Metha, S.J. and Showalter, J.P. (1976). Manometric studies of the human pylorus. *Gastroenterology*, 70, 477–80
78. McShane, A.J., O'Morain, C., Lennon, J.R., Coakely, J.B. and Alton, B.G. (1980). Atraumatic non-distorting pyloric sphincter pressure studies. *Gut*, 21, 826–8
79. White, C.M., Poxon, V. and Alexander-Williams, J. (1981). A study of motility in the normal gastroduodenal region. *Dig. Dis. Sci.*, 26, 609–16
80. Eyre-Brook, I.A., Lindhardt, G.E., Smallwood, R.H. and Johnson, A.G. (1983). Human antroduodenal motility: studies with impedance electrodes. *Dig. Dis. Sci.*, 28, 1106–15
81. Fisher, R.S. and Cohen, S. (1973). Pyloric sphincter dysfunction in patients with gastric ulcer. *N. Engl. J. Med.*, 288, 273–6
82. Valenzuela, J.E. and Defilippi, C. (1976). Pyloric-sphincter studies in peptic ulcer patients. *Am. J. Dig. Dis.*, 21, 229–32
83. Munk, J., Gannaway, R.M., Hoare, M. and Johnson, A.G. (1977). The direct measurement of pyloric diameter and tone in man and their response to cholecystokinin. In Duthie, H.L. (ed.) *Gastrointestinal Motility in Health and Disease*, pp. 349–56. (Lancaster: MTP Press)
84. Bass, P., Code, C.F. and Lambert, E.H. (1961). Motor and electric activity of the duodenum. *Am. J. Physiol.*, 201, 287–91
85. Bortoff, A. and Davis, R.S. (1968). Myogenic transmission of antral slow waves across the gastroduodenal junction *in situ*. *Am. J. Physiol.*, 215, 889–98

86. Duthie, H.L., Kwong, N.K., Brown, B.H. and Whittaker, G.E. (1971). Pacesetter potential of the human gastroduodenal junction. *Gut*, **12**, 250–6
87. Reinke, D.A. Rosenbaum, A.H. and Bennett, D.R. (1967). Patterns of dog gastrointestinal contractile activity monitored *in vivo* with extraluminal force transducers, *Am. J. Dig. Dis.*, **12**, 113–41
88 Johnson, A.G. (1979). Peptic ulcer and the pylorus. *Lancet*, **i**, 710–12
89. Kelly, K.A. and Code, C.F. (1977). Duodenal-gastric reflux and slowed gastric emptying by electrical pacing of the canine duodenal pacesetter potential. *Gastroenterology*, **72**, 429–33
90. Munk, J.F. and Johnson, A.G. (1980). Effects of duodenal and antral pacing on pyloric reflux in the cat. In Christensen, J. (ed.) *Gastrointestinal Motility*, pp. 173–5. (New York: Raven Press)
91. Alvarez, W.C. (1925). Reverse peristalsis in the bowel: a precursor of vomiting. *J. Am. Med. Assoc.*, **85**, 1051–4
92. Weisbrodt, N.W. and Christensen, J. (1972). Electrical activity of the cat duodenum in fasting and vomiting. *Gastroenterology*, **63**, 1004–10
93. Lumsden, K. and Holden, W.S. (1969). The act of vomiting in man. *Gut*, **10**, 173–9
94. Ehrlein, H.J. (1981). Retroperistalsism and duodenogastric reflux in dogs. *Scand. J. Gastroenterol*, **16**, (Suppl. 67), 29–32
95. Eyre-Brook, I.A., Read, N.W., Brownson, A. and Johnson, A.G. (1984). The influence of chenodeoxycholic acid on fasting antroduodenal motility and reflux. *Br. J. Surg.*, **71**, 900

4
Drug-induced mucosal damage

M. J. S. LANGMAN

INTRODUCTION

In attempting to determine the presence and strength of any causal relationship between drug exposure and mucosal damage, evidence can be drawn from several sources.

Experimental data

Animal and tissue experiments

A variety of animal models have been used in which the responses to drug treatment are examined, either alone or in combination with other stressful influences. Using such models, it is generally possible to demonstrate damage, usually as gastroduodenal erosions, and these can be quantified to give dose–response curves. Comparisons can then be attempted between drugs. Usually, aspirin can be shown to produce more erosive damage in these model systems than other non-steroidal anti-inflammatory drugs, and it has been suggested that differences can be detected between others, such as indomethacin and tiaprofenic acid. Data must however be interpreted cautiously. Simple milligram-for-milligram comparisons may be irrelevant; anti-inflammatory potency will usually provide better standardization. Even then direct transfer of findings to man may result in erroneous conclusions. Firstly, dissolution characteristics could alter the amounts of drug to which the mucosa is directly exposed, and secondly variations in metabolic rates could pronouncedly alter the circulating concentrations of drugs. Thirdly, the choice of experimental animal can influence the severity, of damage, either through inherent species variations in mucosal sensitivity, or in the capacity to remove xenobiotics. The rat, for example, has a very high metabolic capacity and hence tissues may be relatively resistant to damage *in vivo*.

Tissue experiments have the virtue that they allow the investigator to isolate specific systems for study, for instance mediating bicarbonate secretion. They may thus give biological plausibility, and may allow the complex inter-relationships between for instance, inhibitory and facilitatory mechanisms to be dissected. However they are unlikely to be useful in supplying critical evidence that an individual biochemical pathway is of prime importance and they do not permit generalization to predict what will necessarily happen *in vivo*.

Human experiments

Typically, drug exposure is followed by searches for mucosal damage either by visual endoscopic means, or by measuring indices of damage, usually by measuring blood loss into the gastric content, or as faecal blood loss by red-cell radiolabelling techniques. Generally, attempts are made to use models which give consistent results and to try to quantitate damage. Again the relevance to gastric and duodenal damage in man is unclear. Clinically, anti-inflammatory drugs are well tolerated, and serious adverse effects, and even minor ones, occur only in a few individuals. Studies in experimental models are unlikely to help in unravelling the problem of individual susceptibility to damage, and automatic acceptance that acute damage models provide morals for chronic clinical disease would be unwise.

Clinical evidence

Safety and tolerance in clinical trials

The one consistent feature of initial clinical-trial data provided at the time of anti-inflammatory drug introduction has been the good safety profiles demonstrated for the gastro-intestinal tract. These findings are often at variance with later clinical perception. Reasons for the differences probably include the small number of subjects included in trials, the lack of concurrent debilitating illness with which impaired mucosal resistance may possibly be associated, and the relatively young age of most patients which may confer resistance to adverse effects. Early clinical data will usually provide a reasonable basis for concluding that a given drug does have the general properties predicted from the results of animal and tissue studies. The results are seldom sufficient in quantity to determine whether the drug is more or less potent than other similar members of the chemical series and they will not be of much value in deciding about drug safety. The reasons for this are that for practical clinical purposes, serious adverse event rates for drugs used in treating chronic inflammatory disease occur with a frequency of less than 1 in 5000 or 10,000 courses. The number of treatment courses prescribed in a country the size of the United Kingdom may be measured in millions per year and so even at the rates suggested the expectation will be of adverse events numbered in the hundreds each year.

Pharmaco-epidemiological evidence

The occurrence of new disease during treatment should always suggest that the treatment may have been the cause. Obtaining proof may be difficult or impossible. Most adverse drug reactions mimic ordinary disease and most treatment is given to elderly people who commonly have secondary diseases. Therefore the development of a secondary illness may represent no more than simple coincidence. Belief in causation will be strengthened by a consistent time relationship between treatment and disease occurrence or by unusual features in the disease. Both of these are uncommon, tissue damage may take a variable amount of time to become evident, and the patterns of damage are limited by the range of reactions available to tissues, such as cholestasis, necrosis or inflammatory reactions in the liver. Return of a reaction on drug re-exposure (challenge) may give convincing evidence but this is seldom in the patients' individual interests because alternative treatments are usually available, and therefore is rarely done.

Spontaneous reports of adverse events, usually to drug regulatory authorities, can act as valuable early-warning systems but, unless the events are unusual in disease pattern, give little help in deciding if a drug is less preferable in practice than other available agents. Comparisons with other members of the same series of compounds are hindered and may be largely invalidated because suspected adverse events are more likely to be reported for new than for established agents. (This is a practice encouraged in the United Kingdom by the printing of a special symbol ▼ in information about new drugs in, for instance, the *British National Formulary*.)

Formal surveillance procedures, in which prescribers are questioned or records are scanned to determine the outcome of treatment, produce more complete information. However it must be remembered that the prescription sets collected are usually still fairly small (perhaps 10,000 or less), that comparative data for other drugs may not be available, and that association does not necessarily imply causation. Nevertheless, surveillance may allow informed guesses at the maximum likely event rates.

When samples of individuals with set diseases are questioned about antecedent drug intake, and the same questions are posed to control individuals, comparisons may allow the calculation of the relative risk (the change, usually increase, in the chances of the set disease in the taker). They may also allow the calculation of the attributable risk (or amount of disease caused) if simultaneously it is possible to obtain information about the total number of prescriptions issued and the total amount of disease in the community. The value of the data depends upon the fairness of the comparisons made and the inherent biases. Those possible have been extensively discussed elsewhere.

All methods of study are complementary: spontaneous reporting suggests the possibility of iatrogenic disease, surveillance can suggest maximum frequency rates, and case control studies, which are only possible once a question has been posed, can quantify the risk.

NON-STEROIDAL INDUCED DAMAGE

Experimental data

Mechanisms have been summarized. Early stages (within minutes) include disruption of the mucus layer, increased mucosal permeability, with acid back diffusion and lowering of the mucosal electrical potential difference. These events favour lysosomal breakdown, and tissue release of destructive free oxygen radicals. Drug accumulation is associated with inhibition of prostaglandin production, and with increased histamine release, although damage results in diminished acid secretion. Vascular endothelial damage also leads to leakage of vascular contents into the tissues. Later stages include inhibition of enzymes involved in mucus glycoprotein formation reduced cellular proliferation, and breakdown of the mucosa[1-3].

For damage to occur it is necessary for the tissues to be exposed to the drug in question which means that it must penetrate in active form the mucus bicarbonate barrier or diffuse from within the vascular compartment and accumulate within the tissues. Aspirin taken as acetylsalicylic acid is unionized but fat-soluble. Therefore the particulate nature of the drug does not confer protective properties, but conversely implies that where in contact with the mucosa a high concentration will occur in relation to lipid membranes and absorption will be facilitated. At alkaline pH (above 4.0) the drug exists in solution as sodium acetylsalicylate, and is not absorbed from the stomach, although it is from the small intestine, and whilst in solution has no damaging effects. A general relationship has also been postulated between the possession of a carboxyl group by a non-steroidal anti-inflammatory drug (NSAID) and liability to accumulate in cells and to cause damage.

A possible correlation has been sought between changes in mucosal prostaglandin content and the earliest evidence of gastric damage using indomethacin and aspirin. Gastric mucosal damage induced by both drugs was associated with a fall in the prostaglandin content, measured as PGE_2 or as 6-keto-$PGF_{1\alpha}$ the stable metabolite of PGI_2. In pigs, the fall in prostaglandin content was preceded by a drop in mucosal potential difference. These findings can be contrasted with others using benoxaprofen where little effect upon overall prostaglandin production was noted by this drug of low acute gastric toxicity[4-9].

A wide range of evidence indicates that prostaglandins can in some way enhance mucosal resistance to damage whether caused by NSAIDs or other agents[7]. This protection can be achieved without inhibiting acid secretion, although potent inhibitors of acid secretion, such as the histamine H_2-receptor antagonists, will also reduce gastric damage, as measured for example by blood loss into the stomach or a reduced frequency of erosions. The easy assumption of a simple relationship between NSAID exposure as harmful through reducing mucosal prostaglandin content, and prostaglandins as restoring protection, may not be justified. Thus adaptive changes can occur which do not seem to be prostaglandin-mediated; for instance, gastric erosions disappear in dogs chronically treated with aspirin, and sodium salicylate-associated protection against necrotic stimuli seems unaffected by indomethacin[10,11].

Aspirin-induced damage can also be reduced or inhibited by anti-oxidant compounds or free-radical scavengers and by allopurinol, presumably because it inhibits the formation of xanthine oxidase-derived superoxide radicals. The occurrence of damage is not critically and simply dependent upon acid production, and this is clearly demonstrated by the propensity of NSAIDs to cause damage in the jejunum and ileum.

The general complexities of the field where, in addition to changes in prostaglandin production and metabolism, and acid secretion, we also have to take account of changes in formation of chemotactic mediators and of alterations in the mucus–bicarbonate barrier, are illustrated by a recent extensive review[7].

Predisposing factors to damage

In general, a relationship has been observed between anti-inflammatory potency and liability to cause damage, and all compounds are usually considered to have the same mechanism(s) of action. However lesions may be found in the stomach, or in the intestine anywhere from the jejunum to the ileum, with variable degrees of necrosis, and penetration up to free perforation. The conditions under which the experiments are conducted, and drug pharmacokinetic aspects would be expected to affect experimental outcome. Fasting tends to promote gastric lesions but to reduce the frequency of intestinal damage, whereas feeding can have the reverse effect. Thus, high dietary lipid intake seemed to reduce the frequency of gastric damage and to exacerbate intestinal damage. Low residue, liquid and milk-based diets have also tended to reduce the frequency of intestinal lesions[12,13]. The mechanisms by which nutritional factors alter susceptibility to damage are unclear. Simple mechanical effects of food intake do not seem likely because cellulose seems to interfere with dietary protective factors. Specific dietary effects, and diet-induced changes in eicosanoid synthesis, in gut motility, in the intestinal flora and in drug pharmacokinetics all seem possible[14,15]. In addition it is clear that, at least in some experiments, drug-induced damage can be made more severe by the simultaneous imposition of stress.

Eicosanoid synthesis

There is evidence that essential fatty acids will protect against both ethanol-induced mucosal necrosis and aspirin-induced damage and that protection is associated with enhanced prostaglandin synthesis[14,15].

Microbial factors

In animals given antibiotics or which were germ-free, lesions following NSAID treatment have been reduced in frequency or have not occurred at all, particularly in the intestine. Protective effects have been less evident in the stomach[16,17].

Pharmacokinetic factors

Unbuffered aspirin is very rapidly absorbed and gastric damage is more quickly evident than with indomethacin which is more slowly absorbed. Although anti-inflammatory potency tends generally to correlate with propensity to cause gastric damage, there may still be differences between drugs. Thus, it has been suggested that azapropazone, although well absorbed, may be an agent which is less prone to cause gastric damage. Whether there are any morals for man seems unclear. In animals there may be significant enterohepatic circulation of indomethacin, and also of other drugs which may in part explain liability to intestinal damage[18]. In man, only about 10% of the ingested dose seems to be excreted in the bile. In animals, intravenously-administered indomethacin may be more toxic to the intestine, and less to the stomach, than the orally-administered drug.

Human experiments

NSAID treatment has typically been shown to be associated with gastrointestinal blood loss as measured by intragastric bleeding, reduction of the transmucosal potential difference (a general index of mucosal integrity) and the development of endoscopically-evident submucosal haemorrhages and mucosal erosions. Such damage is easily demonstrated when unbuffered aspirin is used, with lesser changes when other NSAIDs, such as indomethacin, are employed, or aspirin is enteric-coated.

The significance of all these sets of data is unclear. Ordinary unbuffered aspirin has a well-deserved reputation for inducing upper gastrointestinal damage which can easily be detected in young volunteer populations. Damage associated with the use of non-aspirin NSAIDs may be slower to develop, and the relevance of short-term experiments conducted in young volunteers for drug use chronically in elderly, often debilitated people is doubtful. Thus blood loss as detected using radiochromium labelling has been found to differ little for piroxicam and placebo (but greatly from aspirin associated loss)[9].

Likewise, the value of endoscopic studies of acute gastric lesions occurring during short courses of NSAID treatment is hard to assess. Even assuming that studies are properly conducted with test and placebo medications it is difficult to say whether the occurrence of gastric erythema (assuming this can be reliably detected anyway) or submucosal haemorrhage carries any particular morals. Numbers of subjects studied are usually small, less than ten per treatment group, yet the disease for which the experiments are modelling may occur with a frequency of less than one in a thousand. It is also unclear whether the lesions detected can be correlated with the occurrence of dyspepsia, or major complications, or neither. Data indicating interference with prostaglandin synthesis lend biological plausibility to the belief that the drugs have an effect, but do not tell us whether it is clinically important. In man as well as in animals it appears that continued aspirin ingestion is associated with gastric adaptation, the numbers of erosions and/or petechial haemorrhages being reduced[9,11,20,21]. By contrast, Caruso and Porro[22] showed a high frequency of gastroduodenal lesions in patients given a variety of NSAIDs; however they included a large number of minor erosive lesions and of reactivated ulcers but only two new ulcers. It is therefore difficult to decide whether these were significant clinical changes in general, given, particularly, the high frequency of relapse in patients with healed ulcers who are not taking NSAIDs.

ADVERSE REACTIONS SURVEILLANCE

Spontaneous reports

The Committee on Safety of Medicines (CSM) receives more reports of adverse effects of NSAIDs than any other group of drugs, and these are more likely to involve the gastrointestinal tract than any other system[23]. Table 4.1 shows the proportions of reports to the CSM of serious reactions attributable to the gastrointestinal tract, and the proportions of individuals who died. It confirms, apart from phenylbutazone and oxyphenbutazone (where use has been restric-

Table 4.1 Percentages of serious reports to the Committee on Safety of Medicines attributable to gastrointestinal reactions, and percentages of these who died*

Drug	Date introduced	Serious gastrointestinal reactions (%), A	Death rate in A (%)
Aspirin	1899	88	37
Phenylbutazone	1952	24	32
Indomethacin	1964	59	39
Oxyphenbutazone	1965	5	23
Ibuprofen	1969	57	13
Naproxen	1973	71	12
Ketoprofen	1973	84	8
Azapropazone	1978	70	15
Diclofenac	1979	56	13
Piroxicam	1980	84	10
Benoxaprofen	1980	34	17

*Data given for all drugs where total reported reactions exceed 200. (After *Update*[23])

ted because of a propensity to cause blood dyscrasias), that there is a general tendency for reactions to be reported for the gastrointestinal tract and with a significant proportion of deaths. Because reports are made spontaneously, and because drugs have been introduced over widely differing periods of time it is unsafe to relate figures to prescription rates. Only a minority, perhaps 10% or less, of adverse events associated with drug therapy are reported, and an equal likelihood for reporting to be similar for all drugs cannot be assumed; thus, reports are more likely to be received for newly introduced than for established agents, a practice encouraged by the placing of the special symbol ▼ beside newly-introduced drugs in the *British National Formulary*. The significant percentages of deaths may in part reflect reporting of the worst adverse events but probably are more strongly associated with the use of NSAIDs in the elderly, death rates with bleeding or ulcer perforation rising steeply in individuals aged 60 or over. Although association does not necessarily imply culpability, taken overall, the data suggest that an important problem exists.

Clinical trial data

Conventionally, all reports of clinical trials include information about the adverse effects of treatment. Generalization to the population at large is likely to be misleading. Clinical trial populations tend to be rigorously selected, and, for instance, to be free of any illness apart from that under consideration. Ordinary populations by contrast include individuals with multiple illnesses, and compromised hepatic, metabolic, and renal excretory mechanisms are common. Adverse effects of treatment are therefore much more likely to occur.

Nevertheless, abdominal pain, indigestion, nausea, vomiting or heartburn have almost universally been reported during short-term trials of NSAIDs. Whether these are predictive of the likelihood of drug-associated ulcer development with or without bleeding or perforation is quite unclear. Logically it might appear appropriate to combine data obtained in all clinical trials of a particular agent and then to compare side-effect profiles with those of other drugs. However the varying treatment regimes and patients groups selected, amongst other unknown factors, make any useful conclusions impossible in trying to examine and compare the frequencies of a single type of adverse event.

Case series

Clinicians have repeatedly brought forward data suggesting that in series of cases of ulcer and of upper gastrointestinal bleeding or perforation, exposure to anti-inflammatory drugs is very common, the high frequency of association suggesting causality to them[24-27]. In interpreting such data it has to be remembered that ulcer is common in the community with a prevalence of approximately 10% in men and 5% in women and that NSAIDs are also widely used so that simple coincidence is possible. Secondly, individuals in whom NSAID treatment is thought necessary may be unduly prone to gastrointestinal damage owing to any cause. Thus there have been suggestions that the individual with rheumatoid arthritis may be unduly prone to peptic ulceration. Thirdly, the method of collection of case series can influence the data obtained. Berkson[29] postulated that individuals with one disease are inherently likely to have a second one detected. The significance of this bias in relation to peptic ulcer associations has been discussed elsewhere in detail, and verified[30]. Fourthly, published case series never represent an unbiased set of available data, but tend to be skewed and to emphasize the unusual. Many of these objections would be reduced in cogency if a single individual disease pattern were to be identified. Initially suggestions were made of an association of NSAID intake with greater curve antral ulcers, and of aspirin intake with acute gastric erosions. However associations for NSAID-induced damage have now been claimed for oesophagitis and ulcer, gastric and duodenal ulcer, and for ileal and colonic ulcer, bleeding or perforation.

Case control studies

Provided a working hypothesis exists, and provided it is possible to study representative individuals with a disease suspected as caused by treatment as well as those in whom the same disease has occurred without any association, and finally, provided a comparable non-diseased control group can be studied then the basis exists for risk calculations. Conventionally, comparison of the proportions of individuals who have, and who have not taken, the drug in question will yield a risk ratio, which if all the initial points above are satisfied, expresses as a multiple the number of times that takers of the drugs are more likely to develop a disease than the unexposed population. A high ratio implying high risk is not however enough in itself to allow us to determine that there is necessarily a large burden of drug-induced disease in the community. To decide what this may be, it is necessary to be able to estimate the total amount of the disease in question. Conventionally this is done by formal calculation of the population attributable risk. A complete picture is then given if the total amount of drug use in the population is known and it is then possible to give the numbers of events per thousand prescriptions or daily doses, as well as any increase in risk by takers.

Little complete information is, in fact, available and most investigators have been content with calculating the proportion of takers and non-takers in disease and control groups.

Aspirin

Available data, mainly from case control studies, allow more or less informed guesses at the overall risk of upper gastrointestinal bleeding. They also give the frequency of drug intake in association with specific lesions and for uncomplicated disease. Figures vary widely and these fluctuations may be owing in part to the varied control groups chosen for study (Table 4.2). There are obvious difficulties in obtaining controls representative of the general population, and the simple assumption that sick controls will satisfy is likely to be ill-founded. Thus the anti-platelet effects of aspirin could reduce the proportions of takers in patients with thromboembolic disease or myocardial infarction, and dyspeptic controls may have been warned against drug use. By contrast, in test groups, aspirin use may have been raised because of drug

Table 4.2   Controls chosen in case control studies of aspirin-associated upper gastrointestinal bleeding

Group	Reference	Study
Kelly	31	Myocardial infarction
Muir and Cossar	32	Patient in the next bed
Muir and Cossar	33	Patient in the next bed
Alvarez and Sumerskill	34	Dyspeptic outpatients
Lange	35	Ulcer patients without bleeding
Brown and Mitchell	36	All other admissions
Allibone and Flint	37	Surgical emergencies
Parry and Wood	38	Other medical inpatients
Levy	39	Hospital inpatients
Coggon et al.	40	Community controls

taking to relieve dyspepsia or other symptoms associated with the lesion in question.

No completely satisfactory control group seems likely to be obtainable nor all biases to be avoided and in consequence the exact risks associated with aspirin intake remain hard to determine.

Upper gastrointestinal bleeding. All investigators have found increases in the test groups and many have divided figures to try to decide if a specific lesion is associated. The value of these figures is doubtful. Most were obtained in an era when full fiber-optic oesophago-gastro-duodenal endoscopy was not practised. Diagnoses of erosive disease were often by exclusion (X-ray negative) and of duodenal ulcer by seeking evidence of radiological deformity although this cannot tell us with any certainty if active duodenal ulceration is present.

Table 4.3 shows the relative risks for aspirin-associated bleeding in retrospective case control analyses in patients with bleeding and in randomized controlled studies of the value of aspirin in preventing thrombo-embolic disease. The retrospective analyses generally show raised risks but not universally, and the figures vary widely. Much of this variation is likely to be owing to the differing indices of aspirin exposure chosen from prolonged

Table 4.3 Risk ratios and powers of studies to detect aspirin-associated bleeding (adapted from Belcon et al.[41])

Study type	Reference	Relative risk	95% confidence interval	Power
Case control studies				
Kelly	31	11.6	3.3–50.3	0.30
Alvarez and Summerskill	34	5.8	2.9–11.8	0.65
Allibone and Flint	37	1.1	0.6–11.8	0.78
Muir and Cossar	32	6.1	3.0–12.3	0.66
Parry and Wood	38	4.6	2.8–7.6	0.98
Levy	39	1.7	1.4–2.2	0.86
Randomized controlled trials				
Elwood and Sweetnam	42	0[a]		Unknown
Elwood et al.	43	1.0[b]	0.3–3.8	0.16
AMIS	44	1.7[c]	1.3–2.1	0.99
Canadian Stroke Study	45	0.2[d]	0.2–2.3	0.07
CDPA	46	1.1–1.9[e]		0.12–0.57
AITIA	47	1.3[f]	0.6–2.7	0.37

End points, aspirin dose (mg):
[a] end point measure not stated, 900.
[b] overt gastrointestinal haemorrhage, 300.
[c] haematemesis, black or bloody stools, 1000.
[d] haematemesis and melaena, 325.
[e] multiple end points, 927.
[f] guiac positive stools, 1300.

heavy intake to acute exposure, to the play of biases in questioning and to the differing controls. Generally these studies seemed to possess the power to detect differences if present, though it should be noted that this could mean the power to detect the effects of biases as well as real differences.

By contrast, the randomized controlled trials showed little in the way of increased risks, but most lacked the necessary power to detect real differences, if present. Nevertheless the differences between the odds ratios obtained in most of the retrospective analyses and in most of the randomized controlled trials are large, and fairly consistently so.

One possible explanation derives from considering the reasons why patients admitted with upper gastrointestinal bleeding may take analgesic agents, and attempting to control for them. We used paracetamol intake as a positive control, reasoning that the drug was likely to be used for much the same purposes as aspirin. Paracetamol is not, however, believed to be harmful to the stomach and so any increase in intake in patients with bleeding relative to controls might be assumed to be consequential and not causal of bleeding. An increase was noted, and Table 4.4 shows the data. The increase became steadily more apparent with intake closely related to the episode of bleeding, as did that for aspirin, but was always less by a factor of about two-fold than for aspirin. We concluded that about one-third of aspirin intake by patients with bleeding was probably non-causal and could be related to ordinary population intake, and that a further one-third, by reference to the paracetamol data, was also non-causal, but occurred because of the presence of the bleeding lesion, and did not cause the bleeding. The final one-third was unexplained and could well be causal. If this were true, then we estimated that about 35 to 45 hospital admissions might occur in regular users per 100 000 such individuals each year, a figure in the same area as calculated by Levy[39] in the United States some ten years earlier of 15 per 100 000. We also concluded (in contrast to Levy) that some risk was attached to casual use, and this might be of the order of one episode per quarter million courses of treatment.

Table 4.4 Aspirin and paracetamol intake in patients with haematemesis and melaena and in matched controls[40]

	Analgesic			
	Aspirin		Paracetamol	
Time period	Relative risk	95% confidence interval	Relative risk	95% confidence interval
Past 48 hours	4.8	2.4–10.7	2.1	1.1–4.1
Past week	3.7	2.2–6.4	1.9	1.2–3.3
In each of last two weeks	3.6	1.3–12.4	1.5	0.7–3.0
Once a week for at least 3 months	2.2	0.7–8.1	1.0	0.4–2.5

Non-bleeding ulcer. It has been repeatedly suggested that analgesic intake, particularly of compound analgesics containing aspirin, is associated with gastric ulcer. In Australia it has been considered that the association could account for a high frequency of gastric ulcer perforation in younger women[48-53]. The significance of the association is unclear. Piper and his colleagues[51] compared aspirin and paracetamol intake in ulcer patients and in community controls and found raised risks for both paracetamol and aspirin for gastric but not for duodenal ulcer. Duggan *et al.,* also in New South Wales, found the same pattern for aspirin, but had too few paracetamol users to allow reasoned conclusions[52]. The main contrast therefore lay between the amount of paracetamol use observed in the gastric ulcer patients. It is not possible to decide therefore whether there was a non-specific association of gastric ulcer with analgesic use or a specific association with aspirin use (Tables 4.5 and 4.6).

Whatever may be the true meaning of the association between aspirin intake

Table 4.5 Analgesic intake of all types according to ulcer diagnosis

Study	Reference	Ulcer (No. cases)	
		Gastric	Duodenal
Piper *et al.*	51		
Nil, rare and occasional		31	60
Heavy		29	7
Duggan *et al.*	52		
Less than 2 doses per week		39	49
Two doses or more per week		25	8

Table 4.6 Heavy analgesic use according to ulcer diagnosis

Study	Reference	Ulcer (No. cases)	
		Gastric	Duodenal
Piper *et al.*	51		
Aspirin* only		5	
Paracetamol only		12	7
Both		12	
Neither		31	60
Duggan *et al.*	52		
Aspirin* only		22	8
No heavy use		65	65

* or compound preparations.

93

and the occurrence of ulcer, no evidence has emerged to suggest that ulcer site, healing or relapse rates are affected by aspirin use.

Corticosteroids

Clinical belief that corticosteroids cause peptic ulcer or its complications is poorly supported. Difficulties of assessment arise because associations may not be so much with corticosteroid use *per se* but with the diseases for which they are used. Cooke[54], and Conn and Blitzer[55] having analysed data obtained in 42 controlled trials of corticosteroid therapy, concluded that no proof of association existed. By contrast, Messer *et al.*[56] who analysed 71 controlled studies which included 3061 patients found an excess of ulcers in those treated, with about a doubling (2.3-fold) of relative risk.

Non-aspirin, non-steroidal anti-inflammatory drugs

Non-steroidal associated dyspepsia is very commonly encountered, but convincing evidence of drug causation of ulcer relapse or of complications is difficult to obtain.

Ulcer complications. In case series, a high proportion of patients with ulcer complications have been found to be taking non-aspirin NSAIDs[25-27]. Most patients with ulcer complications are, however, elderly and it is therefore unsafe to conclude that the drugs caused the disease because the elderly are also the group most likely to be taking non-aspirin NSAIDs. Individual data sets nevertheless contain persuasive evidence that non-aspirin NSAID use is unduly common.

Examination of the extensive series of clinical trials of non-aspirin NSAIDs has helped little to resolve the problem. Firstly, most comparisons have been between one drug and another, and therefore no baseline expectation exists. Secondly, ulcer complications generally occur quite rarely. Therefore an increase from a baseline of one episode per 2000 patient-years of experience in the ordinary population (i.e. some 30 000 episodes of bleeding or perforation for a 60 million population each year) to one every 500 years, a four-fold increase, would be well-nigh undetectable.

The same is likely to be true of surveillance studies. If, say, the outcome of 10 000 courses of treatment is examined, then assuming an average prescription duration of one month this means just over 800 patient-years of experience. Again this is likely to be too few to yield useful data and therefore reassurance offered by such studies[57,58], may be of limited value.

Retrospective case control studies allow the possibility of examining the outcome of tens of thousands of treatment courses by concentrating on the individuals with complications and ignoring those without. The methods however are vitally dependent on collecting an unbiased patient sample and a comparable set of controls.

Using this method we have compared the frequency of non-aspirin NSAID intake in patients admitted with bleeding ulcers (gastric or duodenal) aged 60 or over in the Nottingham area with the frequency of drug use in matched hospital inpatient and population controls. Table 4.7 shows the outcome. Drug

Table 4.7 Outcome of questioning about non-aspirin, NSAID intake by patients with upper gastrointestinal bleeding and by controls (after Somerville et al.[59])

Study	Controls	
	Hospital inpatient	Community
A. All subjects combined*		
Takers (80)	33	34
Non-takers (150)	197	173
Total (230)	230	207
Users (%) 35	14	16
Relative risk (controls compared with patients with bleeding)	3.8	2.7
95% confidence limits	2.2–6.4	1.7–4.4
B. Separated by ulcer diagnosis		
Gastric ulcer only (n = 113)		
Relative risk	3.7	2.8
95% confidence limits	1.9–7.5	1.5–5.4
Duodenal ulcer only (n = 117)		
Relative risk	2.7	2.7
95% confidence limits	1.4–5.5	1.3–5.8

* Number of patients with bleeding in parentheses.

use was more common in both gastric and duodenal ulcer patients admitted with haematemesis or melaena than in either of the controls. The risk was increased by about three-fold for both types of ulcer and for both men and women[59].

Though increased, the relative risk is not particularly large, indicating that as individuals those who are taking non-aspirin NSAIDs are not very likely to come to harm. It is possible however to calculate a population-attributable risk, and this is of the order of 20% suggesting that one-fifth of all bleeding in the over-sixties is caused by non-aspirin NSAIDs, or about 2000 episodes in the United Kingdom each year. The discrepancy between the low relative risk and the large number of attributable episodes can be explained by the large scale of non-aspirin NSAID use, now about 24 million prescriptions each year. This indicates that only one in ten thousand users may actually come to harm each year.

Ulcer occurrence. Arthritic patients commonly complain of dyspepsia, and ulcers are often detected in them. Disease is commonly attributed to non-aspirin NSAID use, but proof is hard to obtain. Thus few of the patients studied prospectively by Caruso and Porro[22] actually developed new ulcers, and rheumatoid patients have been thought to be especially likely to develop ulcers anyway. Clinch and his colleagues[60] found a raised frequency of non-aspirin NSAID use in elderly patients who proved to have ulcers at endoscopy compared with those who were ulcer-negative, and Duggan and his associates in New South Wales[52] found a greater frequency of drug use in gastric (but not duodenal) ulcer patients than in matched controls. The failure to find an association with duodenal ulcer is puzzling (assuming that clinical evidence from the United Kingdom, in particular, is correct in suggesting associations for gastric and duodenal ulcer). One possible explanation might be the relative youth of the duodenal ulcer patients in Australia. In the United Kingdom, the association for duodenal ulcer has been detected in the elderly. In this context it is noteworthy that duodenal ulcer mortality, and also perforation rates, have risen markedly in recent years in elderly women in the United Kingdom whereas they have fallen often quite pronouncedly in the remainder (Table 4.8).

Table 4.8 Percentage change in admission rates with gastric and duodenal ulcer in England and Wales[61] between 1958–62 and 1978–82

Sex	Age (years)	Duodenal ulcer	Gastric ulcer
Men	15–44	− 62	− 86
	45–64	− 50	− 72
	65 +	− 13	− 51
Women	15–44	− 36	− 25
	45–64	+ 38	− 39
	65 +	+ 145	+ 20

Oesophageal stricture Two sets of studies have shown a raised frequency of non-aspirin NSAID use in patients with oesophageal stricture compared with controls (Table 4.9). The relative risk would seem to be of the same order as for ulcer bleeding.

Table 4.9 Oesophageal stricture and use of NSAIDs

Study	Reference		Cases	Controls
Wilkins *et al.*	62	Total	53	165
		Takers (%)	49	12
Heller *et al.*	63	Total	76	76
		Takers (%)	29	13

Lower bowel disease   The withdrawal of osmotically-released indomethacin (Osmosin) from the United Kingdom market following the reporting of colonic perforation prompted the study of the possible association between non-steroidal use and lower bowel disease[64-68]. Reports have accumulated suggesting associations with ileal ulcer and stricture and inflammation with blood and protein loss[66,67]. In addition, a retrospective case control study has indicated that takers of NSAIDs may be between two and three times as liable to lower bowel perforation and bleeding as are non-takers[68]. The mechanisms are unclear, but the lesions clearly cannot be acid-mediated. Non-steroidal use seems to make synthetic probe molecules more likely to cross the mucosal barrier in the small bowel, an effect which is quite consistently detectable. Experimental animal data confirm that intestinal lesions can be produced by NSAIDs.

Ulcerative colitis   Use of fenamates has been associated with diarrhoea, with enterocolitis, and with stimulation of intestinal secretion[69], while sulphasalazine may rarely cause paradoxical exacerbation of colitis. Indomethacin suppositories have been claimed to cause rectal ulceration, and flurbiprofen and indomethacin to cause reversible electrophysiological and histological changes[70]. There is no reason to believe that these are specific drug effects which are not shared by other NSAIDs. Laxative actions mediated by effects on electrolyte transport have also been described[71] for NSAIDs.

Exacerbation of colitis has been associated particularly with use of para-cetamol, rather than aspirin[72]. This rather surprising association has yet to be proved to be causal rather than consequential.

CONCLUSIONS

The spectrum of NSAID-associated damage is wide and no part of the gut seems immune. Damage to the large bowel clearly cannot be acid-mediated but the simple assumption of prostaglandin mediation may be incorrect. Use of NSAIDs is clearly associated, and in part causally, with the occurrence of ulcer complications probably both gastric and duodenal, with oesophageal stricture and with large bowel damage. NSAIDs probably also cause ulcers to develop and the elderly may be especially prone. Decisions about disease frequency and importance are dependent upon carefully-controlled studies: careful experimental design and analysis are crucial if the correct conclusions are to be drawn.

REFERENCES

1. O'Laughlin, J.C., Hoftiezer, J.W. and Ivey, K.J. (1981). Effect of aspirin on the human stomach in normals; endoscopic comparisons of damage produced one hour, 24 hours and 2 weeks after administration. *Scand. J. Gastroenterology*, **16**, (Suppl. 67), 211–14
2. Lanza, F.L., Royer, G.L. and Nelson, R.S. (1980). Endoscopic evaluation of the effects of aspirin, buffered aspirin and enteric coated aspirin on gastric and duodenal mucosa. *New Engl. J. Med.*, **303**, 136–40
3. Rainsford, K.D. (1984). Mechanisms of gastrointestinal ulceration by non steroidal anti-inflammatory/analgesic drugs. In Rainsford, K.D. and Velo, G.P. (eds.) *Advances in Inflammation Research Side Effects of Anti-inflammatory/Analgesic drugs*, Volume 6. (New York: Raven Press)
4. Hunt, J.N. and Franz, D. (1981). Effect of prostaglandin E_2 on gastric mucosal bleeding caused by aspirin. *Dig. Dis. Sci.*, **26**, 301–5
5. Aly, A., Selling, J.A., Hogan, D.L., Isenberg, J.I., Koss, M.A. and Johansson, C. (1985). Gastric and duodenal prostaglandin E_2 (PGE_2) in humans: effect of luminal acidification (H^+) and indomethacin (I). *Gastroenterology*, **88**, A1305
6. Rainsford, K.D. and Willis, C. (1982). Relationship of gastric mucosal damage induced in pigs by anti-inflammatory drugs to their effects on prostaglandin production. *Dig. Dis. Sci.*, **27**, 624–35
7. Hawkey, C.J. and Rampton, D.S. (1985). Prostaglandins and gastrointestinal mucosa: are they important in its function, disease or treatment? *Gastroenterology*, **89**, 1162–88
8. Rainsford, K.D. (1982). A profile of the gastric ulcerogenic activity of benoxaprofen compared with other non-steroidal anti-inflammatory drugs in rats, stressed or given alcohol, and in pigs. *Eur. J. Rheumatol. Inflammation*, **5**, 148–54
9. Whittle, B.J.R. (1977). Mechanisms underlying gastric mucosal damage induced by indomethacin and bile salts and the actions of prostaglandins. *Br. J. Pharmacol.*, **60**, 455–60
10. Robert, A. (1981). Gastric cytoprotection by sodium salicylate. *Prostaglandins*, **2**, 139–45
11. Ligumsky, M., Hansen, D. and Kauffman, G.L. (1982). Salicylate blocks indomethacin- and aspirin-induced cyclo-oxygenase inhibition in rat gastric mucosa. *Gastroenterology*, **83**, 1043–6
12. Sato, H., Guth, P.H. and Grossman, M.I. (1982). Role of food in gastrointestinal ulceration produced by indomethacin in the rat. *Gastroenterology*, **83**, 210–15
13. Quevauviller, A. and Fauquet, J.P. (1970). Influence du taux de lipides dans le régime sur la sensibilité du rat à l'ulcère gastrique expérimental par la phenylbutazone. *C.R. Acad. Sci. D (Paris)*, **270**, 421–4
14. Tarnawski, A., Hollander, D., Stachura, J., Krause, W.I., Dadufalza, V., Gergely, H. and Zipser, R.D. (1985). Can arachidonic acid (prostaglandins precursor) protect the gastric mucosa against aspirin injury? Macroscopic, histologic, ultrastructural and functional time sequence analysis. *Gastroenterology*, **88**, 1610A
15. Tarnawski, A., Hollander, D., Krause, W.J., Stachura, J., Zipser, R.D., Gergely, H. and Dadufalza, V. (1985). Is linoleic acid (dietary essential fatty acid – EFA) cytoprotective for the gastric mucosa? *Gastroenterology*, **88**, 1610A
16. Robert, A. and Asano, T. (1977). Resistance of germ-free rats to indomethacin-induced intestinal lesions. *Prostaglandins*, **14**, 333–41
17. Kent, T.H., Cardelli, R.M. and Stamler, S.W. (1969). Small intestine ulcers and intestinal flora in rats given indomethacin. *Am. J. Pathol.*, **54**, 237–45
18. Duggan, D.E., Hooke, K.F., Noll, R.M. and Kwan, K.C. (1975). Enterohepatic circulation of indomethacin and its role in intestinal irritation. *Biochem. Pharmacol.*, **25**, 1749–54
19. Pitts, N.E. and Proctor, R.R. (1978). Summary: efficacy and safety of piroxicam. *Royal Society of Medicine International Congress and Symposium Series*, **1**, 97–108
20. Robert, A., Nezamis, J.E., Lancaster, C., Davis, J.P., Field, S.O. and Hanchar, A.J. (1983). Mild irritants prevent gastric necrosis through 'adaptive cytoprotection' mediated by prostaglandins. *Am. J. Physiol.*, **245**, G113

21. Graham, D.Y., Smith, J.L. and Dobbs, S.M. (1983). Gastric adaptation occurs with aspirin administration in man. *Dig. Dis. Sci.*, **28**, 1–6
22. Caruso, D. and Porro, G.B. (1980). Gastroscopic evaluation of anti-inflammatory drugs. *Br. Med. J.*, **i**, 75–8
23. Update, C.S.M. (1986). Non-steroidal anti-inflammatory drugs and serious gastrointestinal reactions—1. *Br. Med. J.*, **292**, 614–15
24. Emmanuel, J.H. and Montgomery, R.D. (1971). Gastric ulcer and anti-arthritic drugs. *Postgrad. Med. J.*, **47**, 227–32
25. Collier, D.St.J. and Pain, J.A. (1985). Non-steroidal anti-inflammatory drugs and peptic ulcer perforation. *Gut*, **26**, 359–63
26. O'Brien, J.D. and Burnham, W.R. (1985). Bleeding from peptic ulcers and use of non-steroidal anti-inflammatory drugs in the Romford area. *Br. Med. J.*, **291**, 1609–10
27. Armstrong, C.P. and Blower, A.L. (1986). Peptic ulcer complications and non-steroidal anti-inflammatory drugs. *Gut*, **27**, A609
28. Kurata, J.H., Elashoff, J.D. and Grossman, M.I. (1982). Inadequacy of the literature on the relationship between drugs, ulcers and gastrointestinal bleeding. *Gastroenterology*, **82**, 373–6
29. Berkson, J. (1946). Limitations of the application of four-fold tables to hospital data. *Biomet. Bull.*, **2**, 17–53
30. Roberts, R.S., Spitzer, W.O., Delmore, T. and Sackett, P.L. (1978). An empirical demonstration of Berkson's Bias. *J. Chronic Dis.*, **31**, 119–28
31. Kelly, J. (1956). Salicylate ingestion: a frequent cause of gastric haemorrhage. *Am. J. Med. Sci.*, **232**, 119–27
32. Muir, A. and Cossar, I.A. (1955). Aspirin and ulcer. *Br. Med. J.*, **ii**, 7–12
33. Muir, A. and Cossar, I.A. (1959). Aspirin and gastric haemorrhage. *Lancet*, **i**, 539–41
34. Alvarez, A.S. and Summerskill, W.H.J. (1958). Gastrointestinal haemorrhage and salicylates. *Lancet*, **ii**, 920–5
35. Lange, H.F. (1957). Salicylates and gastric haemorrhage. 2. Manifest bleeding. *Gastroenterology*, **33**, 778–88
36. Brown, R.K. and Mitchell, N. (1956). The influence of some of the salicyl compounds (and alcoholic beverages) on the natural history of peptic ulcer. *Gastroenterology*, **31**, 196–203
37. Allibone, A. and Flint, F.J. (1958). Bronchitis, aspirin, smoking and aetiology of peptic ulcer. *Lancet*, **ii**, 179–82
38. Parry, D.J. and Wood, P.H.N. (1967). Relationship between aspirin taking and gastroduodenal haemorrhage. *Gut*, **8**, 301–7
39. Levy, M. (1974). Aspirin use in patients with major upper gastrointestinal bleeding and peptic ulcer disease. *New Engl. J. Med.*, **290**, 1158–62
40. Coggon, D., Langman, M.J.S. and Spiegelhalter, D. (1982). Aspirin, paracetamol and haematemesis and melaena. *Gut*, **23**, 340–4
41. Belcon, M.C., Rooney, P.J. and Tugwell, P. (1985). Aspirin and gastrointestinal haemorrhage: a methodologic assessment. *J. Chronic Dis.*, **38**, 101–11
42. Elwood, P.C. and Sweetnam, P.M. (1979). Aspirin and secondary mortality from myocardial infarction. *Lancet*, **ii**, 1313–15
43. Elwood, P.C., Cochrane, A.L., Barr, M.L., Sweetnam, P.M., Williams, G. and Welsley, E. *et al.* (1984). A randomized controlled trial of acetylsalicylic acid in the secondary prevention of mortality from myocardial infarction. *Br. Med. J.*, **i**, 436–40
44. Aspirin myocardial infarction study research group. (1980). A randomized controlled trial of aspirin in persons recovered from myocardial infarction. *J. Am. Med. Assoc.*, **243**, 661–9
45. The Canadian Co-operative Study Group. (1978). A randomized trial of aspirin and sulfinpyrazone in threatened stroke. *New Engl. J. Med.*, **299**, 53–8
46. The Coronary Drug Project Research Group (1976). Aspirin in coronary heart disease. *J. Chronic Dis.*, **29**, 625–42
47. Fields, W.S. and Lemak, N.A. (1977). Controlled trial of aspirin in cerebral ischemia (AITIA Study). *Stroke*, **8**, 301–15

48. Billington, B.P. (1965). Observations from New South Wales on the changing incidence of gastric ulcer in Australia. *Gut*, **6**, 121–33
49. Cameron, A.J. (1975). Aspirin and gastric ulcer. *Mayo Clinic Proc.*, **50**, 565–75
50. Gillies, N.A. and Skyring, A. (1969). Gastric and duodenal ulcer. The association between aspirin ingestion, smoking and family history of ulcer. *Med. J. Australia*, **2**, 280–5
51. Piper, D.W., McIntosh, J.H., Ariotti, D.E., Fenton, B.H. and McLennan, R. (1981). Analgesic ingestion and chronic peptic ulcer. *Gastroenterology*, **80**, 427–32
52. Duggan, J.M., Dobson, A.J., Johnson, H. and Fahey, P. (1986). Peptic ulcer and non-steroidal anti-inflammatory agents. *Gut*, **27**, 929–33
53. Duggan, J.M. (1976). Aspirin in chronic gastric ulcer: an Australian experience. *Gut*, **17**, 378–84
54. Cooke, A.R. (1967). Corticosteroids and peptic ulcer: is there a relationship. *Am. J. Dig. Dis.*, **12**, 323–9
55. Conn, H.O. and Blitzer, B.L. (1976). Non association of adrenocorticosteroid therapy and peptic ulcer. *New Engl. J. Med.*, **294**, 473–9
56. Messer, J., Reitman, D., Sacks, H.S., Smith, H. and Chalmers, T.C. (1983). Association of adrenocorticosteroid therapy and peptic ulcer disease. *New Engl. J. Med.*, **309**, 21–9
57. Jick, H., Feld, A.D. and Perera, D.R. (1985). Certain non-steroidal anti-inflammatory drugs and hospitalization for upper gastrointestinal bleeding. *Pharmacotherapy*, **5**, 289–94
58. Inman, W.H.W. (1984). Non-steroidal anti-inflammatory drugs. *PEM News* (August), **2**, 4–10
59. Somerville, K.W., Faulkner, G. and Langman, M.J.S. (1986). Non-steroidal anti-inflammatory dru;3s and bleeding peptic ulcer. *Lancet*, **i**, 462–4
60. Clinch, D., Banerjee, A.K., Ostick, G. and Levy, D.W. (1983). Non-steroidal anti-inflammatory drugs and gastrointestinal adverse effects. *J. R. Coll. Physicians (London)*, **17**, 228–30
61. Walt, R., Katschinski, B., Logan, R., Ashley, J. and Langman, M.J.S. (1986). Rising frequency of ulcer perforation in elderly people in the United Kingdom. *Lancet*, **i**, 489–92
62. Wilkins, W.E., Ridley, R.G. and Pozniak, A.L. (1984). Benign stricture of the oesophagus: role of non-steroidal anti-inflammatory drugs. *Gut*, **25**, 478–80
63. Heller, S.R., Fellows, I.W., Ogilvie, A.L. and Atkinson, M. (1982). Non-steroidal anti-inflammatory drugs and benign oesophageal stricture. *Br. Med. J.*, **285**, 167–8
64. Day, T.K. (1983). Intestinal perforation associated with osmotic slow release indomethacin capsules. *Br. Med. J.*, **287**, 1671–2
65. Schwartz, H.A. (1981). Lower gastrointestinal side effects of non-steroidal anti-inflammatory drugs. *J. Rheumatol.*, **6**, 952–4
66. Bjarnason, I., Lang, J., Gumpel, M.J., Levi, A.J. and Price, A.B. (1986). Nonsteroidal anti-inflammatory drugs (NSAIDs) and intestinal pathology. *Gastroenterology*, **90**, 134–7
67. Bjarnason, I., Zanelli, G., Prousa, P., Gumpel, J.W. and Levi, A.J. (1986). Complications of non-steroidal anti-inflammatory drug (NSAID) induced small intestinal inflammation in man: bleeding and protein loss. *Gastroenterology*, **90**, 1347
68. Langman, M.J.S., Morgan, L. and Worrall, A. (1985). Use of anti-inflammatory drugs by patients admitted with small or large bowel perforations and haemorrhage. *Br. Med. J.*, **290**, 347–9
69. Hall, R.I., Petty, A.H., Cobden, I. and Lendrum, R. (1983). Enteritis and colitis associated with mefenamic acid. *Br. Med. J.*, **287**, 1182
70. Rampton, D.S. and Sladen, G.E. (1981). Prostaglandin synthesis inhibitors in ulcerative colitis: flurbiprofen compared with conventional treatment. *Prostaglandins*, **21**, 417
71. Gullikson, G.W., Sander, M. and Bass, P. (1982). Laxative-like effects of non-steroidal anti-inflammatory drugs on intestinal fluid movements and mucosal integrity. *J. Pharmacol. Exptl. Therapeut.*, **220**, 236–42
72. Rampton, D.S., McNeill, N.I. and Sarner, M. (1983). Analgesic ingestion and other factors preceding relapse in ulcerative colitis. *Gut*, **24**, 187–8

5
Bacteria and gastroduodenal inflammation

B. J. RATHBONE, J. I. WYATT and R. V. HEATLEY

The stomach and upper gut are normally sterile with only transient flora appearing following ingestion of food. The gastric defences including acid, mucus, lysozyme and immunoglobulins protect the upper gut from bacterial colonization. With decreasing gastric acidity, which occurs normally with ageing and with conditions such as pernicious anaemia and following gastric surgery, the stomach may become colonized with faecal as well as oral bacteria[1]. Patients with hypochlorhydria are also more susceptible to enteric infections such as cholera and salmonellosis[2].

At the turn of the century, bacteria were isolated from peptic ulcers in patients with normal as well as diminished gastric acidity. This led to much study and debate as to the role these bacteria might have in the pathogenesis of ulcers, but by the 1940s bacteria were not considered to play an important part. The recent rediscovery and isolation of spiral bacteria from gastric mucosa in the majority of patients with chronic gastritis has rekindled interest in the possible role of bacteria in the pathogenesis of peptic ulcer disease.

HISTORICAL ASPECTS

Bottcher[3] has been credited with the first demonstration of bacterial colonization of gastric ulcers in 1874[4] and the subsequent early work has been well summarized by Ivy et al[5]. In 1888, Letulle[6] reported that the oral or

101

parenteral administration of *Staphylococcus pyogenes* to guinea pigs resulted in gastric ulcers. Similar results were reported with other bacteria including dysentery organisms, pyogenic streptococci and lactobacilli. The implication from these reports was that infection may be an occasional or accessory cause of ulceration. The subsequent work mainly concentrated on two organisms, a colonic *Bacillus* and a specific strain of *Streptococcus*.

Whereas the above work reported acute lesions, Turck[7] claimed that chronic ulcers could be produced in 100% of dogs after they had been fed colonic bacilli daily for several months. The photographs illustrating these lesions however showed only non-specific gastric and duodenal changes[4]. Completely negative results were obtained when these experiments were repeated[8]. When rabbits were injected with the bacillus, gastric and duodenal lesions occurred within 24 hours but histological examination revealed that they had an embolic aetiology.

Streptococci

The role of streptococci in ulceration was championed by Rosenow[9-12], who demonstrated that streptococci isolated from humans, especially those with ulceration, produced gastric ulcers when injected into laboratory animals. Rosenow maintained that the *Streptococcus* initiating gastric ulceration had a selective affinity for gastric mucosa where it produced local destruction of the glandular tissue, which was then digested by the acid gastric juice. He postulated that an acute lesion so produced may be made chronic by the constant discharge into the blood of the specific organisms lurking in distant foci. That injection of streptococci produced ulcers and the selective localization of organisms isolated from ulcer patients to the stomach following injection, was confirmed by other workers[13-15].

In 1930 Saunders[16] isolated an alpha-*Streptococcus* from human peptic ulcers and demonstrated specific agglutinins to this organism which were present in higher titres in ulcer patients compared to controls with other streptococcal infection. Attempts to produce ulcers in animals by injection of the specific organism however were unsuccessful. Saunders suggested that the lesions produced by Rosenow were owing to an anaphylactic shock-type reaction to foreign protein present in the broths injected into animals. Celler and Thalhimer[17] isolated a non-haemolytic *Streptococcus* from human ulcers and like Saunders[16] failed to produce ulcers when they injected it into animals.

Streptococci can thus be isolated from many ulcers in the stomach and duodenum and when injected into animals have often been associated with acute lesions of the gastric mucosa. These short-lived lesions, however, bear little relation to the ulcer crater seen in human peptic ulcer disease.

Fungi

Of more relevance to chronic ulcers are the reports of *Candida albicans* colonizing human peptic ulcers[18-21]. The literature supports *Candida* being a secondary invader of ulcers, particularly in debilitated patients, where it may prolong the life of the ulcer and on occasion cause complications. In two cases, both alcoholics, reported by Peters *et al.*[18], fungal invasion of the ulcer, eroding the wall of a major artery, was thought to have precipitated their death. Currently, there is no good evidence to support *Candida* having a role in the pathogenesis of peptic ulcers in healthy subjects.

Little further interest in microorganisms and any role they may have in the aetiology of ulcers occurred until the 1980s. Warren[22] and Marshall[23] described and isolated gastric spiral bacteria associated with active chronic gastritis. Independently, Steer[24] in a scanning electron microscopy study of gastro-duodenal mucosa and Rollason *et al.*[25] in a retrospective study of gastric biopsies also reported these bacteria on gastric-type epithelium. The organisms described by these three groups of workers had been observed previously, but their potential significance was not appreciated.

Spiral organisms

Bizzozero[26] in 1893 noted the presence of spirochaetes in the gastric glands and parietal cells of six dogs he examined. Salomon[27] then reported similar organisms in the gastric mucosa of cats and rats. Human spirochaetes were first reported in necrotic material at the surface of ulcerating carcinomas and in gastric secretion[28,29]. Doenges[30] in a histological study of 242 autopsy stomachs using haematoxylin and eosin staining of sections found spirochaetes present in 43% of cases. The organisms occurred predominantly in the glandular lumen but were seen also in the parietal cells. Autolysis made detailed assessment of the gastric histology impossible. To avoid this, Freedburg and Barron[31] studied gastric resection specimens using haematoxylin and eosin, and a silver stain, which they found best for identifying the bacteria. Overall, 37.1% of their 35 patients were positive for the spirochaetes. However, in many cases bacteria were seen only after examining multiple sections. The organisms were mostly associated with gastric ulcers and gastric carcinoma. In 13 duodenal ulcer patients with associated chronic gastritis, only two were positive. In an attempt to confirm the presence of spirochaetes in gastric mucosa, Palmer[32] studied 1180 suction biopsies (mostly from the gastric body) from 1000 patients using haematoxylin and eosin stains. He reported no spirochaetes or any structure which could reasonably be of spirochaetal nature.

After these studies, no further mention of gastric epithelial bacteria occurred until 1975, when bacteria were described on the lumenal surface of epithelial cells of gastric ulcer patients[33,34]. The bacteria were seen to have at least one filum and to be deep to the mucus layer, with the gastric epithelial cells having a diminished mucus content compared to those from a normal stomach. Electron micrographs illustrated phagocytosed bacteria within polymorphonuclear leukocytes, and the absence of the bacteria from areas of intestinal metaplasia was noted. Attempted culture of gastric biopsies resulted in a growth of *Pseudomonas aeruginosa* which was almost certainly a contaminant from the endoscope.

Fung *et al.*[35] in 1979 correlating endoscopic, histological and ultrastructural appearances of chronic gastritis described and demonstrated bacteria in the crevices between surface mucus cells and in gastric pits. It was noted that many of these bacteria abutted directly onto the plasmalemma of the epithelial cell, but were never seen within the cell and were thus assumed to be of little significance.

In 1980 Warren[22] noted that the majority of endoscopic biopsies from patients with gastritis and peptic ulceration were colonised with curved *Campylobacter*-like organisms. These organisms were poorly stained by haematoxylin and eosin, but seen easily with the Warthin–Starry silver stain. A prospective study was set up and attempts made to culture the organisms from gastric biopsies using non-selective and standard *Campylobacter* media for 48 hours. No growth was observed until the 35th biopsy was incubated during an Easter holiday and was thus examined after five days' incubation. A heavy growth of *Campylobacter*-like organisms was found on the nonselective media. When other biopsies were also incubated for three to four days, a similar growth of Gram-negative bacteria were seen[36]. Independently, in 1983 Rollason *et al.*[25] in a retrospective study of endoscopic gastric biopsies, described spiral bacteria in association with chronic superficial and chronic atrophic gastritis. Steer[24] continuing his morphological studies of gastroduodenal mucosa in peptic ulceration also submitted a paper in 1983 describing the scanning electron microscopy appearance of bacteria in patients with ulcer-associated chronic gastritis.

CAMPYLOBACTER PYLORIDIS

The *Campylobacter*-like organism isolated by Warren and Marshall and independently described by Rollason *et al.* and by Steer was officially named *Campylobacter pyloridis*[37] but is now being altered to *Campylobacter pylori*[38]. It is now apparent that *C. pylori* is a coloniser of gastric epithelium world-wide[39–50] (Table 5.1). It is consistently associated with mucosal inflammation and is rarely seen adhering to normal gastric mucosa (Table 5.1). The differences in the prevalence of *C. pylori* may be partly attributable to varying methods of detection of the bacteria and to differences in histological criteria necessary for the diagnosis of chronic gastritis. The type of gastritis is of importance,

Table 5.1 Prevalence of *C. pylori* in chronic gastritis and peptic ulcer disease in different countries. Figures in parentheses refer to population size

Country	Normals	Gastritis	Gastric ulcer	Duodenal ulcer	Reference
Australia	0%(21)	96%(54)	68%(40)	90%(70)	39
Holland	7%(15)	89%(35)	67%(3)	100%(9)	40
UK	11%(119)	71%(86)	57%(21)	78%(32)	41
Yugoslavia	0%(8)	52%(62)	83%(6)	71%(28)	42
Spain	10%(10)	91%(33)	– 86%(28)* –		43
USA	11%(37)	63%(96)	54%(28)	60%(25)	44
Canada	0%(26)	60%(10)	43%(42)	27%(26)	45,46
Japan	– 65%** –		– 100%* –		47
Hong Kong	40%	78%	– 80%* –		48
Italy	31%	43%	79%(14)	71%(28)	49
Peru	–	100%(103)	–	–	50

*Figures published do not differentiate between gastric and duodenal ulcers.
**Overall prevalence in endoscopy patients, not taking into account histology.

since *C. pylori* is rarely observed on mucosa from patients with bile reflux gastritis[51] or pernicious anaemia[52]. In the latter group of patients however, there may be a tendency to underestimate colonisation, owing to the high prevalence of intestinal metaplasia, on which *C. pylori* is never found[53].

Attention has focussed on the association between *C. pylori* and the presence of gastric and duodenal ulceration (Table 5.1). The association is however less strong than that with mucosal inflammation in the stomach. It is recognised that antral gastritis commonly accompanies peptic ulceration[54,55], especially duodenal ulceration, and this may well account for the prevalence of *C. pylori* in peptic ulcer disease. In those gastric ulcer patients not colonised by *C. pylori* there is frequently another aetiological factor precipitating ulceration, such as ingestion of non-steroidal anti-inflammatory agents[56]. In colonised ulcer patients, both the gastritis and *C. pylori* persist after treatment with most ulcer-healing agents, with the notable exception of bismuth compounds[57,58].

Histological identification of *C. pylori*

Campylobacter pylori can be readily detected in routinely processed gastric biopsies and, owing to their characteristic S-shaped morphology and position, are unlikely to be confused with other bacteria. They are present, often in very considerable numbers, adhering to the luminal aspect of the gastric epithelium of the surface, gastric pits (foveolae), and also free within the surface mucus, where they tend to be orientated in parallel. Because of their faint haematoxyphilia, the organisms may be seen in haematoxylin and eosin-stained sections. The Warthin–Starry silver stain demonstrates the bacteria well, and has been used by most workers. This is a time-consuming and sometimes

105

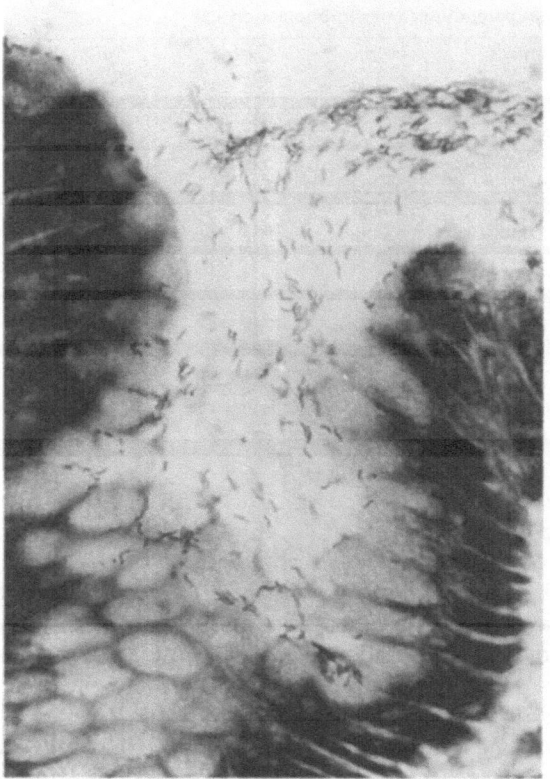

Figure 5.1 *Campylobacter pylori* on gastric mucosa: the bacteria are present on the surface of the epithelial cells, especially in the regions of inter-cellular junctions, and tend to show parallel orientation in the overlying mucus. (Modified Giemsa original magnification × 320)

unpredictable technique, and more recently phase-contrast microscopy[59], fluorescent staining with Acridine Orange[60], and a modification of the Giemsa stain[61] (Figure 5.1) have been recommended as alternatives.

The mucosa-associated curved bacteria can be confirmed as *C. pylori* by immunohistochemistry using a polyclonal rabbit antibody raised against the organism[62] but this step is not necessary for routine detection.

The presence of *C. pylori* in our series of 268 non-ulcer dyspepsia patients is shown in Table 5.2, using the Whitehead classification for chronic gastritis[63]. The bacteria are seen in all grades of superficial and atrophic gastritis, but do not colonize areas of intestinal metaplasia. They are significantly associated with the activity of the gastritis (Table 5.3), characterized by neutrophils within the epithelium[63]. Surface *C. pylori* are also frequently associated with depletion

Table 5.2 Prevalence of gastric antral and body *C. pylori* colonization according to the presence of histological chronic gastritis in 268 dyspeptic patients

Presence of chronic gastritis	C. pylori colonization of antral and body biopsies		
	Both	One	None
Antrum and body	97	11	11
Antrum only	25	6	1
Body only	0	0	6
Both normal	0	0	111

Table 5.3 Prevalence of *C. pylori* colonization in patients with chronic gastritis according to the activity of the gastritis

Gastritis	C. pylori	
	Positive	Negative
Active	198	23
Inactive	33	22

of neutral cytoplasmic mucin in the gastric epithelial cell[64]. They are commonly present on morphologically-normal body type mucosa when inflammation involves only the antrum[65]. We have seen no patients with gastric *C. pylori* colonization and a histologically-normal gastric antrum and body.

Campylobacter pylori also occur in the duodenum in duodenitis and in association with duodenal ulceration in up to 90% of cases[56]. Foci of gastric epithelial metaplasia are usually present in the duodenal mucosa in active duodenitis[66], and *C. pylori* occurs in these sites only, sparing the intestinal epithelium as they do in the stomach[67].

Campylobacter pylori – bacteriology

Since the original isolation of *C. pylori*, culture techniques have been improved[68]. Biopsies can be transported to the laboratory in a small quantity of sterile saline[36]. Provided biopsies are kept at 4°C, a delay of up to five hours does not seem to affect the isolation of *C. pylori*. Biopsies treated in a ground glass grinder appear to yield a heavier growth of organisms than minced biopsies. Although *C. pylori* will grow on simple 7% blood agar plates at 37°C, Goodwin *et al.* found brain–heart infusion agar with 7% horse blood, 1% Isovitalex, vancomycin 6 mg/litre, nalidixic acid 20 mg/litre, and amphotericin 2 mg/litre to be the most satisfactory medium with contaminants inhibited almost completely[68]. The most effective incubation atmosphere is an anaerobic gas mixture.

Table 5.4 Summary of *C. pylori* biotyping compared to *C. jejuni*

Characteristic	C. pylori	C. jejuni
Oxidase	+	+
Catalase	+	+
Indole	−	−
Nitrate reduction	−	+
Hydrogen sulphide	+	±
Hippurate hydrolysis	+	+
Urease	+	−
Glucose (acid)	−	−
Growth at 42°C	±	±
Nalidixic acid sensitivity	−	+

Campylobacter pylori are microaerophilic, Gram-negative, oxidase- and catalase-positive bacteria and although now included in the Genus *Campylobacter*, they differ from other *Campylobacter* species in a number of ways. The biotyping and growth characteristics of *C. pylori*[56] and *C. jejuni*[69] are summarized in Table 5.4. One of the most remarkable features of *C. pylori* is its powerful urease activity[40], which is not seen with other *Campylobacter* affecting man, and unlike the urease activity of *Proteus* does not require induction. So marked is the ability to hydrolyse urea that gastric colonization can be diagnosed by the urease activity of homogenized gastric biopsies[70] or a [^{13}C]urea breath test[71]. Luck and Seth[72] in 1924 described the presence of considerable urease activity in the stomach. That the urease might be bacterial in origin was suggested by Lieber and Lefevre[73] who demonstrated that the hypoacidity found in many patients with uraemia could be reversed with antibiotic therapy. This view was opposed by Mossberg *et al.*[74]. Studies using conventional and germ-free animals however confirmed that the gastric urease in animals was bacterial in origin[75], although it was not until 1982 that the urease-positive human bacteria were identified.

Using polyacrylamide gel electrophoresis, *C. pylori* protein bands have been demonstrated to differ from those of *Campylobacter* reference strains[41]. The major cellular fatty acids are also different to those of other *Campylobacter*[76]. Unlike all previously-known *Campylobacter*, *C. pylori* lacks methylated menaquinone-6 and it shows phosphatase activity in the phenolphthalein phosphate test[77]. The DNA base-pair ratio is however in the *Campylobacter* range (guanine + cytosine 36%)[39]. Thus, although it is generally convenient to include *C. pylori* as a *Campylobacter* for classification purposes at present, studies of cistron similarities will confirm whether or not it represents a new bacterial Genus[77].

In vitro, *C. pylori* antibiotic susceptibilities are in general similar to those of other *Campylobacter* and are summarized in Table 5.5[78,79]. One exception, which is useful in identification, is the resistance of *C. pylori* to nalidixic acid, which is not seen with other similar organisms.

Table 5.5   *In vitro C. pylori* drug susceptibilities

Drug	MIC_{50} (mg/litre)	MIC_{90} (mg/litre)	Range (mg/litre)
Penicillin	0.06	0.25	0.015–1.0
Amoxycillin	0.06	0.12	0.015–0.25
Erythromycin	0.12	0.25	0.06–0.25
Kanamycin	2.0	2.0	1.0–4.0
Gentamicin		1.0	0.5–1.0
Tetracycline	0.12	0.12	0.06–0.25
Chloramphenicol	4.0	8.0	2.0–8.0
Metronidazole	0.5	4.0	0.5–4.0
Tinidazole	0.5	4.0	0.5–32
Cephalexin	2.0	8.0	0.5–8.0
Cefotaxime	0.5	1.0	0.12–1.0
Cephalothin	0.5	2.0	0.5–2.0
Cefoxitin	0.12	0.12	0.015–0.5
Nalidixic acid	32	64	1.0–64
Sulphamethoxazole	128	> 256	32 to > 256
Trimethoprim	512	1024	256–1024
Ranitidine	64	128	64–128
Cimetidine	400	800	200–1600
Bismuth citrate	8.0	16	4.0–32
Bismuth tartrate	8.0	16	2.0–32
Omeprazole	–	–	> 1000

Like certain other spiral bacteria seen in animals, *C. pylori* appears especially adapted to the ecological niche provided by intestinal mucus. Studies by Hazell and Lee[80] show that *C. pylori* is extremely flexible and will rapidly corkscrew though a viscous environment which would severely impede the movement of more conventional rod-shaped organisms.

Whilst culturing gastric biopsies for *C. pylori*, a curved rod has also been identified in a small number of patients and called gastric *Campylobacter*-like organism type 2 (GCLO-2)[81]. Their biotyping[81] and cellular fatty acid profile[77] resembles that of *C. jejuni*, indicating that it is a true *Campylobacter* and not related to *C. pylori*.

Campylobacter pylori – immunology

Aspects of both the systemic and local immune response to *C. pylori* have been investigated. Serum antibodies against gastric *Campylobacters* have been demonstrated by complement fixation[82], haemagglutination[83], bacterial agglutination[82] and ELISA (enzyme-linked immunosorbent assay) techniques[84–87]. Each show raised levels of antibody in patients colonized by *C. pylori* compared with normal, especially in those studies where a normal gastric mucosa is confirmed histologically.

109

The ELISA assay enables the immune response to be studied according to the class of antibody produced. Patients with *C. pylori* have significantly-raised serum IgG and IgA to *C. pylori*, but IgM is found to be similar in bacteria positive and negative patients. This pattern of response is in keeping with the view that bacterial colonization, once established, persists for long periods. There is little antigenic cross-reactivity with other *Campylobacter* species, and an ELISA assay using a sonicate of bacteria as antigen appears to be specific[85,87]. A rabbit polyclonal antibody reported by Steer and Newell[62] against *C. pylori* does not cross-react with *C. jejuni* and by immunoelectron microscopy the antibody recognizes sites on the cell membrane and flagellae. We have also developed a rabbit antibody using a different antibody preparation and found it to cross-react with other *Campylobacter*. Interestingly, a common *Campylobacter* antibody used for fluorescent identification of the bacteria in stools reacts with *C. pylori*[88].

Antigenic differences between strains are being recognized, which may correspond to differences in the relative proportions of outer membrane proteins identified by polyacrylamide gel electrophoresis, or to varying surface proteins in different strains[89].

Local production of anti-*C. pylori* antibody by gastric mucosa in tissue culture occurs with mucosa from gastritic patients, but not with normal tissue[90]. Bacterial coating *in vivo* by host antibody can be demonstrated by immunohistochemistry (Figure 5.2), where the class of antibody involved varies with the activity of the gastritis[63]. Uncoated bacteria were invariably present deep in the gastric pits, an observation which may explain their ability to persist in the stomach despite the immune response of the host.

Campylobacter pylori – electron microscopy

Campylobacter pylori has distinctive ultrastructural characteristics. It has a smooth surface with 4–6 polar sheathed flagellae[76] each with a terminal bulb, not found in other *Campylobacter*, and ultrastructurally resembles members of the Genus *Spirillum* more closely than *Campylobacters*[91].

In the gastric mucosa, *C. pylori* are localized predominantly in the gutters between adjacent epithelial cells, where they adhere to microvilli[80]. At sites of close contact with the bacterium, shallow cup-shaped elevations form in the epithelial cells which are morphologically similar to the adherence pedestals of enteropathogenic *E. coli* [64]. The plama membranes of the mucus-secreting cells are intact but indented, with the number of microvilli considerably depleted[64]. The population density of the bacteria correlates with the presence[63] and number of polymorph leukocytes in the epithelium[92], and the organisms have been seen in phagocytic vacuoles, suggesting that they can attract and activate polymorphs[93].

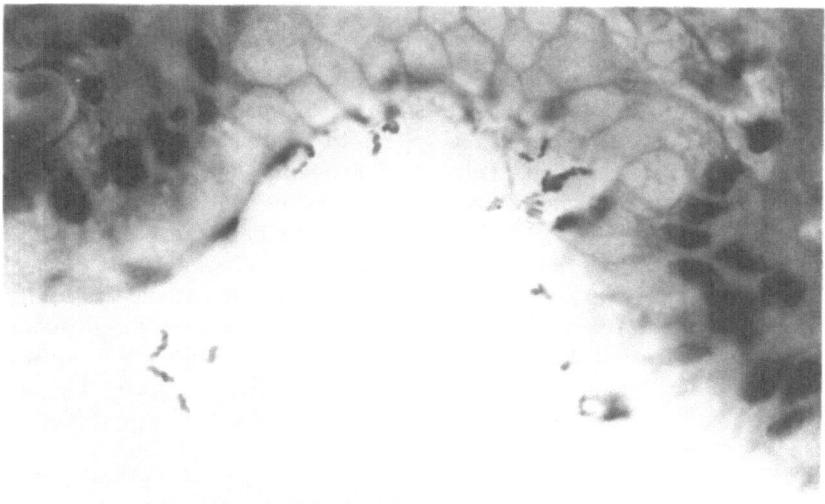

Figure 5.2 Surface of gastric mucosa stained by the indirect immunoperoxidase technique for IgA. *Campylobacter pylori* are labelled by anti-IgA indicating *in vivo* adsorption of host IgA on the bacteria surface. (Original magnification × 320)

Evidence for *C. pylori* pathogenicity

Once established, *C. pylori* colonization appears to be long-term. At present, the data supporting a pathogenic role for *C. pylori* in human disease rely on its strong association with chronic gastritis, the effects of *C. pylori* ingestion in a normal volunteer and the results of treatment studies.

The association with gastritis is particularly strong with non-autoimmune, type-B gastritis. Patients with autoimmune gastritis[52] and with bile reflux gastritis[51] have a much lower level of *C. pylori* colonization, suggesting that the bacteria are not simply commensals in the inflamed stomach.

When a volunteer (Barry Marshall) known to have normal gastric histology, ingested live *C. pylori* following a dose of cimetidine, a variety of non-specific symptoms occurred[94]. Histology performed 10 days' post-ingestion, showed the presence of spiral organisms on the epithelium, diminished intracellular mucus, and polymorph infiltration of the mucosa. At electron microscopy, the microvilli were depleted. A repeat biopsy four days' later showed no organisms or polymorphs present. The mucus content of the epithelial cells had improved, but was not normal and the ultrastructural changes remained. No serological response to the organisms was seen.

In the past, cases of presumed infective gastritis have been reported in a number of volunteers undergoing gastric juice studies when the same unsterilized equipment was used[95,96]. It has been suggested that these cases might have been owing to *C. pylori*[94,97] and retrospective analysis of the available biopsy material has shown *C. pylori* colonization, confirming that this may indeed have been the infective agent[94].

In vitro studies have shown *C. pylori* to be sensitive to a number of antibiotics[76,79,98] and tests using ulcer-healing agents have shown susceptibility to bismuth but relative insensitivity to cimetidine, ranitidine, carbenoxalone, sucralfate and omeprazole[79,98]. Bismuth salts have been used for many years in the treatment of dyspepsia and peptic ulceration although their mechanism of action has not been clear. Well-known is the anti-spirochaeteal activity of bismuth and the recent studies demonstrating reduced relapse rates in duodenal ulcer patients treated with bismuth compounds[99–101], raising the possibility that it acts by an antibacterial mechanism. The antibiotic sensitivities are of considerable interest in view of studies reporting ulcer healing with metronidazole[102,103] and furazolidone[104,105].

Only now are the preliminary results of prospective treatment studies appearing. Bismuth alone has been reported to eradicate *C. pylori* in the majority of patients treated[57,58,106–108]. Similar results were also seen in a small number of patients treated with amoxycillin[106] but not erythromycin[57,108]. In patients where eradication of *C. pylori* has been achieved, there was histological improvement with a decrease in the polymorphonuclear and mononuclear cellular infiltrate. Follow-up of these patients has, however, shown a significant relapse rate[57,58,106]. Restricted endonuclease analysis of the bacterial DNA before treatment and after relapse in these patients, shows that the same strain is involved, suggesting relapse rather than re-infection[107]. A combination of bismuth and antibiotic has also been used in treatment and appears to result in a lower relapse rate than bismuth alone as judged by assessment one month after treatment[106]. Studies where H_2-receptor antagonists, sucralfate, Pyrogastrone and Misoprostil have been investigated, show no alteration in *C. pylori* colonization nor improvement in gastritis[57,106,107,109].

Although increasing evidence supports *C. pylori* having a pathogenic role, the natural history of the organism and mechanisms of pathogenicity remain unclear. Based on their own studies and the reports of infectious gastritis, Marshall *et al.*[94] proposed that initial infection with *C. pylori* may result in an acute gastrointestinal disturbance (epigastric discomfort, nausea and vomiting) in approximately 50% of cases. Those patients who do not clear the organism develop the histological picture of chronic gastritis with lymphocytes largely replacing the acute inflammatory cells. This period is associated with achlorhydria lasting between 3 and 12 months, which resolves as the inflammation of the gastric body subsides. Once acid secretion has returned and chronic inflammation persists, the patients then have the potential for developing peptic ulcers.

In the duodenum, the presence of metaplastic gastric epithelium is associated both in man[110] and experimental animals[111] with a high gastric acid output. We have found that active duodenitis usually occurs in those patients with both gastric metaplasia and *C. pylori* colonization of the stomach, implying the combination of hyperacidity and *Campylobacter*-associated gastritis is necessary for duodenal inflammation to occur. Within the duodenum, polymorph infiltration occurs preferentially in sites of gastric metaplasia[112] where surface *C. pylori* are often present[67].

At the ultrastructural level, cytopathic effects of colonization are seen: depletion of microvilli, disruption of submembranous cytoskeletal supporting microfilaments and the formation of adherence pedestals[64]. There is little to suggest that the organisms invade and as yet there are no studies which examine toxin production. One hypothesis put forward to explain pathogenecity concerns the remarkable urease activity of *C. pylori*. Hazell and Lee[113] suggest that the rapid hydrolysis of urea at intercellular junctions results in impaired passage of hydrogen ions from the gastric glands through the mucus to the lumen and permits back diffusion. The possible mechanisms they suggest for this include direct toxicity of ammonia as well as alteration of the mucosal-charge gradient and paracellular permeability which would all affect the gastric $Na^+ - K^+$ ATPase pump system.

Fox *et al.*[114] suggested the ferret may be a potential animal model for evaluating the cause and importance of *Campylobacter*-like organism-associated gastritis and ulceration in man. They identified a urease-positive *Campylobacter*-like organism in 3 of 17 ferret stomachs examined, one of the bacteria-positive ferrets having gastric ulceration. We were able to isolate a similar urease-positive bacterium from ferrets and found them to be biochemically and immunologically different to *C. pylori*. Unlike Fox *et al.* we isolated the organism from all of the 17 ferrets we studied and found no association with significant gastric inflammation[115]. This raises doubts both about the suitability of the ferret as a model and also the role of the bacterial urease in causing inflammation.

Whatever the exact mechanism of pathogenicity, *C. pylori* can only on present information be viewed as an aggressive factor. These organisms disturb enterocyte mucus production which is thought important in gastric mucosal protection. A diminution in quantity or quality of this mucus layer would be expected to increase the possibility of damaging luminal factors gaining access to the epithelium. Further work is clearly required to clarify whether this is the major activity in producing damage by *C. pylori*.

CONCLUSION

Despite all the work at the turn of the century into possible bacterial causes of peptic ulceration, the only organism now thought to have a possible role, *Campylobacter pylori*, was not isolated until 1982. *Candida albicans* appears to be a secondary colonizer of ulcers particularly in debilitated patients where it may be important in perpetuating ulcers and occasionally causing invasion.

The description and isolation of *C. pylori* has stimulated considerable interest worldwide. Present evidence from morphological, serological and therapeutic studies strongly implicates *C. pylori* in its unique ecological niche in the stomach, in the pathogenesis of active chronic gastritis. The role in gastric and duodenal ulcers is less clear.

Research over the next few years will hopefully answer many questions about *C. pylori* and human disease, in particular its mode of transmission and its role in ulceration. Chronic indolent infection by this highly-adapted organism may prove to be the common denominator linking gastro-duodenal inflammation and ulceration.

REFERENCES

1. Hill, M. (1986). Bacterial factors. In Losowsky, M.S. and Heatley, R.V. (eds) *Gut Defences in Clinical Practice*, pp. 147–54. (Edinburgh: Churchill Livingstone)
2. Elder, J.B. (1986). Gastric acid. In Losowsky, M.S. and Heatley, R.V. (eds) *Gut defences in clinical practice*, pp. 1–8. (Edinburgh: Churchill Livingstone)
3. Bottcher, H. (1874). Zur Genese des perforierten Magengeschwurs. *Dorpat. Med Ztschr.*, **5**, 148
4. Bolton, C. (1913). *Ulcer of the Stomach.* (London: Edward Arnold)
5. Ivy, A.C., Grossman, M.I. and Bachrach, W.H. (1950). *Peptic Ulcer*, 1st edn. (Philadelphia: The Blakiston Company)
6. Letulle, M. (1888). Origine infectieuse de certains ulcères simples de l'estomac ou du duodenum. *Soc. Med. D. Hôp. de Paris*, **5**, 360–87
7. Turck, F.B. (1906). Ulcer of the stomach: pathogenesis and pathology: experiments in producing artifical gastric ulcer and genuine induced peptic ulcer. *J. Am. Med. Assoc.*, **46**, 1753–63
8. Gibelli, C. (1908–10). Contributo critico sperimentale all'eziologia dell ulcera gastrica in rapporto coi traumi. *Arch. Internat. Chir.*, **4**, 127–71
9. Rosenow, E.C. (1913). The production of ulcer of the stomach by injection of streptococci. *J. Am. Med. Assoc.*, **61**, 1947–50
10. Rosenow, E.C. (1916). The causation of gastric and duodenal ulcer by streptococci. *J. Infect. Dis.*, **19**, 333–63
11. Rosenow, E.C. (1923). Etiology of spontaneous ulcer of stomach in domestic animals. *J. Infect. Dis.*, **32**, 384–99
12. Rosenow, E.C. (1923). The specificity of the *Streptococcus* of gastroduodenal ulcer and certain factors determining its localization. *J. Infect. Dis.* **33**, 248–68
13. Hardt, L.L.J. (1916). Contributions to the physiology of the stomach: XXXIII. The secretion of gastric juice in cases of gastric and duodenal ulcers. *Am. J. Physiol.*, **40**, 314–31
14. Haden, R.L. (1925). The elective localization of bacteria in peptic ulcer. *Arch. Int. Med.*, **35**, 457–71

15. Nickel, A.C. and Hufford, A.R. (1928). Elective localization of streptococci isolated from cases of peptic ulcer. *Arch. Int. Med.*, **41**, 210–30
16. Saunders, E.W. (1930). The serologic and etiologic specificity of the alpha *Streptococcus* of gastric ulcer. *Arch. Int. Med.*, **45**, 347–82
17. Celler, H.L. and Thalhimer, W. (1916). Experimental studies of the etiology of gastric and duodenal ulcer. *Med. Record*, **90**, 389
18. Peters, M., Weiner, J. and Whelan, G. (1980). Fungal infection associated with gastro-duodenal ulceration: endoscopic and pathologic appearances. *Gastroenterology*, **78**, 350–54
19. Katzenstein, A.A. and Maksem, J. (1979). Candidal infection of gastric ulcers. *Am. J. Clin. Pathol.*, **71**, 137–141
20. Mohtashemi, H. and Davidson, F.Z. (1973). Candidiasis and gastric ulcer. *Dig. Dis.*, **18**, 915–19
21. Minoli, G., Terruzzi, V., Butti, G., Frigerio, G. and Rossini, A. (1982). *Gastrointest. Endoscopy*, **28**, 59–61
22. Warren, J.R. (1983). Unidentified curved bacilli on gastric epithelium in active chronic gastritis. *Lancet*, **i**, 1273
23. Marshall, B. (1983). Unidentified curved bacilli on gastric epithelium in active chronic gastritis. *Lancet*, **i**, 1273–5
24. Steer, H.W. (1984). Surface morphology of the gastroduodenal mucosa in duodenal ulceration. *Gut*, **25**, 1203–10
25. Rollason, T.P., Stone, J. and Rhodes, J.M. (1984). Spiral organisms in endoscopic biopsies of the human stomach. *J. Clin. Pathol.*, **37**, 23–26
26. Bizzozero, G. (1893). Ueber die schlauchformigen Drüsen des magendarmkanals und die Beziehungen ihres epithels zu dem Oberflachenepithel der Schleimhaut. *Arch, fuer Mikr. Anat.*, **42**, 82–152
27. Salomon, H. (1896). Ueber das Spirillum des Saugetiermagens und sein Verhalten zu den Belegzellen. *Centralbl. fuer Bakt.*, **19**, 433–42
28. Luger, A. (1917). Ueber Spirochaeten und fusiforme Bazillen im Darm, mit einem Beitrag zur Frage der Lamblien-enteritis. *Wein. Klin. Wochenschr.*, **52**, 1643–7
29. Krienitz, W. (1906). Ueber das Auftreten von Mageninhalt bei Carcinoma Ventriculi. *Dtsch. Med. Wochenschr.*, **22**, 872
30. Doenges, J.L. (1939). Spirochaetes in the gastric glands of *Macacus rhesus* and of man without related disease. *Arch. Path.* **27**, 469–77
31. Freedburg, A.S. and Barron, L.E. (1940). The presence of spirochaetes in human gastric mucosa. *Am. J. Dig. Dis.*, **7**, 443–5
32. Palmer, E.D. (1954). Investigation of the gastric mucosa spirochetes of the human. *Gastroenterology*, **27**, 218–20
33. Steer, H.W. and Colin-Jones, D.G. (1975). Mucosal changes in gastric ulceration and their response to carbenoxolone sodium. *Gut*, **16**, 590–7
34. Steer, H.W. (1975). Ultrastructure of cell migration through the gastric epithelium and its relationship to bacteria. *J. Clin. Pathol.*, **28**, 639–46
35. Fung, W.P., Papadimitriou, J.M. and Matz, L.R. (1979). Endoscopic, histological and ultrastructural correlations in chronic gastritis. *Am. J. Gastroenterol.*, **71**, 269–79
36. Marshall, B.J., Royce, H., Annear, D.I., Goodwin, C.S., Pearman, J.W., Warren, J.R. and Armstrong, J.A. (1984). Original isolation of *Campylobacter pyloridis* from human gastric mucosa. *Microbiol. Lett.*, **25**, 83–8
37. Anon. (1985). Validation of publication of new names and new combinations previously effectively published outside the IJSB. *Int. J. Syst. Bacteriol.*, **85**, 223–5
38. Marshall, B.J. and Goodwin, C.S. (1987). Revised nomenclature for *C. pyloridis. Int. J. Syst. Bacteriol.*, **37**, 68
39. Marshall, B.J. and Warren, J.R. (1984). Unidentified curved bacilli in the stomach of patients with gastritis and peptic ulceration. *Lancet*, **i**, 1311–15
40. Langenberg, M.-L., Tytgat, G.N.J., Schipper, M.E.I., Rietra, P.J.G.M. and Zanen, H.C. (1984). *Campylobacter*-like organisms in the stomach of patients and healthy individuals. *Lancet*, **i**, 1348
41. Pearson, A.D., Bamforth, J., Booth, L., Holdstock, G., Ireland, A., Walker, C., Hawtin, P.

and Millward-Sadler, H. (1984). Polyacrylamide gel electrophoresis of spiral bacteria from the gastric antrum. *Lancet*, **i**, 1349–50

42. Kalenic, S., Faliseva, V., Scukanec-Spoljar, M. and Vodopija, I. (1985). *Campylobacter pyloridis* in the gastric mucosa of patients with gastritis and peptic ulcer. In Pearson, A.D., Skirrow, M.B. and Lior, H. (eds.) Campylobacter. *III. Proceedings of the Third International Workshop on* Campylobacter *Infections*, p. 193. (London: Public Health Laboratory Service)

43. Lopez-Brea, M., Jimenez, M.L., Blanco, M. and Pajares, J.M. Isolation of *Campylobacter pyloridis* from patients with and without gastroduodenal pathology. In Pearson, A.D., Skirrow, M.B. and Lior, H. (eds) Campylobacter. *III. Proceedings of the Third International Workshop on* Campylobacter *Infections*, pp. 193–4. (London: Public Health Laboratory Service)

44. Pettross, C.W., Cohen, H., Appleman, M.D., Valenzuela, J.E. and Chandrasama, P. (1986). *Campylobacter pyloridis:* relationship to peptic disease, gastric inflammation and other conditions. *Gastroenterology*, **90**, 1585

45. Bohnen, J., Krajden, S., Kempston, J., Anderson, J. and Karmali, M. (1985). *Campylobacter pyloridis* in Toronto. In Pearson, A.D., Skirrow, M.B. and Lior, H. (eds) Campylobacter. *III. Proceedings of the Third International Workshop on* Campylobacter *Infections*, pp. 175–7. (London: Public Health Laboratory Service)

46. Drumm, B., O'Brien, A., Cutz, E. and Sherman, P. (1986). *Campylobacter pyloridis* are associated with primary antral gastritis in the paediatric population. *Gastroenterology*, **90**, 1399

47. Ishii, E., Inoue, H., Tsuyuguchi, T., Shimoyama, T., Tanaka, T., Wada, M., Kishi, T., Masui, M., Tamura, T., Yanagase, Y. and Shoji, K. (1985). *Campylobacter pyloridis* in cases of stomach diseases in Japan. In Pearson, A.D., Skirrow, M.B. and Lior, H. (eds.) Campylobacter. *III. Proceedings of the Third International Workshop on* Campylobacter *Infections*, pp. 179–80. (London: Public Health Laboratory Service)

48. Hui, W.M., Lam, S.K., Ho, J., Chan, P.Y., Lui, I., Lai, C.L., Lok, A. and Ng, M.M.T. (1986). *Campylobacter*-like organisms do not affect the healing of gastric ulcers. *Gastroenterology*, **90**, 1468

49. Marcheggianao, A., Iannoni, C., Agnello, M., Paoluzi, P. and Pallone, F. (1986). *Campylobacter*-like organisms (CLOs), gastritis and peptic ulcer. *Gastroenterology*, **90**, 1533

50. Barreda, C., Gilman, R.H., Leon-Barua, R., Koch, J., Quevedo, N., Ramirez-Ramos, A., Recavarren, S., Rodriguez, C., Spira, W.M. and Stephensen, C. (1985). Differential colonisation of the stomach by *Campylobacter pyloridis* studied by a novel sheathed brush. In Pearson, A.D., Skirrow, M.B. and Lior, H. (eds.) Campylobacter. *III. Proceedings of the Third International Workshop on* Campylobacter *Infections*, p. 192. (London: Public Health Laboratory Service)

51. Dixon, M., O'Connor, H.J., Axon, A.T.R., King, R.F.G.J. and Johnston, D. (1986). *Campylobacter*-like organisms and reflux gastritis. *J. Clin. Pathol.*, **39**, 531–4

52. O'Connor, H.J., Axon, A.T.R., Dixon, M.F. (1984). *Campylobacter*-like organisms unusual in type A (pernicious anaemia) gastritis. *Lancet*, **ii**, 1091

53. Meyrick Thomas, J. (1984). *Campylobacter*-like organisms in gastritis. *Lancet*, **ii**, 1217

54. Schrager, J., Spink, R. and Mitra, S. (1967). The antrum in patients with duodenal and gastric ulcers. *Gut*, **8**, 497–508

55. Earlam, R.J., Amerigo, J., Kakavoulis, T. and Pollock, D.J. (1985). Histological appearances of oesophagus, antrum and duodenum and their correlation with symptoms in patients with a duodenal ulcer. *Gut*, **26**, 95–100

56. Marshall, B.J., McGechie, D.B., Rogers, P.A. and Glancy, R.J. (1985). Pyloric *Campylobacter* infection and gastroduodenal disease. *Med. J. Australia*, **142**, 439–44

57. Jones, D.M., Eldridge, J., Whorwell, P.J. and Miller, J.P. (1985). The effects of various anti-ulcer regimens and antibiotics on the presence of *Campylobacter pyloridis* and its antibody. In Pearson, A.D., Skirrow, M.B. and Lior, H. (eds) Campylobacter. *III. Proceedings of the Third International Workshop of* Campylobacter *Infections*, p. 161. (London: Public Health Laboratory Service)

58. Marshall, B.J., McGechie, D.B., Armstrong, J.A. and Francis, G. (1985). The antibacterial

action of bismuth: early results using antibacterial regimens in the treatment of duodenal ulcer. In Pearson, A.D., Skirrow, M.B. and Lior, H. (eds) Campylobacter. *III. Proceedings of the Third International Workshop on* Campylobacter *Infections*, pp. 165–6. (London: Public Health Laboratory Service)

59. Pinkard, K.J., Harrison, B., Capstick, J.A., Medley, G. and Lambert, J.R. (1986). Detection of *Campylobacter pyloridis* in gastric mucosa by phase contrast microscopy. *J. Clin. Pathol.*, **39**, 112–13

60. Walters, L.L., Budin, R.E. and Paull, G. (1986). Acridine-orange to identify *Campylobacter pyloridis* in formalin fixed, paraffin-embedded gastric biopsies. *Lancet*, **i**, 42

61. Gray, S.F., Wyatt, J.I. and Rathbone, B.J. (1986). Simplified techniques for identifying *Campylobacter pyloridis*. *J. Clin. Pathol.* , **39**, 1279–80

62. Steer, H.W. and Newell, D.G. (1985). Immunological identification of *Campylobacter pyloridis* in gastric biopsy tissue. *Lancet*, **ii**, 38

63. Wyatt, J.I., Rathbone, B.J. and Heatley, R.V. (1986). Local immune response to gastric *Campylobacter* in non-ulcer dyspepsia. *J. Clin. Pathol.*, **39**, 863–70

64. Goodwin, C.S., Armstrong, J.A. and Marshall, B.J. (1986). *Campylobacter pyloridis*, gastritis, and peptic ulceration. *J. Clin. Pathol.*, **39**, 353–65

65. Rathbone, B.J., Wyatt, J.I., Worsley, B.W., Trejdosiewicz, L.K., Heatley, R.V. and Losowsky, M.S. (1985). Immune response to *Campylobacter pyloridis*. *Lancet*, **i**, 1217

66. Hanson, M., Sircus, W. and Ferguson, A. (1981) Duodenal mucosal architecture in non-specific and ulcer-associated duodenitis., *Gut*, **22**, 637–41

67. Johnston, B.J., Reed, P.I. and Hali, M. (1986). *Campylobacter*-like organisms in duodenal and antral endoscopic biopsies: relationship to inflammation. *Gut*, **27**, 1132–7

68. Goodwin, C.S., Blincow, E.D., Warren, J.R., Waters, T.E., Sanderson, C.R. and Easton, L. (1985). Evluation of cultural tenchniques for isolating *Campylobacter pyloridis* from endoscopic biopsies of gastric mucosa. *J. Clin. Pathol.*, **38**, 1127–31

69. Cowna, S.T. and Steel, K.J. (1974). *Manual for the Identification of Medical Bacteria*, 2nd Edn, pp. 119–20. (Cambridge: Cambridge University Press)

70. McNulty, C.A.M. and Wise, R. (1985). Rapid diagnosis of *Campylobacter* associated gastritis. *Lancet*, **i**, 1443–4

71. Graham, D.Y., Klein, P.D., Evans, D.G. Opekun, A.R., Evans, D.G., Alpert, L.C., Lobb, K.W. and Boutton, T.W. (1986). Rapid noninvasive diagnosis of gastric *Campylobacter* by a ^{13}C-urea breath test. *Gastroenterology*, **90**, 1435

72. Luck, J.M. and Seth, T.N. (1924). Gastric urease. *Biochem. J.*, **18**, 1227–31

73. Lieber, C.S. and Lefevre, A. (1959). Ammonia as a source of gastric hypoacidity in patients with uremia. *J. Clin. Invest.* **38**, 1271–7

74. Mossberg, S.M., Thayer, W.R. and Spiro, H.M. (1963). Azotemia and gastric acidity: the effect of intravenous urea on gastric acid and gastric ammonium production in man. *J. Lab. Clin. Med.*, **61**, 469–75

75. Delluva, A.M., Markley, K. and Davies, R.E. (1968). The absence of gastric urease in germ-free animals. *Biochim. Biophys. Acta*, **151**, 646–50

76. Goodwin, C.S., McCulloch, R.K., Armstrong, J.A. and Wee, S.H. (1985). Unusual cellular fatty acids and distinctive ultrastructure in a new spiral bacterium (*Campylobacter pyloridis*) from the human gastric mucosa. *J. Med. Microbiol.*, **19**, 257–67

77. Goodwin, S., Blincow, E., Armstrong, J., McCulloch, R., Collins, D. (1985). *Campylobacter pyloridis* is unique: GCLO-2 is an ordinary *Campylobacter. Lancet*, **ii**, 38–9

78. Goodwin, S. and Blincow, E. (1985). Cimetidine and ranitidine activity against *Campylobacter pyloridis* and other *Campylobacters*. In Pearson, A.D., Skirrow, M.B. and Lior, H. (eds) Campylobacter. *III. Proceedings of the Third International Workshop on* Campylobacter *Infections*, pp. 167–9. (London: Public Health Laboratory Service)

79. McNulty, C.A.M., Dent, J. and Wise, R. (1985). Susceptibility of clinical isolates of *Campylobacter pyloridis* to 11 antimicrobial agents. *Antimicrob. Agents Chemother.*, **28**, 837–8

80. Hazell, S.L. and Lee, A. (1986). *Campylobacter pyloridis* and gastritis: association with intercellular spaces and adaption to an environment of mucus as important factors in colonization of the gastric epithelium. *J. Infect. Dis.*, **153**, 658–63

117

81. Kasper, G. and Dickgiesser, N. (1985). Isolation from gastric epithelium of *Campylobacter*-like bacteria that are distinct from '*Campylobacter pyloridis*'. *Lancet*, **i**, 111–2
82. Jones, D.M., Lessells, A.M. and Eldridge, J. (1984). *Campylobacter*-like organisms on the gastric mucosa: culture, histology, and serological studies. *J. Clin. Pathol.*, **37**, 1002–6
83. Marshall, B.J., McGechie, D.B., Francis, G.J. and Utley, P.J. (1985). Pyloric *Campylobacter* serology. *Lancet*, **ii**, 281
84. Kaldor, J., Tee, W., McCarthy, P., Watson, J. and Dwyer, B. (1985). Immune response to *Campylobacter pyloridis* in patients with peptic ulceration. *Lancet*, **i**, 921
85. Booth, L., Holdstock, G., MacBride, H., Hawtin, P., Gibson, J.R., Ireland, A., Bamforth, J., DuBoulay, C., Lloyd, R.S. and Pearson, A.D. (1986). Clinical importance of *Campylobacter pyloridis* and associated serum IgG and IgA antibody responses in patients undergoing upper gastrointestinal endoscopy. *J. Clin. Pathol.*, **39**, 215–19
86. Rathbone, B.J., Wyatt, J.I., Worsley, B.W., Shires, S.E., Trejdosiewicz, L.K., Heatley, R.V. and Losowsky, M.S. (1986). Systemic and local antibody response to gastric *Campylobacter pyloridis* in non-ulcer dyspepsia. *Gut*, **27**, 642–7
87. Rathbone, B.J., Wyatt, J.I., Tompkins, D., Heatley, R.V. and Losowsky, M.S. (1986). Diagnostic ELISA for gastric *Campylobacter pyloridis* infection using serum samples. *Gut*, **27**, 607 (Abstract)
88. Price, A.B., Levi, J., Dolby, J.M., Dunscombe, P.L., Smith, A., Clarke, J. and Stephenson, M.L. (1985). *Campylobacter pyloridis* in peptic ulcer disease: microbiology, pathology, and scanning electron microscopy. *Gut*, **26**, 1183–8
89. Newell, D.G. (1985). The outer membrane proteins and surface antigens of *Campylobacter pyloridis*. In Pearson, A.D., Skirrow, M.B. and Lior, H. (eds) Campylobacter. *III. Proceedings of the Third International Workshop on* Campylobacter *Infections*, pp. 199–200. (London: Public Health Laboratory Service)
90. Rathbone, B.J., Wyatt, J.I., Tompkins, D., Heatley, R.V. and Losowsky, M.S. (1986). *In vitro* production of *Campylobacter pyloridis* specific antibodies by gastric mucosal biopsies. *Gut*, **27**, 607 (Abstract)
91. Jones, D.M., Curry, A. and Fox, A.J. (1985). An ultrastructural study of the gastric *Campylobacter*-like organism '*Campylobacter pyloridis*'. *J. Gen. Microbiol.*, **131**, 2335–41
92. Steer, H.W. (1985). The gastroduodenal epithelium in peptic ulceration. *J. Pathol.*, **146**, 355–62
93. Shousha, S., Bull, T.B. and Parkins, R.A. (1984). Gastric spiral bacteria. *Lancet*, **ii**, 101
94. Marshall, B.J., Armstrong, J.A., McGechie, D.B. and Glancy, R.J. (1985). Attempts to fulfil Koch's postulates for pyloric *Campylobacter*. *Med. J. Australia*, **142**, 436–9
95. Ramsay, E.J., Carey, K.V., Peterson, W.L., Jackson, J.J., Murphy, F.K., Read, N.W., Taylor, K.B., Trier, J.S. and Fordtran, J.S. (1979). Epidemic gastritis with hypochlorhydria. *Gastroenterology*, **76**, 1449–57
96. Gledhill, T., Leicester, R.J., Addis, B., Lightfoot, N., Barnard, J., Viney, N., Darkin, D. and Hunt, R.H. (1985) Epidemic hypochlorhydria. *Br. Med. J.*, **290**, 1383–6
97. Rathbone, B.J., Wyatt, J.I., Worsley, B.W., Trejdosiewicz, L.K., Heatley, R.V. and Losowsky, M.S. (1985). Epidemic hypochlorhydria. *Br. Med. J.*, **ii**, 52–3
98. Lambert, J.R., Hansky, J., Davidson, A., Pinkard, K. and Stockman, K. (1985). *Campylobacter*-like organisms (CLO) – *in vivo* and *in vitro* susceptibility to antimicrobial and antiulcer therapy. *Gastroenterology*, **88**, 1462
99. Shreeve, D.R., Klass, H.J. and Jones, P.E. (1983). Comparison of cimetidine and tripotassium dicitrato bismuthate in healing and relapse of duodenal ulcers. *Digestion*, **28**, 96–101
100. Lee, F.I., Samloff, I.M. and Hardman, M. (1985). Comparison of tri-potassium di-citrato bismuthate tablets with ranitidine in healing and relapse of duodenal ulcers. *Lancet*, **i**, 1299–1302
101. Hamilton, I., O'Connor, H.J., Wood, N.C., Bradbury, I., and Axon, A.T.R. (1986). Healing and recurrence of duodenal ulcer after treatment with tri-potassium dicitrato bismuthate (TBD) tablets or cimetidine. *Gut*, **27**, 106–110
102. Shirokova, K.I., Filomonov, R.M. and Poliakova, L.V. (1981). Metronidazole in the treatment of peptic ulcer. *Klinikal Medicine (Mosk.)*, **59**, 48–50

103. Quintero Diaz, M. and Sotto Escobar, A. (1986). Metronidazole versus cimetidine in treatment of gastroduodenal ulcer. *Lancet*, **i**, 907
104. Zhi-Tian, Z., Zeng-Ying, W., Ya-Xian, C., Yi-Nung, L., Qiong-Fang, L., San-Ren, L. and Zhao-Min, X. (1985). Double-blind short-term trial of furazolidone in peptic ulcer. *Lancet*, **i**, 1048—9
105. Huai-Yu, Z., Guozhen, L., Jundong, G., Zhi, Y., Shaowu, S., Linsheng, L., Youmao, D. and Fuzu, Y. (1985). Furazolidone in peptic ulcer. *Lancet*, **ii**, 276—7
106. Tytgat, G.N.J., Rauws, E.A.J., Langenberg, M.-L. and Houthoff, H.J. (1986). *Campylobacter pyloridis*: the Amsterdam study. *Dig. Dis. Sci.*, **31**, 149S
107. O'Morain, C., Humphries, H., Dooley, C., Sweeney, E. and Keane, C. (1986). A controlled randomised trial to determine the effect of treatment of *Campylobacter pyloridis* in peptic disease. *Dig. Dis. Sci.*, **31**, 152S
108. McNulty, C.A.M., Gearty, J.C., Crump, B., Davis, M., Donovan, I.A., Melikian, V., Lister, D.M. and Wise, R. (1986). *Campylobacter pyloridis* and associated gastritis: investigator blind, placebo controlled trial of bismuth salicylate and erythromycin ethylsuccinate. *Br. Med. J.*, **293**, 645—9
109. Wyatt, J.I., Rathbone, B.J. and Heatley, R.V. (1986). *Campylobacter pyloridis* and cimetidine. *Gut*, **27**, A607
110. Patrick, W.J.A., Denham, D. and Forrest, A.P.M. (1974). Mucous change in the human duodenum: a light and electron microscopic study and correlation with disease and gastric acid secretion. *Gut*, **15**, 767—76
111. Rhodes, J. (1964). Experimental production of gastric epithelium in the duodenum. *Gut*, **5**, 454—8
112. Shousha, S., Spiller, R.C. and Parkins, R.A. (1983). The endoscopically abnormal duodenum in patients with dyspepsia: biopsy findings in 60 cases. *Histopathology*, **7**, 23—34
113. Hazell, S.L. and Lee, A. (1986). *Campylobacter pyloridis*, urease, hydrogen ion back diffusion, and gastric ulcers. *Lancet*, **ii**, 15—17
114. Fox, J.G., Edrise, B.M., Cabot, E.B., Beaucage, C., Murphy, J.C. and Prostak, K.S. (1986). *Campylobacter*-like organisms isolated from gastric mucosa of ferrets. *Am. J. Vet. Res.*, **47**, 236—9
115. Rathbone, B.J., West, A.P., Wyatt, J.I., Johnson, A.W., Tompkins, D.S. and Heatley, R.V. (1986). *Campylobacter pyloridis*, urease, and gastric ulcers. *Lancet*, **ii**, 400—1

6
Mucus and gastroduodenal mucosal protection

L. A. SELLERS and A. ALLEN

MUCUS *IN VIVO*

A layer of water-insoluble mucus gel, adherent to the gastroduodenal mucosal surface acts as a protective barrier between a susceptible epithelium and the aggressive factors in luminal juice. An understanding of the structure and properties of this adherent mucus gel secretion is the key to elucidating the role of mucus in gastroduodenal mucosal protection and changes in the mucus barrier associated with ulcer pathogenesis. The adherent mucus can be observed *in situ* on unfixed mucosal sections as a thin layer of translucent gel which completely covers the mucosal surface[1,2]. In the stomach and duodenum the mucus layer is continuous but of variable thickness ranging between 50 to 450 μm on human stomach (median thickness 180 μm) and 10 to 400 μm on rat stomach or duodenum (median thickness 70 μm and 80 μm respectively). The thickness of the adherent mucus layer is the result of a dynamic balance between new secretion from the epithelium and erosion at the luminal aspect of the mucus layer (Fig. 6.1). Mucus erosion results from the mechanical forces associated with the digestive processes and mucolysis by proteolytic enzymes, in particular pepsin.

The extracellular adherent mucus gel layer, although clearly visible on unfixed mucosal sections is either absent or very much reduced on mucosal sections that have been fixed and stained for histological observation. An explanation for this effect is that mucus is 95% water and fixatives such as

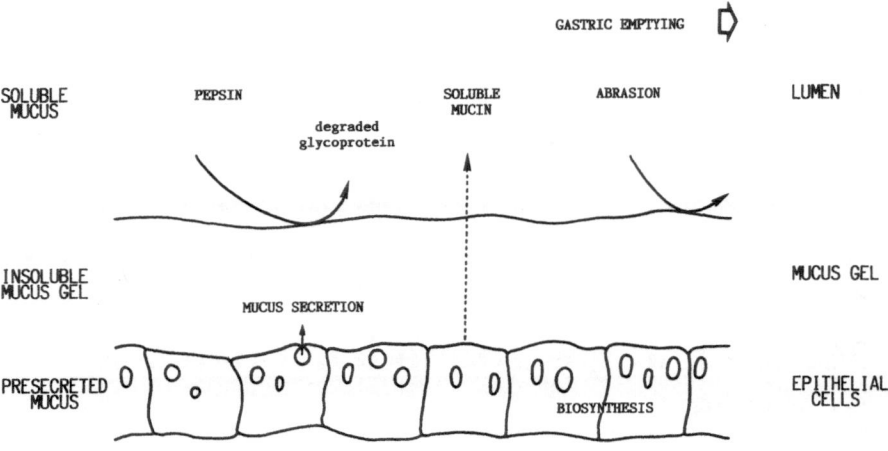

Figure 6.1 A diagrammatic representation of the dynamics of the adherent mucus gel layer *in vivo*

ethanol and glutaraldehyde will dehydrate mucus causing denaturation and an overall shrinkage of the gel[3]. In contrast, presecreted mucus contained within intracellular vesicles remains after histological processing to give the mucus-secreting epithelia its characteristic neutral mucin and basophilic staining properties[4,5]. Stimulation of the various mucus-secreting cell types (surface epithelial and mucus neck cells of the stomach and Brunner's glands of the duodenum) by prostaglandins results in the release of mucus stores increasing the thickness of the barrier by up to three-fold[2,6,7]. Luminal mucus, since it mixes freely with the gastric juices, is unlikely to have significant protective functions, although a plentiful output of soluble mucus will act as a lubricant preventing excessive depletion of the adherent mucus gel layer and damage to the mucosa from mechanical forces.

ADHERENT MUCUS GEL

The rheological properties of adherent mucus obtained from the human stomach, pig stomach and pig duodenum as measured by mechanical spectroscopy are characteristic of a weak, viscoelastic gel that is water-insoluble[8]. The adherent mucus is a relatively stable gel and will only show flow characteristics over a relatively long time scale of 0.5 to 1 hour. The mucus gel is resistant to a variety of mucosal damaging agents: for example prolonged exposure of gastric or duodenal mucus to hypertonic sodium chloride, ethanol (up to 40% v/v), bile or acid (pH 1) does not alter its measured mechanical properties. The absence of effect of acid on gastroduodenal mucus gel structure is again supported by observations *in vivo* in the rat, where topical hydrochloric acid at pH 2 produces no significant change in gel thickness[3].

A complete breakdown of gel structure to that of a viscous solution for both gastric and duodenal mucus occurs after exposure to proteolytic enzymes (pepsin or papain) or reducing agents (N-acetylcysteine or mercaptoethanol)[8]. The time-course of collapse of mucus gel structure on incubation in 0.2 M mercaptoethanol shows short-term resistance to mucolysis, with no evidence of any change in gel structure within the first 50–60 min of reduction at 37°C. These results are again supported by direct observation of the adherent mucus on rat mucosal sections *in vitro* that show the thickness of the gel to be unchanged after incubation in N-acetylcysteine (20% w/v) for 30 min at 37°C. Further exposure to the reducing agent, however, results in a progressive loss of mechanical structure (over 1–2 h) resulting in a system characteristic of a viscous liquid (after 2 h at 37°C).

Enzymes such as pepsin and papain of comparatively large molecular weight cannot penetrate the mucus gel unlike mercaptoethanol but act only at the surface of the sample[8]. The result is a progressive reduction in size of the gel sample with no change in its overall mechanical properties. The effectiveness of the mucus barrier *in vivo* to proteolytic attack will thus depend on two factors: firstly, the depth or thickness of the adherent mucus layer and secondly the integrity of its structure. Although luminal pepsin cannot diffuse through the mucus, adherent to the mucosal surface, it will continually hydrolyse the mucus gel at its luminal aspect to release degraded glycoprotein into the lumen (Figure 6.1). There is evidence that pepsin erodes the mucus barrier both in experimental animal models and in man[3,9,10]. Instillation of pepsin (2 mg ml^{-1}) into the rat stomach results in a five-fold increase in the amount of glycoprotein present in the luminal juice with respect to a steady release of approximately 100 μg glycoprotein per hour in pH 2.2 acid controls[11]. The adherent mucus layer following pepsin treatment under these conditions changes from a continuous, translucent layer to one which is granular in appearance with areas of discontinuity. Focal epithelial damage and bleeding is also associated with pepsin damage under these conditions. Evidence for peptic erosion of the mucus barrier in man is seen following insulin stimulation when there is a parallel increase in pepsin activity and luminal mucin glycoprotein content in the gastric washouts from duodenal ulcer patients[10]. This rise in both pepsin and luminal mucin glycoprotein content is absent in vagotomized patients.

Native mucus *in vivo* is a heterogeneous material and contains besides the mucin glycoprotein secretion, material from sloughed epithelial cells, bacteria, digested food, plasma proteins, digestive enzymes, secretory IgA and bile[12]. The molecules responsible for the viscous and gel-forming properties of mucus secretions are the glycoproteins or mucins[13], which constitute between 1 and 10% by weight of the gel; the major constituent of mucus is water (up to 95%)

and the remaining solids are proteins, nucleic acids and lipids. It has been suggested that some of the non-covalently bound proteins associated with the mucin glycoproteins may be involved in determining its viscous behaviour and addition of serum albumin to solutions of pig gastric mucin has been shown to enhance the solution viscosity of the mixture[14]. Other preparations in which non-covalently bound proteins have been removed from the mucin glycoprotein have shown consistently that their removal increases viscosity, suggesting that proteins interfere with, rather than enhance, mucin glyco-protein interactions[13]. Rheological studies on pig gastrointestinal mucus gels also support this latter view. Pure glycoprotein gels formed by concentrating the purified mucin to the same concentration found within the native secretion, can reproduce the viscoelastic characteristics of the respective native secretion, indicating that other components within the native gel are not involved in gel formation[8,15]. In particular, non-mucin components have been shown to be detrimental to gel formation and the stability of the gel matrix. For example, mucus obtained by scraping the surface of the pig small intestinal mucosa contains relatively large amounts of soluble protein and unlike the other gastrointestinal mucus secretions, substantial amounts of insoluble material (86% by volume of the gel compared to 30% for gastric) which can be removed by an initial centrifugation step. Interestingly, the native small intestinal mucus gel is of poorer quality than the other gastrointestinal secretions and shows unique instability on exposure to acid (pH 2.0) or concentrated salt solutions (2.0 M sodium chloride, 8.0 M urea or 6.0 M guanidinium chloride)[15]. The explanation for the collapse of gel structure under these denaturing conditions appears to be related to the presence of this excessive amount of non-mucin glycoprotein material in native small intestinal mucus, since the corresponding reconstituted gel is of better quality and unaffected by the above solvents[15]. However, it remains to be seen whether lipids or proteins are important for conferring on the gel *in vivo* particular physiological functions. In this respect, it has been proposed that a phospholipid monolayer associated with mucus establishes a hydrophobic lining over the gastric mucosa which impedes the diffusion of hydrogen ions[16]. Neutral lipids, glycolipids and phospholipids are associated with gastric mucus glycoprotein preparations and it has been claimed that their presence hinders the rate of diffusion of hydrogen ions through mucus[17] and the actual degradation of the mucus barrier itself.

MUCIN GLYCOPROTEIN STRUCTURE

Mucus glycoproteins from the gastrointestinal tract are large molecules (2×10^6 to 45×10^6 molecular weight)[13,18] containing over 60% by weight of carbohydrate. A basic structural unit of a mucus glycoprotein, often referred to as a subunit, is a protein core to which are attached many oligosaccharide side-chains (Figure 6.2). The sugar side-chains are linked to the polypeptide core by O-glycosidic bonds between N-acetylgalactosamine and serine or threonine[19,20,21]. Approximately 30% of the amino acid residues (most of the serine and threonine) bear an oligosaccharide chain which may be branched. These project from the protein core to produce a close packing of the oligosaccharide side-chains forming a sheath of carbohydrate around the protein backbone. An analogy to a bottle brush is sometimes made with this subunit structure where the 'bristles' represent the carbohydrate chains and the 'wire' the protein core.

The constituent sugars of mucus glycoproteins are galactose, N-acetyl-galactosamine, N-acetylglucosamine, fucose and sialic acid. The sugar chains can also carry ester sulphate groups and this together with sialic acid gives the carbohydrate chains a negative charge. There are considerable variations in the structure of the carbohydrate chains in glycoproteins from different regions of the gastrointestinal tract in the same species, as well as interspecies differences[13,22]. The molar ratio of the five different sugars characteristic of these molecules can vary considerably, and in some glycoproteins one or more of these sugars may be absent[23]. However, several commonly-occurring sugar substructures have been identified and there appears to be a degree of con-cordance between these regions in several species. A feature common to many of these mucus glycoproteins is that they are ABH antigens for the ABO blood group system, the structure of the terminal portions of their carbohydrate side-chains being the same as those of the blood group antigens on the surface of red blood cells[24]. The ABH antigenic activity of human mucus glycoproteins from all regions of the orogastrointestinal tract is thus reflected in the structure of their carbohydrate chains, which end in either N-acetylgalactosamine (A secretor) or galactose (B secretor), or with just the terminal fucose α-2-galactose (H secretor). About 20% of people are non-secretors where the carbohydrate chains of the glycoproteins end in a single galactose without the terminal fucose residue, but these non-secretors do not seem in any way disadvantaged in the formation of a viable mucus secretion.

Despite the variation in the size of the carbohydrate side-chains attached to the protein core (the sugar chains will exist in all stages of completeness), the sequence of the sugars and their linkages are the same for a given glycoprotein, although it is possible that chains with different sequences may also occur. Glycoproteins from human[25] or pig[26] gastric mucus have branched chains that are up to 19 sugar residues in length joined by 10 or so different glycosidic linkages and about 150 of these chains on a subunit of 5×10^5 molecular weight. Human and rat colonic mucus have branched complex chains consisting of up to 12 sugars[27,28]. In overall composition the glycoprotein from pig gastric and pig colonic mucus are very similar except for a greater amount of negatively-charged sialic acid residues on the colonic glycoprotein[29]. Pig

Each glycoprotein subunit has a bottle-brush type structure. Mucus is a polymer of glycoprotein subunits.

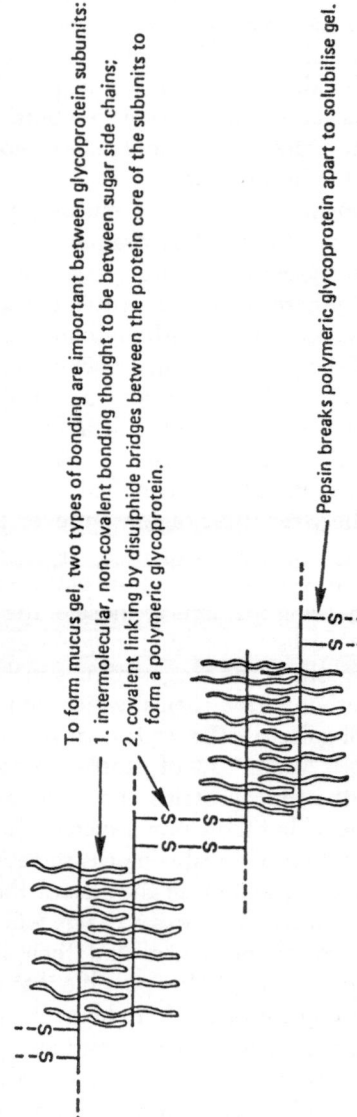

CARBOHYDRATE CHAINS

PROTEIN CORE

GLYCOSYLATED   NON-GLYCOSYLATED
PROTEIN CORE   PROTEIN CORE

Mucus gels are formed from these glycoprotein molecules

To form mucus gel, two types of bonding are important between glycoprotein subunits:

1. intermolecular, non-covalent bonding thought to be between sugar side chains;
2. covalent linking by disulphide bridges between the protein core of the subunits to form a polymeric glycoprotein.

Pepsin breaks polymeric glycoprotein apart to solubilise gel.

Figure 6.2   A diagrammatic representation of mucin glycoprotein structure and formation of mucus gel

small intestinal mucus glycoprotein differs markedly in composition from the other two glycoproteins in that it contains a much higher proportion of N-acetylgalactosamine, is heavily charged and has side-chains which are relatively short with an average of no more than seven sugar residues per chain[30]. Detailed analysis of the carbohydrate from duodenal mucus glycoproteins has not yet been performed.

The most common amino acids found in mucus glycoproteins are serine and threonine[19]. Their levels are considerably higher than those found in most proteins and this is associated with their involvement in the O-glycosidic linkage of the protein core to the carbohydrate side-chains[20]. The carbohydrate side-chains can be packed very close together; for example, in pig gastric mucus, one in three or four amino acids on the protein core must carry a chain averaging 15 sugar residues in length. The proline content of mucus glycoproteins is also high and this amino acid may be involved in maintaining a particular conformation in the protein core that will enable the close packing of the large carbohydrate side-chains. With such a protective sheath of carbohydrate, the protein backbone buried inside is protected from attack by proteolytic enzymes. However, in addition to the heavily glycosylated protein core there are regions of protein that are susceptible to enzymic digestion (Figure 6.2).

Several gastrointestinal mucus glycoproteins isolated by non-degradative methods and purified free of all non-covalently bound protein have an extra portion of protein not found in the same glycoprotein isolated by proteolysis[31]. Pig gastric mucus glycoprotein exposed to pepsin, papain, trypsin or Pronase loses 51% of the original amino acid content by weight (less than 5% by weight of the glycoprotein molecule) without any loss of carbohydrate[32]. This is equivalent to approximately 750 amino acid residues and of composition comparable to that of an average globular protein. There is evidence for similar naked, non-glycosylated regions of the protein in glycoproteins from human gastric mucus[33], pig small intestinal[30] and colonic mucus[29] and human[34] and rat small intestinal mucus[35]. It is these non-glycosylated regions of the glycoprotein that are found to be rich in cysteine residues (about 39 per glycoprotein molecule in pig gastric mucus) and therefore have the potential for disulphide bridge formation. Considerable evidence shows that the glycoprotein subunits are linked together through these disulphide bridges to form the polymeric structure of the glycoprotein[36] (Figure 6.2). Since these disulphide bridges are located in regions of the protein core that are accessible to proteolytic attack (non-glycosylated) then either proteolysis of the peptide or reduction of the interchain disulphide bridges themselves will split the glycoprotein polymeric structure into 'digested subunits' and 'subunits' respectively. There is a substantial reduction in the cysteine content of the proteolytically digested glycoprotein compatible with the removal of the interchain disulphide bridges between the glycoprotein subunits. In pig gastric mucus the proteinase-susceptible non-glycosylated protein region has a molecular weight of about 120 000 daltons and contains a discrete 70 000 molecular weight protein joined to the rest of the mucin glycoprotein molecule by disulphide bridges (one '70 000' protein component per polymer)[37]. Polymeric structures formed from glycoprotein subunits, joined by disulphide bridges, have been shown for pig small intestinal[38], duodenal[8] and colonic mucus[29] and for human gastric[37] and small intestinal mucus[39].

Associated with proteolysis and reduction is a marked decrease in molecular weight of the glycoprotein molecules corresponding to the destruction of the polymeric structure into subunits. For example there is a four-fold drop in molecular weight following reduction of pig gastric mucus glycoprotein[36]. The purified undegraded glycoprotein has a molecular weight of at least 2×10^6 (dependent upon extraction media) and on the basis of these results the polymeric glycoprotein structure consists of on average four 'bottle brush' subunits of equal size (5×10^5 molecular weight) which are joined by disulphide bridges located on non-glycosylated regions of the protein core[13]. The 70 000 molecular weight protein is also associated with this polymeric structure[37].

MUCIN GLYCOPROTEIN STRUCTURE AND FORMATION OF MUCUS GEL

A major structural feature of mucus glycoproteins, shown to be essential for gel formation, is the covalent, polymeric structure which confers the necessary three-dimensional arrangement for formation of the gel network[8,36]. A comparison of the gastrointestinal mucus gels, both native and reconstituted, with other biopolymer systems shows they have true gel-like structures. This contrasts with the fully reduced and proteolytically digested mucus preparations which show viscoelastic–liquid characteristics typical of those seen in an entangled polymer system[40]. Mechanical spectroscopy measurements made on preparations of mucus gel that have been incubated with 0.2 M mercaptoethanol for times shorter than that required for complete collapse of gel structure, show mechanical properties that are intermediate between those of the native and fully reduced gels[8,41]. All the gastrointestinal mucus glycoproteins have covalent, polymeric molecular sizes of at least 2×10^6. In contrast, following exhaustive reduction or proteolysis, there is a drastic reduction in size consistent with the breakdown of the polymeric structure into subunits. To determine quantitatively the amount of polymeric and subunit glycoprotein within mucus, the samples may be fractionated by gel filtration on Sepharose CL-2B (Figure 6.3). All native mucus preparations show a large glycoprotein peak eluting in the excluded volume, whereas following complete reduction, the glycoprotein-positive peak elutes into the included

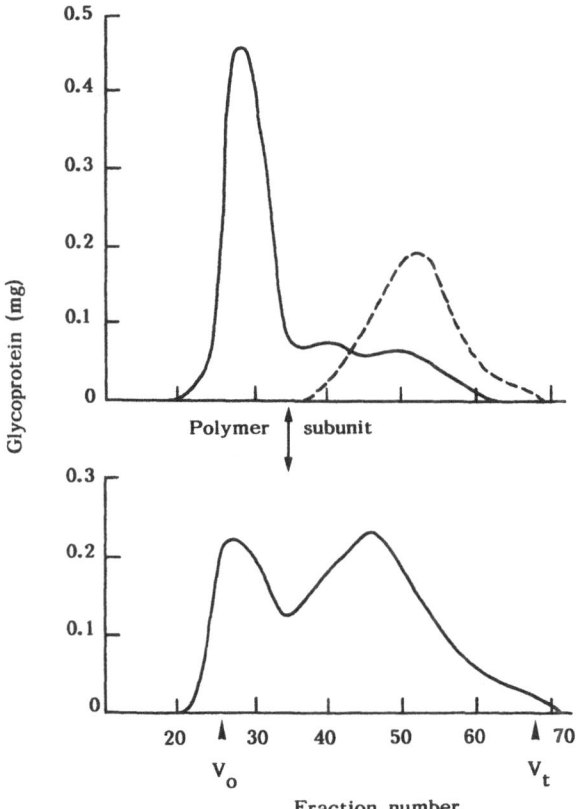

Figure 6.3 Analysis by gel filtration on Sepharose CL-2B of gastric mucus glycoprotein purified from the adherent mucus gel of resected antral mucosa. The top figure shows the elution profiles obtained for mucus glycoprotein from 'normal' gastric mucosa (pancreato-duodenectomy) (————) or after the glycoprotein has been completely digested with pepsin (–––––). In 'normal' mucus gel, 67% of the total glycoprotein content is excluded by the column or is in its polymeric form; pepsin digestion breaks the polymeric glycoprotein into subunits that are partially included on Sepharose CL-2B. The bottom figure shows that only 35% of the total glycoprotein in adherent mucus from gastric ulcer patients is excluded or in the polymeric form

volume of the Sepharose CL-2B column approximately midway between the exclusion and inclusion limits. These gel-filtration results are typical for all mucus preparations from the pig gastrointestinal tract showing clear separation of polymeric glycoprotein (excluded) from subunit glycoprotein (included) by this method (Figure 6.3). Glycoprotein samples from partially-reduced samples of mucus, however, elute as a continuum from the excluded into the included volume of the column indicating incomplete reduction of the glycoprotein.

129

The proportion of the total mucus glycoprotein that is excluded by the column is seen to decrease progressively with increasing time of reduction. The time-course for this observed shift in the size of the glycoprotein (from excluded to included material) is similar for pig gastric and duodenal mucus on reduction, and in both cases the decrease in the amount of polymeric glycoprotein is accompanied by a parallel collapse in the mechanical properties of the gel. The ratio of the 'gel-like' to the 'liquid-like' properties of the mucus samples gives an overall indication of the quality of the gel, and when this value is plotted against the length of time for which the mucus sample has been exposed to the reducing agent, the rate of collapse of gel structure on reduction can be quantified. For reduced mucus gel samples, a linear relationship is observed between the quality of the gel (indicative of gel strength) and the amount of polymeric glycoprotein remaining in the reduced mucus (Figure 6.4). These relationships for native and reconstituted samples of gastric, duodenal and colonic mucus emphasize the direct correlation between polymeric structure and the ability of the glycoprotein to form a gel[41].

A model for gel formation in pig gastric mucus has been proposed based on physical studies[42] and supported by electron microscopy studies[43,44]. Analytical ultracentrifugation and viscosity studies have shown that in dilute solution the polymeric glycoprotein from pig gastric mucus of 2×10^6 molecular weight is a highly expanded, hydrated, roughly spherical molecule occupying a large solution volume and at a concentration of about 20 mg ml^{-1}, the glycoprotein molecules fill the whole of the volume of solution and the probability of intermolecular interaction becomes appreciable. It is above this concentration that the viscosity of the glycoprotein solution is seen experimentally to rise asymptotically, owing to increasing intermolecular interactions as the hydrodynamic domains of the glycoprotein molecules overlap. These inter-molecular, non-covalent interactions increase until, at about 50 mg ml^{-1}, the glycoprotein solution assumes the characteristics of the native mucus gel taken directly from the pig gastric mucosal surface. The concentration of the glycoprotein in the native secretion is 50 mg ml^{-1} and when this gel is compared by mechanical spectroscopy with that reconstituted from the purified gastric mucus glycoprotein, at the same concentration, their mechanical spectra are identical[8]. Very similar mechanical spectra are also obtained for native and reconstituted pig duodenal mucus[8] and native and reconstituted pig colonic mucus[15]; good evidence that all these mucus gels have the same basic structure and the glycoprotein molecules alone can reproduce the gel-forming properties of the native mucus secretions.

Information about the nature of the interactions between the polymeric glycoprotein units in the gel can be obtained again from mechanical spectroscopy[40,41]. By comparison of the behaviour of pig gastrointestinal mucus gels (gastric, duodenal and colonic) with the flow curves for a purely entangled

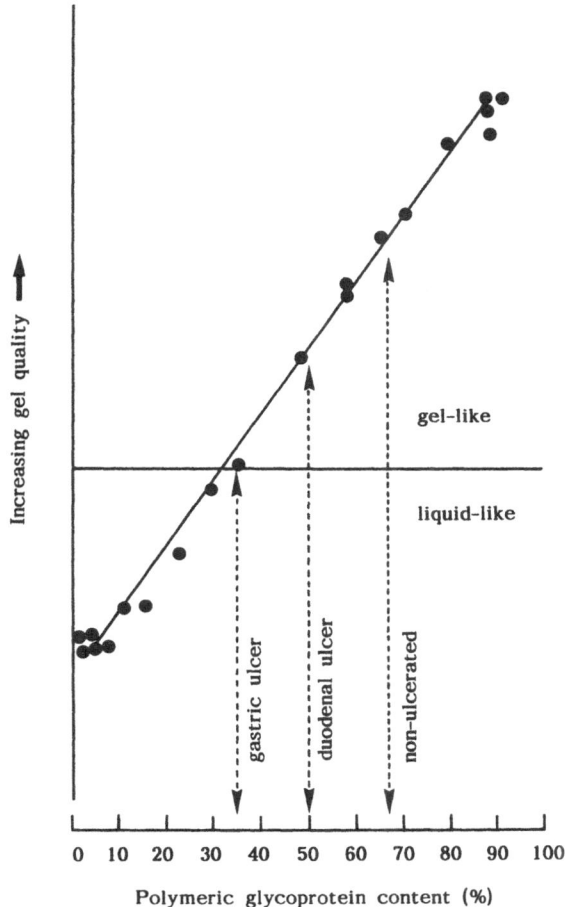

Figure 6.4 Correlation between gel quality (strength) and the proportion of glycoprotein in polymeric form in adherent gastric mucus. The points were obtained by reducing pig gastric mucus with 0.2 M mercaptoethanol for varying times (between 0 and 4 h) at 37°C. The quality of the gel sample was determined by mechanical spectroscopy. The amount of polymeric glycoprotein within mucus was calculated from the percentage of the total glycoprotein content that was excluded from Sepharose CL-2B (see Figure 6.3). The amount of polymeric glycoprotein in adherent gastric mucus obtained from non-ulcerated stomachs and those from patients suffering from gastric or duodenal ulcer was 67%, 35% and 50%, respectively, of the total glycoprotein. 'Normal' human and pig gastric mucus have the same structure. Therefore this is evidence that adherent gastric mucus from gastric ulcer and to a lesser extent duodenal ulcer patients is a weaker gel than that from non-ulcerated stomachs

131

system such as hyaluronate, it is immediately evident that the time-scale of intermolecular association between the glycoprotein molecules is longer than would be anticipated for simple polymer entanglement; evidence for some further form of interaction over and above this. What gives rise to these non-covalent interactions is unknown but since interactions similar to those occurring between intact molecules can form between proteolytically-digested subunits, in which most of the accessible protein core has been lost, there is good evidence to suggest that these presumed gel-forming interactions are between the carbohydrate side-chains (Figure 6.2). The denaturants, 2.0 M sodium chloride, 6.0 M guandinium chloride and 8.0 M urea do not disrupt gel structure which also supports the proposal that it is the carbohydrate rather than the protein that is involved in the gel-forming, non-covalent interactions.

While pig gastric, duodenal and colonic mucus glycoproteins all show evidence for positive interactions on gel formation, there are wide differences in their carbohydrate composition and sugar-chain length as discussed earlier. This suggests that the carbohydrate chains, although primarily involved in the glycoprotein–glycoprotein interactions can vary considerably without qualitative changes in gel structure. In disease therefore, differences in the carbohydrate composition of the gastrointestinal mucus glycoproteins are unlikely to affect their overall gel-forming abilities. However, precise carbohydrate structures are probably very important for other properties such as conferring on the mucus secretion its individual characteristics of permeability, antigenicity, stability to enzymic digestion, etc.

IMPAIRMENT OF THE MUCUS BARRIER IN PEPTIC ULCER DISEASE

Changes in the structure of the adherent mucus gel layer that would be predicted to impair its protective efficacy have been shown to occur in peptic ulcer disease. The protective properties of the adherent mucus barrier depend on its ability to form a stable, water-insoluble gel. Structural studies on gastrointestinal mucus already discussed, have shown that gel formation is absolutely dependent on the polymeric structure of the component glycoproteins[41]. There is a direct correlation between the relative amount of polymeric glycoprotein to lower molecular size subunit and the strength and overall stability of the gel sample as measured by rheological methods (Figure 6.4). Analysis of mucus glycoprotein from gastrectomy specimens shows 67%, 50% and 35% polymeric glycoprotein occurs in the adherent gel lining the gastric mucosa of non-ulcerated patients, duodenal ulcer patients and gastric ulcer patients respectively[45] (Figure 6.3). These groups were statistically different from one another and in fact there was no overlap in the patients' samples for gastric ulcer and those from normal, non-ulcerated mucosa. Combining these data with those from the rheological studies on isolated mucus, it can be seen that a very much structurally weaker adherent mucus barrier covers the mucosa of gastric ulcer and to a lesser extent duodenal ulcer patients than compared to the normal adherent gel (Figure 6.4).

Studies in the rat animal model have shown a defect in the polymeric structure of the glycoprotein in adherent mucus, similar to that seen in man, which has been associated with aspirin ulceration[46]. A natural variation occurs in the percentage of glycoprotein that is in the polymeric form in non-ulcerated rats. After inducing chronic gastric ulceration with aspirin, a strong inverse correlation is observed between the severity of ulceration and the amount of mucin that was polymerized prior to ulceration. Therefore this pre-existent, potential weakness in the mucus barrier of individual rats can be related to the susceptibility of the stomach to chronic ulceration. Further evidence for a disrupted mucus layer in ulcer disease comes from the observation of unfixed sections of gastric mucosa[47]. In non-ulcerated stomachs, a layer of translucent gel with a median thickness of 180 μm is observed, while in duodenal ulcer patients there is a significant decrease to a median of 120 μm. Adherent mucus over the antral mucosal surface of gastric ulcer patients is markedly more heterogeneous than that from non-ulcerated stomachs owing to mixing of mucus with cellular material, making accurate thickness readings impossible. The reason for the disruption of the mucus barrier is unknown but in part could reflect pepsin degradation since similar observations have been reported in the rat after topical exposure of the gastric mucosa to elevated levels of luminal pepsin[9]. Other possible explanations for the decreased quality of the mucus layer particularly in gastric ulcer disease could be inflammation and increased cell-shedding associated with gastritis[48]. This could cause disruption of the adherent mucus layer and the increased cell turnover will release lysosomal proteases which could digest the mucus barrier at its mucosal surface.

An impairment of the gastric mucus barrier in peptic ulcer disease is not necessarily a primary effect, and in fact evidence suggests that it may well be in part secondary to changes in the relative amounts of different pepsins present in gastric juice[49]. Pepsin-3 is the major pepsin in man, and pepsin-1 accounts for only 3.6% of total pepsin activity in non-ulcer controls. However, in gastric and duodenal ulcer patients, pepsin-1 accounts for 23% and 16.5%, respectively, of the total pepsin activity present[50,51]. The ulcer-associated pepsin, pepsin-1, has been shown to digest mucus more readily than pepsin-3, both at the optimum pH 2.0 (two-fold greater activity) and at higher pH values, where the difference is even more exaggerated (at pH 4 there is a six-fold greater activity)[49]. Similarly, gastric juice from duodenal ulcer patients digests mucus more readily than that from non-symptomatic controls both at the optimum pH of 2 and markedly at higher pH values, e.g. pH 4. Thus the raised concentration of pepsin-1 in the gastric juice of peptic ulcer patients would be expected to increase breakdown of the mucus barrier under conditions likely to pertain in the higher pH conditions of the duodenal bulb as well as at the lower pH conditions of the stomach.

There is evidence from many workers that changes in the carbohydrate composition and/or structure of the mucus glycoproteins occur in gastroduodenal disease states. Comparisons have been made of the ratios of the glycoprotein sugars in gastric washouts from ulcer patients and control subjects[52-54]. Although the results have been conflicting and often negative, in one investigation there was less glycoprotein-bound sialic acid in the gastric juice from ulcer patients compared with controls[55]. In a study of gastric washouts, where the glycoprotein had been purified by equilibrium density-gradient centrifugation[56], there was an increase, compared with control subjects, in total mucus glycoprotein in the juice from patients with gastric ulcer but not in gastric juice from those with duodenal ulcers. In both groups of patients, the ratio of the sugars compared with control subjects was the same. These studies were performed on the luminal glycoprotein content which may, or may not, reflect changes in structure of the glycoprotein forming the adherent mucus layer, the more functionally important glycoprotein in terms of mucosal protection.

It is not clear how, or whether, small changes in the carbohydrate structure of mucin glycoproteins, associated with peptic ulcer disease affect the properties of the adherent mucus gel. As indicated above, the carbohydrate side-chains of the component glycoproteins can vary considerably in both length and composition without seemingly affecting the ability to form a gel. One aspect where the carbohydrate might play an important role in mucosal protection is interaction with bacteria. Recently *Campylobacter pylori* has been implicated in inducing gastritis and gastric ulceration[57]. Although there are no experimental studies, it might be expected that interaction between these organisms and mucus gel would be important for their colonization of the gastric mucosal surface. One important factor is whether *Campylobacter pylori* bind to mucus and whether changes in carbohydrate structure, such as those demonstrated in peptic ulcer disease, affect this adhesion. In this respect it is interesting that pig gastric mucus binds to cholera toxin and prevents its attachment to the cell surface[58].

THE ROLE OF MUCUS IN MUCOSAL PROTECTION AGAINST ACID

The adherent mucus gel layer, although stable and structurally unaffected by exposure to pH 1, is 95% solution and hydrogen ions have been shown to diffuse through it quite rapidly. In fact the rate of diffusion is only about four-fold slower than the rate of diffusion through an equivalent volume of unstirred solution[59,60]. At these rates, acid in the lumen will equilibrate across the thin mucus layer in a matter of minutes. Histamine stimulation of acid in man can cause acute mucosal lesions, while increased back diffusion of acid in response to mucosal damaging agents also occurs very rapidly, within 2 or 3 min[61,62]. From these observations, it can be concluded that the gel matrix, or for that matter lipid components within it[17,63], are unlikely to provide *in vivo* an effective permeability barrier between acid in the lumen and the epithelium. Further, even when mixed with substantial amounts of mucosal tissue, the mucus gel does not have significant buffering capacity to be able to neutralize the luminal acid[64]. So how is the acid-sensitive gastroduodenal epithelium protected from acid by the adherent mucus covering?

A role of gastric mucus in protection against acid was suggested by Hollander[65] and Heatley[66] who emphasized its function as a mixing barrier ensuring that any mucosal alkaline secretion was retained in a relatively high concentration at the mucosal surface so neutralizing acid diffusing in from the lumen. Heatley postulated the need for a pH gradient from the lumen (acid) to the mucosal surface (neutrality), since gastric mucus gel does not provide an impenetrable barrier to hydrogen ions. There is now good experimental evidence for this so called 'mucus–bicarbonate barrier' (Figure 6.5) (see Chapter 7).

THE ROLE OF MUCUS IN MUCOSAL PROTECTION AGAINST PEPSIN

The mucus gel, while readily permeable to lower molecular weight ions, solutes and solvents, at least up to the size of vitamin B_{12} (molecular weight 1346), is not permeable to large-sized proteins, e.g. myoglobin (molecular weight 17 500)[67]. Therefore pepsin in the lumen (molecular weight 35 000) cannot diffuse through the continuous layer of adherent mucus gel and attack the underlying mucosal cells. Pepsin, however, as discussed above, will readily dissolve the mucus barrier *in vivo* to produce soluble, degraded mucus glycoprotein which will be released into the lumen[8,31], and in the rat gastric damage model will produce epithelial damage and mucosal bleeding[9]. Since a layer of mucus gel is observed over the undamaged mucosa *in vivo*[1,2] it can be deduced that a dynamic balance must exist whereby secretion maintains that portion of the expendable mucus barrier lost through peptic digestion. There is little or no mucus within the gastric glands and these cells appear to be resistant to their own secretions[68]. It is interesting that erosion of the mucosal surface, induced both naturally or experimentally, is a phenomenon of the epithelial cell layer and not the gastric glands, in keeping with the sensitivity of the former to damage by acid and pepsin. While mucus is absent

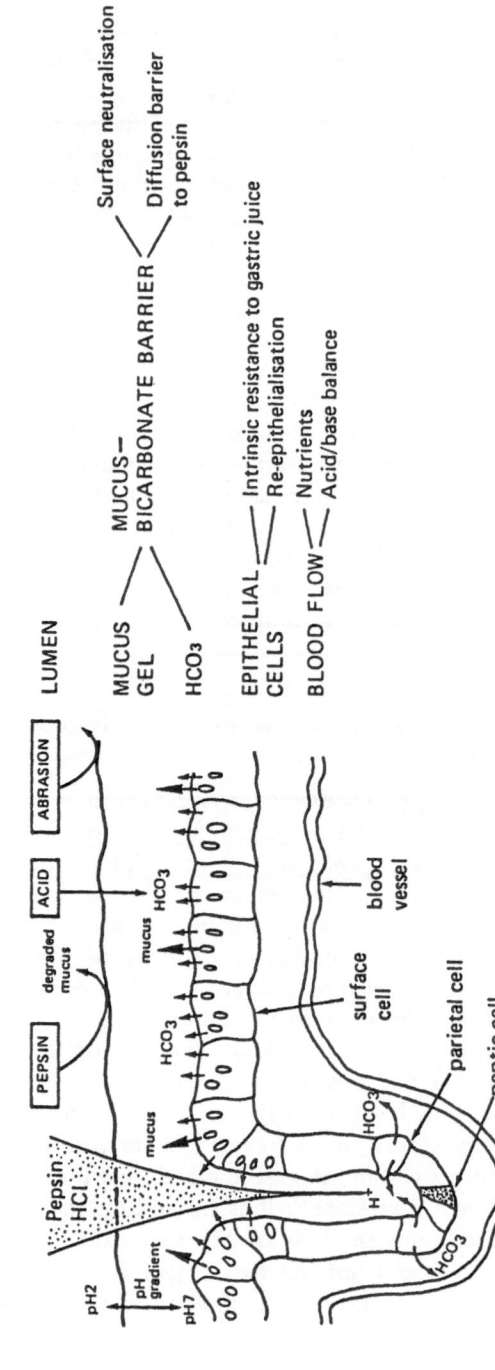

Figure 6.5 Mucosal protection against endogenous aggressors acid and pepsin

from within the gastric glands, it is observed to form a continuous cover over the whole gastric mucosa[1,2]. A plausible explanation of how pepsin and acid gain rapid access from the glands through this mucus barrier into the lumen, is that hydraulic pressure created in the gastric glands during secretion forces acid and pepsin through the gel. Once the secretion of acid and pepsin has finished, the mucus gel may then reseal, an assumption consistent with its visco-elastic gel properties[8].

THE ROLE OF MUCUS IN ETHANOL-INDUCED GASTRIC MUCOSAL DAMAGE

Noxious agents that damage the gastroduodenal mucosa can be divided into two groups: the endogenous aggressors originating naturally within the lumen and exogenous damaging agents administered by man to himself or experimental animals. Natural defence mechanisms have presumably evolved against the former aggressors, acid and pepsin (Figure 6.5) and not necessarily against 'man-made' exogenous damaging agents such as ethanol (Figure 6.6) and non-steroidal anti-inflammatory drugs. Therefore experimental models using mucosal damaging agents, such as ethanol, may not necessarily reflect the sequence of changes in mucosal defences that precede peptic ulcer disease. The mucus barrier, as already discussed, is readily permeated by acid and similarly cannot provide a diffusion barrier to the exogenous damaging agents such as ethanol, non-steroidal anti-inflammatory drugs, high concentrations of bile salts and hypertonic saline. Once in contact with the mucosa, all these

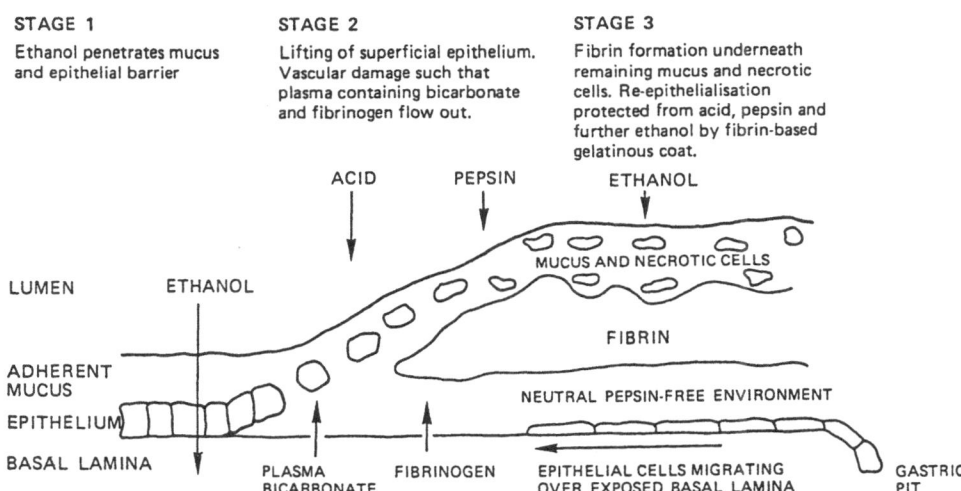

Figure 6.6 Mucosal response to acute ethanol injury and subsequent protection

agents cause destruction of the epithelial cells and in severe cases vascular damage, haemorrhage and visible lesions[69,70]. After acute damage, confined to the epithelial layer, complete repair will occur through replacement of the necrotic cells by preformed cells migrating from the gastric pits[69,71–73] (see Chapter 8). This process of re-epithelialization has been studied *in vitro* in frog and guinea-pig as well as *in vivo* in rat and man[74–77]. Re-epithelialization is rapid, often complete within 1 h and explains why epithelial damage is not always seen on mucosa surveyed some time after exposure to damaging agents. A prerequisite for the re-epithelialization process to occur would be a near neutral, pepsin-free environment. More severe damage will extend deeper into the mucosa beneath the epithelial layer causing hyperemia, haemorrhage as well as destruction of pit cells and lamina propria thus preventing re-epithelialization. The healing process following such damage will take days to complete and involve inflammation and associated healing processes[73].

Histological studies following acute but extensive gastric mucosal damage by high concentrations of ethanol in the rat show a massive release of a gelatinous material, the composition of which has been assigned primarily to mucus and necrotic cells[69,72,73]. This coat, which forms over the newly re-epithelialized mucosa is dependent upon a blood supply for formation, and studies have also noted fibrin (from dimensions on electron micrographs) at the damaged mucosal surface[75]. Recent studies using unfixed mucosal sections from this ethanol damage model have shown the thickness of the gelatinous coat to be much greater (1–2 mm) and far more heterogeneous and 'sloppy' than the stable adherent mucus layer observed on undamaged rat gastric mucosa (median thickness $70 \mu m$)[78]. It is interesting to note that in the same animal preparation, maximal stimulation of mucus secretion by intact epithelium with prostaglandin analogues results in only a three-fold increase in the thickness of adherent mucus gel[7]. Clearly from the dimensions of the gelatinous coat formed in response to acute ethanol damage, mucin glycoprotein can only be one constituent of what, presumably, must be a composite gel. Using a peroxidase–antiperoxidase stain for fibrinogen, thick bands of fibrinogen-positive material (which are poorly stained by PAS for mucin) are present in the gel coat, indicating substantial fibrin deposition. These bands are devoid of cells, although many exfoliated cells are found above these fibrin bands mixed with material that is strongly PAS-positive. Thus a gelatinous fibrin-based coat with mucus and sloughed necrotic cells forms over the re-epithelializing mucosa[78] (Figure 6.6). Measurement of plasma coagulation times *in vitro* suggest that the mucus remaining after acute ethanol damage may play a role as a template for the formation of the fibrin gel *in vivo*. Fibrin clot formation has been shown to take approximately 100 sec, but is virtually instantaneous in the presence of rat and pig gastric mucus gel[78].

The thick fibrin-based gelatinous coat with essentially unlimited neutralizing capacity from the plasma exudate should be quite effective in protecting re-epithelialization from acid and pepsin in the lumen. It will create a 10 times thicker unstirred layer to support surface neutralization of acid and provide a substantial permeability barrier to pepsin. The gelatinous coat has also been shown to have protective properties against ethanol, not shown by the normal adherent mucus layer. Thus in contrast to the mucus barrier on undamaged mucosa, this fibrin-based gelatinous coat protects the newly regenerated epithelium from further damage on re-exposure to ethanol[79]. If the gelatinous coat is removed from the surface, the epithelium regains its original sensitivity to ethanol damage. The preservation of the fibrin gelatinous coat but not adherent mucus in histologically-fixed sections is further evidence for its resistance to ethanol.

Studies have shown that the mechanism of damage differs between that caused by acid, pepsin or the exogenous damaging agent ethanol. In contrast to exogenous damaging agents and acid, the adherent mucus layer does provide a physical barrier to pepsin. Pepsin can only cause mucosal damage by progressively hydrolysing the mucus gel layer and subsequently the underlying epithelial barriers, a very different mechanism from ethanol which rapidly penetrates the mucus barrier to cause gross epithelial damage. In the case of the natural aggressor acid, damage is prevented by neutralization from mucosal bicarbonate. It thus seems reasonable to conclude that the mucus bicarbonate barrier can provide initial protection against acid and pepsin but provides little or no defence to ethanol or other damaging agents which can diffuse through the mucus gel. Following acute ethanol damage, the rat gastric mucosa is protected against further mucosal damage by a most effective gelatinous coat of fibrin with mucus and necrotic cells which also provides a microenvironment conducive to re-epithelialization. It remains to be seen whether such a protective coat is formed in other situations of acute mucosal damage in animal models and in man, although recent work shows that a 'mucoid cap' formed in response to topical hypertonic saline protects the repairing mucosa from further exposure to this damaging agent[80].

ULCER THERAPY

An alternative approach to the inhibition of gastric secretion by histamine H_2-receptor antagonists, omeprazole, or antacids is to enhance the mucosal defence mechanisms. In the healthy stomach or duodenum, evidence supports an important role for the adherent mucus gel in protecting the underlying mucosa from the endogenous aggressors acid and pepsin in gastric juice. Therefore, mucosal defences could be enhanced by agents that stimulate secretion of the mucus barrier or that bind to mucus, strengthening its barrier properties and reducing its degradation by pepsin. Prostaglandins have been found to be potent stimulants of both mucus secretion and biosynthesis[81,82] and intragastric instillation of 16,16-dimethyl-PGE$_2$ or misoprostil[7] has been shown to significantly increase mucus gel thickness both in the rat and frog[1,2,6]. Such a thicker gel creates an increased unstirred layer to sustain surface neutralization of acid and an increase in the permeability barrier to pepsin. Another agent, carbenoxolone, has been reported to stimulate mucus biosynthesis measured by incorporation of radiolabelled glycoprotein precursors[83] but it does not increase the thickness of the adherent gastric mucus layer[84].

Various anti-ulcer agents which are thought to exert their action at least in part, by adhering to and reinforcing the mucus barrier, include natural clays (smecta)[85], colloidal bismuth salts (De-Nol)[86], sulphated carbohydrates (sucralfate)[87] and polyacrylates (carbomer)[88]. Furthermore, many of these agents have intrinsic anti-pepsin activity. Smecta, an insoluble double silicate of aluminium and magnesium has been shown to bind to mucus and *in vivo* will form a layer over the rat stomach equivalent to the thickness of the adherent mucus gel itself. At an acid pH, colloidal bismuth compounds form a precipitate which has been shown to form a layer over the surface of the stomach and the ulcer base. Sucralfate, a basic aluminium salt of sucrose octasulphate, increases mucus viscosity and inhibits peptic degradation. It also selectively binds to exposed protein at the ulcer site, thereby simulating the barrier functions of adherent mucus. Polyacrylates have been shown to interact with mucus in solution to produce a dramatic increase in viscosity. Such a non-acid anti-secretory approach could be particularly useful in maintenance therapy following administration of H$_2$-receptor blockers. The association of peptic ulcer with the chronic use of non-steroidal anti-inflammatory drugs is well documented and co-administration of a mucosal protective agent could well mitigate such side-effects.

References

1. Kerss, S., Allen, A. and Garner, A. (1982). A simple method for measuring thickness of the mucus gel layer adherent to rat, frog and human gastric mucosa: influence of feeding prostaglandin, N-acetylcysteine and other agents. *Clin. Sci.*, **63**, 187–95
2. McQueen, S., Hutton, D., Allen, A. and Garner, A. (1983). Gastric and duodenal surface mucus gel thickness in rat: effects of prostaglandins and damaging agents. *Am. J. Physiol.*, **8**, 388–94
3. Allen, A., Hutton, D.A., Leonard, A.J., Pearson, J.P. and Sellers, L.A. (1986). The role of mucus in the protection of the gastroduodenal mucosa. *Scand. J. Gastroenterol.*, **21**, (Suppl. 125), 71–7
4. Filipe, M.I. (1979). Mucins in the human gastrointestinal epithelium: a review. *Invest. Cell Pathol.*, **2**, 195–216
5. Neutra, M.R. and Forstner, J.F. (1987). Gastrointestinal mucus: synthesis, secretion and function. In Johnson, L.R. (ed.) *Physiology of the Gastrointestinal Tract*, 2nd Edn., pp. 975–1009. (New York: Raven Press)
6. Bickel, M. and Kauffman, G.L. (1981). Gastric mucus gel thickness: effect of distension, 16,16-dimethyl prostaglandin E$_2$ and carbenoxolone. *Gastroenterology*, **80**, 770–75

7. Sellers, L.A., Carroll, N.J.H. and Allen, A. (1986). Misoprostil-induced increases in adherent gastric mucus thickness and luminal mucus output. *Dig. Dis. Sci.*, **31**, (Suppl. 2), 91S–95S

8. Bell, A.E., Sellers, L.A., Allen, A., Cunliffe, W.J., Morris, E.R. and Ross-Murphy, S.B. (1985). Properties of gastric and duodenal mucus: effect of proteolysis, disulphide reduction, bile, acid, ethanol and hypertonicity on mucus gel structure. *Gastroenterology*, **88**, 269–80

9. Leonard, A. and Allen, A. (1986). Gastric mucosal damage by pepsin. *Gut*, **27**, A1236–7

10. Younan, F., Pearson, J.P., Allen, A. and Venables, C.W. (1982). Gastric mucus degradation *in vivo* in peptic ulcer patients and the effects of vagotomy. In Chantler, E.N., Elder, J.B. and Elstein, M. (eds) *Mucus in Health and Disease*, pp. 235–7. (New York: Plenum Press)

11. Allen, A., Bennett, M.K., Leonard, A.J. and Sellers, L.A. (1987). Pepsin and ethanol damage: two different mechanisms of response by the rat gastric mucosa. *J. Physiol*, **391**, 69P

12. Forstner, J.F. (1978). Intestinal mucins in health and disease. *Digestion*, **17**, 234–63

13. Allen, A. (1981). Structure and function of gastrointestinal mucus. In Johnson, L.R. (ed.) *Physiology of the Gastrointestinal Tract*, Vol. 1, pp. 617–39. (New York: Raven Press)

14. List, S.J., Findlay, B.P., Forstner, G.G. and Forstner, J.F. (1978). Enhancement of the viscosity of mucin by serum albumin. *Biochem. J.*, **175**, 565–71

15. Sellers, L.A., Allen, A., Morris, E.R. and Ross-Murphy, S.B. (1983). Rheological studies on pig gastrointestinal mucous secretion. *Biochem. Soc. Trans.*, **11**, 763–4

16. Lichtenberger, L.M., Richards, J.E. and Hills, B.A. (1985). Effect of 16,16-dimethyl prostaglandin E₂ on the surface hydrophobicity of aspirin-treated canine gastric mucosa. *Gastroenterology*, **88**, 308–14

17. Sarosiek, J., Slomiany, A., Takagi, A. and Slomiany, B.L. (1984). Hydrogen ion diffusion in dog gastric mucus glycoprotein: effect of associated lipids and covalently bound fatty acids. *Biochem. Biophys. Res. Commun.*, **118**, 523–31

18. Carlstedt, I., Sheehan, J.K., Corfield, A.P. and Gallagher, J.T. (1985). Mucous glycoproteins: a gel of a problem. In Campbell, P.N. and Marshall, R.D. (eds) *Essays in Biochemistry*, Vol. 20, pp. 40–76. (New York: Academic Press)

19. Gottschalk, A., Bargava, A.S. and Murty, V.L.N. (1972). Submaxillary gland glycoproteins. In Gottschalk, A. (ed.) *Glycoproteins, their Composition, Structure and Function*, pp. 810–29. (Amsterdam: Elsevier)

20. Carlson, D.M. (1977). Chemistry and biosynthesis of mucin glycoproteins. In Elstein, M. and Parke, D.V. (eds) *Mucus in Health and Disease*, pp. 251–73. (New York: Plenum Press)

21. Horowitz, M.I. (1977). Gastrointestinal glycoproteins. In Horowitz, M.I. and Pigman, W. (eds) *The Glycoconjugates*, Vol. 1, pp. 189–213. (New York: Academic Press)

22. Hounsell, E.F., Lawson, A.M. and Feizi, T. (1982). Structural and antigenic diversity in mucin carbohydrate chains. In Chantler, E.N., Elder, J.B. and Elstein, M. (eds.) *Mucus in Health and Disease*, pp. 39–41. (New York: Plenum Press)

23. Clamp J.R. (1978). Chemical aspects of mucus. *Br. Med. Bull.*, **34**, 25–7

24. Watkins, W.M. (1966). Blood group substances. *Science*, **152**, 172–81

25. Schrager, J. and Oates, M.D.G. (1974). The isolation and partial characterisation of a glycoprotein isolated from human gastric aspirates and from extracts of gastric mucosa. *Biochim. Biophys. Acta*, **372**, 183–95

26. Slomiany, B.L. and Meyer, K. (1972). Isolation and structural studies of sulphated glycoproteins of hog gastric mucosa. *J. Biol. Chem.*, **247**, 5062–70

27. Podolsky, D.K. (1985). Oligosaccharide structures of human colonic mucin. *J. Biol. Chem.*, **260**, 8262–71

28. Murty, V.L., Downs, F.J. and Pigman, W. (1978). Rat colonic mucus glycoprotein. *Carbohydrate Res.*, **61**, 139–45

29. Marshall, T. and Allen, A. (1978). Isolation and characterisation of the high molecular weight glycoproteins from pig colonic mucus. *Biochem. J.*, **173**, 569–78

30. Mantle, M. and Allen, A. (1981). Isolation and characterisation of the native glycoprotein from pig small intestinal mucus. *Biochem. J.*, **195**, 267–75

31. Allen, A. (1978). Structure of gastrointestinal mucus glycoproteins and the viscous and gel-forming properties of mucus. *Br. Med. Bull.*, **34**, 28–33

32. Scawen, M. and Allen, A. (1977). The action of proteolytic enzymes on the glycoprotein from pig gastric mucus. *Biochem. J.*, **163**, 363–8

33. Pearson, J.P., Allen, A. and Venables, C.W. (1980). Gastric mucus: isolation and polymeric structure of the undegraded glycoprotein: its breakdown by pepsin. *Gastroenterology*, **78**, 709–15
34. Mantle, M., Forstner, G. and Forstner, J. (1984). Biochemical characterization of the component parts of human intestinal mucin from patients with cystic fibrosis. *Biochem. J.*, **224**, 345–54
35. Fahim, R.E.F., Forstner, G.G. and Forstner, J.F. (1983). Heterogeneity of rat goblet-cell mucin before and after reduction. *Biochem. J.*, **209**, 117–24
36. Snary, D., Allen, A. and Pain, R.H. (1970). Structural studies on gastric mucoproteins. Lowering of molecular weight after reduction with 2-mercaptoethanol. *Biochem. Biophys. Res. Commun.*, **40**, 844–51
37. Pearson, J.P., Allen, A. and Parry, S. (1981). A 70,000 molecular-weight protein isolated from purified pig gastric mucus glycoprotein by reduction of disulphide bridges and its implication in the polymeric structure. *Biochem. J.*, **197**, 155–62
38. Mantle, M., Mantle, D. and Allen, A. (1981). Polymeric structure of pig small intestinal mucus glycoprotein. Dissociation by proteolysis or by reduction of disulphide bridges. *Biochem. J.*, **195**, 277–85
39. Mantle, M., Forstner, G.G. and Forstner, J.F. (1984). Antigenic and structural features of goblet-cell mucin of human small intestine. *Biochem. J.*, **217**, 159–67
40. Bell, A.E., Allen, A., Morris, E.R. and Ross-Murphy, S.B. (1984). Functional interactions of gastric mucus glycoprotein. *Int. J. Biol. Macromol.*, **6**, 309–15
41. Sellers, L.A., Allen, A., Morris, E.R. and Ross-Murphy, S.B. (1987). Mucus glycoprotein gels: role of glycoprotein polymeric structure and carbohydrate side-chains in gel-formation. *Carbohydrate Res.* (In press)
42. Allen, A., Pain, R.H. and Robson, T. (1976). Model for the structure of the gastric mucus gel. *Nature (London)*, **264**, 88–9
43. Hallett, P., Rowe, A.J. and Harding, S.E. (1984). A highly expanded spheroidal conformation for a mucin from a cystic fibrosis patient: new evidence from electron microscopy. *Biochem. Soc. Trans.*, **12**, 878–9
44. Harding, S.E., Rowe, A.J. and Creeth, J.M. (1983). Further evidence for a flexible and highly expanded spheroidal model for mucus glycoproteins in solution. *Biochem. J.*, **209**, 893–6
45. Younan, F., Pearson, J., Allen, A. and Venables, C. (1982). Changes in the structure of the mucus gel on the mucosal surface of the stomach in association with peptic ulcer disease. *Gastroenterology*, **82**, 827–31
46. Bagshaw, P.F., Munster, D.J. and Wilson, J.G. (1987). Molecular weight of gastric mucus glycoprotein is a determinant of the degree of subsequent aspirin induced chronic gastric ulceration in the rat. *Gut*, **28**, 287–93
47. Allen, A., Ward, R., Cunliffe, W.J., Hutton, D.A., Pearson, J.P. and Venables, C.W. (1985). Changes in adherent mucus gel and pepsinolysis in peptic ulcer patients. *Dig. Dis. Sci.*, **30**, 365
48. Lipkin, M. (1981). Cell turnover in gastrointestinal mucosa. In Harmon, J.W. (ed.) *Basic Mechanisms of Gastrointestinal Mucosal Cell Injury and Protection*, pp. 31–48. (Baltimore, London: Williams & Wilkins)
49. Pearson, J.P., Ward, R., Allen, A., Roberts, N.B. and Taylor, W.H. (1986). Mucus degradation by pepsin: comparison of mucolytic activity of human pepsin 1 and pepsin 3: implications in peptic ulceration. *Gut*, **27**, 243–8
50. Walker, V. and Taylor, W.H. (1980). Pepsin 1 secretion in chronic peptic ulceration. *Gut*, **21**, 766–71
51. Roberts, N.B., Sheers, R. and Taylor, W.H. (1981). Pepsin 1 secretion in normal human subjects. *Clin. Sci.*, **61**, 37
52. Glass, G.B.J. and Slomiany, B.L. (1977). Derangements in gastrointestinal injury and disease. In Elstein, M. and Parke, D.V. (eds.) *Mucus in Health and Disease*, pp. 311–47. (New York: Plenum Press)
53. Roberts, S.H., Heffermann, C. and Douglas, A.P. (1975). The sialic acid and carbohydrate content and the synthesis of glycoprotein from radioactive precursors by tissues of the normal and diseased upper intestinal tract. *Clin. Chim. Acta*, **63**, 121–8

54. Schrager, J. and Oates, M.D.G. (1978). Human gastrointestinal mucus in disease states. *Br. Med. Bull.*, **34**, 79–82
55. Domschke, W., Domschke, S., Classen, M. and Demling, L. (1972). Some properties of mucus in patients with gastric ulcer. Effect of treatment with carbenoxolone sodium. *Scand. J. Gastroenterol.*, **7**, 647–51
56. Roberts-Thompson, J.C., Clarke, A.E., Maritz, V.M. and Denborough, M.A. (1975). Gastric glycoproteins in chronic peptic ulcer. *Austral. N. Z. J. Med.*, **5**, 507–14
57. Rathbone, B.J., Wyatt, J.I. and Heatley, R.V. (1986). *Campylobacter pyloridis* – A new factor in peptic ulcer disease? *Gut*, **27**, 635–41
58. Strombeck, D.R. and Harrold, D. (1974). Binding of cholera toxin to mucins and inhibition by gastric mucin. *Infect. Immun.*, **10**, 1266–72
59. Pfeiffer, C.J. (1981). Experimental analysis of hydrogen ion diffusion in gastrointestinal mucus glycoprotein. *Am. J. Physiol.*, **240**, 176–82
60. Williams, S.E. and Turnberg, L.A. (1980). Retardation of acid diffusion by pig gastric mucus: a potential role in mucosal protection. *Gastroenterology*, **79**, 299–304
61. Katz, D., Siegel, H.I. and Glass, G.B.J. (1969). Acute gastric mucosal lesions produced by augmented histamine test. *Am. J. Dig. Dis.*, **14**, 447–55
62. Davenport, H.W. (1967). Physiological structure of gastric mucosa. In Code, C.F. (ed.) *Handbook of Physiology. Alimentary Canal*, Vol. II, pp. 759–79. (Baltimore: Williams & Wilkins)
63. Hills, B.A., Butler, B.D. and Lichtenberger, L.M. (1983). Gastric mucosal barrier: hydrophobic lining to the lumen of the stomach. *Am. J. Physiol.*, **244**, G561–8
64. Bell, A.E. and Allen, A. (1982). Gastrointestinal mucus, electrolytes and mucosal protection. In Case, R.M., Garner, A., Turnberg, L. and Young, J. (eds.) *Electrolyte and Water Transport across Gastrointestinal Epithelia*, pp. 253–5. (New York: Raven Press)
65. Hollander, F. (1954). Two-component mucous barrier. Its activity in protecting gastro-duodenal mucosa against peptic ulceration. *Arch. Intern. Med.*, **93**, 107–29
66. Heatley, N.G. (1959). Mucosubstance as a barrier to diffusion. *Gastroenterology*, **37**, 313–18
67. Allen, A (1981). The structure and function of gastrointestinal mucus. In Harmon, J.W. (ed.) *Basic Mechanisms of Gastrointestinal Mucosal Cell Injury and Protection*, pp. 351–67. (Baltimore: Williams & Wilkins)
68. Sanders, M.J., Aayalon, A., Roll, M. and Soll, A.H. (1985). The apical surface of canine chief cell monolayers resists H^+ back diffusion. *Nature (London)*, **313**, 82–4
69. Morris, G.P. and Wallace, J.L. (1981). The roles of ethanol and of acid in the production of gastric mucosal erosions in rats. *Virchow's Arch. (Cell Pathol.)*, **38**, 23–38
70. Robert, A. (1979). Cytoprotection by prostaglandins. *Gastroenterology*, **77**, 761–7
71. Lacy, E.R. and Ito, S. (1982). Microscopic analysis of ethanol damage to rat gastric mucosa after treatment with a prostaglandin. *Gastroenterology*, **82**, 619–25
72. Lacy, E.R. and Ito, S. (1984). Rapid epithelial restitution of the rat gastric mucosa after ethanol injury. *Lab. Invest.*, **51**, 573–83
73. Silen, W. and Ito, S. (1985). Mechanisms for rapid re-epithelialisation of the gastric mucosal surface. *Ann. Rev. Physiol.*, **47**, 217–29
74. Baskin, W.N., Ivey, K.J., Krause, W.J., Jeffrey, G.E. and Gemmell, R.T. (1976). Aspirin induced ultrastructural changes in human gastric mucosa. Correlation with potential differences. *Ann. Intern. Med.*, **85**, 299–303
75. Lacy, E.R. and Ito, S. (1984). Ethanol-induced insult to the superficial rat gastric epithelium: a study of damage and rapid repair. In Allen, A., Flemström, G., Garner, A., Silen, W. and Turnberg, L.A. (eds) *Mechanisms of Mucosal Protection in the Upper Gastrointestinal Tract*, pp. 49–54. (New York: Raven Press)
76. Rutten, M.J. and Ito, S. (1984). Luminal acid effects on reconstitution of damaged guinea pig gastric mucosa *in vitro*. In Allen, A., Flemström, G., Garner, A., Silen, W. and Turnberg, L.A. (eds) *Mechanisms of Mucosal Protection in the Upper Gastrointestinal Tract*, pp. 41–7. (New York: Raven press)
77. Svanes, K., Ito, S., Takeuchi, K. and Silen, W. (1982). Restitution of the surface epithelium of *in vitro* frog gastric mucosa after damage with hyperosmolar sodium chloride: morphologic and physiologic characteristics. *Gastroenterology*, **82**, 1409–26

143

78. Sellers, L.A., Allen, A. and Bennett, M.K. (1987). Formation of a fibrin based gelatinous coat over repairing rat gastric epithelium after acute ethanol damage: interaction with adherent mucus. *Gut*, **28**, 835–43
79. Lacy, E.R. (1985). Gastric mucosal resistance to a repeated ethanol insult. *Scand. J. Gastroenterol.*, **20**, 63–72
80. Wallace, J.L. and Whittle, J.R. (1986). The role of extracellular mucus as a protective cap over gastric mucosal damage. *Scand. J. Gastroenterol.*, **21** (Suppl. 125), 79–84
81. Allen, A., Garner, A., Hunter, A.C. and Keogh, J.P. (1987). The gastroduodenal mucus barrier and the place of eicosanoids. In Hillier, K. (ed.) *Eicosanoids and the Gastrointestinal Tract*. (Lancaster: MTP Press) (In press)
82. Jentjens, T., Smits, A.L. and Strong, G.J. (1984). 16,16-dimethyl prostaglandin E_2 stimulates galactose and glucosamine but not serine incorporation in rat gastric mucous cells. *Gastroenterology*, **87**, 409–16
83. Parke, D.V. (1978). Pharmacology of mucus. *Br. Med. Bull.*, **34**, 89–94
84. McQueen, S., Allen, A. and Garner, A. (1984). Measurement of gastric and duodenal mucus gel thickness. In Allen, A., Flemström, G., Garner, A., Silen, W. and Turnberg, L.A. (eds) *Mechanisms of Mucosal Protection in the Upper Gastrointestinal Tract*, pp. 215–21. (New York: Raven Press)
85. Allen, A. and Leonard, A. (1985). Mucus structure. *Gastroenterol. Clin. Biol.*, **9**, 9–12
86. Salmon, P.R., Brown, P., Williams, R. and Read, A.E. (1974). Evaluation of colloidal bismuth (De-Nol) in the treatment of duodenal ulcer employing endoscopic selection and follow up. *Gut*, **15**, 189–93
87. Nagashima, R. (1981). Development and characteristics of sucralfate. *J. Clin. Gastroenterol.*, **3**, 103–10
88. Foster, S.N.E., Allen, A. and Pearson, J.P. (1985). Mechanism for the mucosal protective action of polyacrylate on the gastric mucus barrier. *Gut*, **26**, A1109

7
Gastroduodenal bicarbonate secretion: its contribution to mucosal defence

J. R. CRAMPTON and W. D. W. REES

INTRODUCTION

For decades physiologists have postulated the existence of non-parietal alkali secretion by gastric mucosa and recent techniques have allowed detailed study of its transport characteristics and regulation. Parallel studies have also advanced our knowledge of bicarbonate secretion by proximal duodenal mucosa. In isolation, this alkali secretion could contribute little to mucosal protection but in combination with the layer of mucus gel that covers the gastroduodenal epithelium it results in a physical barrier that separates the epithelial cells from luminal acid.

The 'mucus–bicarbonate' barrier produced by bicarbonate secretion into mucus gel is thought to form a first-line defence against the potentially damaging luminal environment. The regulation of this barrier in health, its contribution to overall mucosal defence and its role in the pathogenesis of peptic ulcer disease however remain uncertain. The present chapter reviews current knowledge on the mechanisms and control of bicarbonate secretion and discusses the likely contribution of the mucus–bicarbonate barrier to gastroduodenal mucosal protection.

HISTORICAL DEVELOPMENT

Both Schierbeck[1] and Pavlov[2] proposed the existence of an alkaline component to gastric secretion but its potential importance was not realized as it was argued that the small amount of alkali produced would have no significant neutralizing effect upon the larger acid component. Furthermore Teorell[3] suggested that the electrolyte and acid content of gastric juice could be equally well explained by a process of back diffusion of hydrogen ions into mucosa from lumen in exchange for sodium ions. These observations held sway for a considerable time although experimental evidence for the existence of back diffusion has always been lacking[4]. In 1952 Hollander[5] produced his two-component hypothesis of gastric acidity and secretion and Heatley[6] took this a stage further in 1959 by suggesting that acid may be neutralized within a surface mucus layer by bicarbonate. Heatley also appreciated that this would create a pH gradient across the mucus layer and protect epithelium from acid, although no means of confirming this was available at the time. The hypothesis of a mucus–bicarbonate barrier was not widely accepted owing to lack of experimental support and it was generally believed that mucosal protection against acid arose from a specialized layer in the gastric epithelial cells, the 'mucosal barrier'[7]. Later Makhlouf[8] demonstrated mathematically how [Na$^+$] and [H$^+$] concentrations of gastric juice could best be explained by the existence of both bicarbonate and acid secretion, the latter varying according to the secretory state of parietal cells and the former remaining relatively constant. It was suggested that bicarbonate secretion occurred from 'non-parietal' cells and served to produce gastric luminal contents from pure parietal cell secretion of 160 mM hydrochloric acid. The work of Flemström et al.[9–12] finally demonstrated the existence of an alkaline secretion by fundic and antral gastric mucosa using isolated pieces of mucosa mounted in chambers. They demonstrated that this secretion occurred by active transport as well as by passive diffusion and in a series of publications, along with Garner[13–16], established the basic mechanisms of bicarbonate secretion. This work has since been confirmed by others in a wide variety of experimental animals. Subsequent studies by these authors and others have also demonstrated bicarbonate secretion by duodenal mucosa[17] and experimental evidence indicates that both gastric and duodenal bicarbonate secretion play an important part in mucosal defence[18–20]. Parallel advances in the physiology and biochemistry of gastroduodenal mucus have improved understanding of how bicarbonate secretion contributes to mucosal defence (see Chapter 6). Work by Allen has indicated that secreted mucus consists of a glycoprotein tetramer[21] which forms a continuous visco-elastic gel on the surface epithelium[22]. The gel layer is in dynamic equilibrium, with secretion by goblet cells and mucus neck cells of gastric glands balanced by erosion by pepsin from the luminal surface. The mucus gel layer exists as a continuous layer on unfixed specimens[23-25] with a variable but measurable thickness (mean thickness in man of 200 μm). Although acting mainly as an unstirred layer of water, the gel is capable of impeding the movement of hydrogen ions some four times more than a similar layer of water[26,27]. The mucus layer is able to support pH gradient owing to bicarbonate secretion neutralizing luminal acid within the gel matrix (Figure 7.1) and this has been confirmed using antimony microelectrodes, *in vitro* and *in vivo*[28,29], both in gastric and duodenal mucosa of a number of animals[28,30,31] as well as in man[29]. The depth of the pH gradient substantially exceeds mucus gel thickness (500 μm compared with 200 μm) implying the existence of an adjacent unstirred layer of gastric juice which contributes to the dimensions of the gradient[32]. The gradient can be enhanced by prostaglandins of the E series[30] which both stimulate bicarbonate[33] and mucus secretion[34]. Conversely the gradient is disrupted by non-steroidal anti-inflammatory drugs and mucolytic agents such as N-acetylcysteine[28]. Recent work has established the presence of the pH gradient in the intact human stomach and duodenum using an endoscopic technique and the characteristics of the gradient in various mucosal diseases are currently being evaluated[35,36].

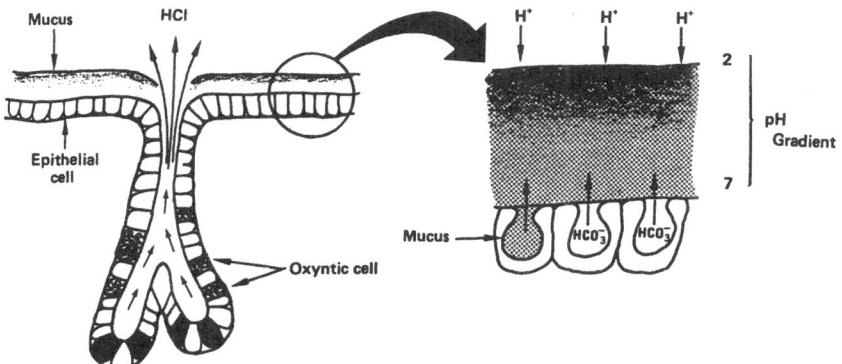

Figure 7.1 Diagram to illustrate the components and site of the 'mucus–bicarbonate' barrier

MECHANISMS OF SECRETION

Gastric bicarbonate

Unlike gastric acid which is produced by parietal cells within gastric glands, alkali secretion is thought to originate from surface epithelial cells and possibly mucus–neck cells. Since there are no direct markers of bicarbonate production, the evidence for the localization of alkali secretion has been inferred indirectly.

The transport mechanism of gastric bicarbonate secretion has been derived from studies using isolated mucosa[10]. Both amphibian and mammalian mucosae have been used and these are stripped of muscularis externa and mounted in a chamber bathed by a separate luminal and serosal side solutions, that on the luminal side being devoid of exogenous buffer. The transmucosal potential difference may be simultaneously measured and pH changes in the luminal solution detected by a pH meter, an autoburette titrating acid equivalent to the amount of alkali secreted. Such a 'pH stat' system strictly measures alkalinization but this is likely to be largely composed of bicarbonate since secretion of other buffering anions has not been demonstrated. Using this experimental method, bullfrog antral mucosa (containing no parietal cells) spontaneously secretes alkali at a rate[9] of 0.3 μmol/cm^2/h but with the fundic mucosa it is necessary to inhibit acid secretion with cimetidine or thiocyanate, when alkalinization occurs at a similar rate[10]. Similar studies have demonstrated alkalinization by rabbit antral and fundic mucosa[37,38].

Bicarbonate secretion has been demonstrated in other animal experimental models, by perfusion of the intact guinea-pig stomach[39,40], in dogs with Heidenhain pouches[14] and also in rats[41] and cats[42]. More recently, gastric bicarbonate secretion has been demonstrated using a variety of techniques in man[43–45].

The animal experiments indicate that gastric alkali secretion is almost entirely active in fundic mucosa although in antral mucosa 30–40% of alkalinization may be owing to passive diffusion through this more leaky epithelium[11]. The active component is identified as that abolished by anoxia and cyanide and also by 2,4-dinitrophenol which implies an ATP-dependent process[10]. Inhibition of carbonic anhydrase with acetazolamide reduces bicarbonate secretion suggesting that carbon dioxide formed within the cells as a result of cellular metabolism is the origin of the secreted anion from fundic mucosa[10]. Replacement of the luminal chloride ions with sulphate reduces bicarbonate secretion[46] and this suggests that gastric bicarbonate secretion occurs via an electroneutral exchange process situated on the apical membrane (Figure 7.2).

Duodenal bicarbonate secretion

The proximal duodenal mucosa has also been examined as an isolated system and can be demonstrated to secrete alkali at rates between two and three times greater than gastric mucosa[47–49]. The rate of alkali secretion is also greater in proximal than distal duodenum[50] implying special adaptation of this region to withstand acid load. As in gastric antrum, a proportion of secretion (approximately 30%) occurs owing to passive diffusion through a paracellular shunt but the majority is owing to active secretion. The relative importance of an electrogenic secretory process and chloride–bicarbonate exchange has been subject to some controversy as different workers have reached disparate

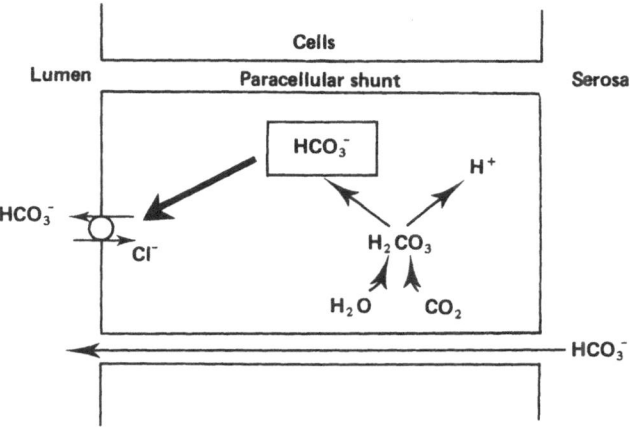

Figure 7.2 Mechanisms of gastric bicarbonate transport

conclusions on the effects of chloride free solutions on secretion[51,52]. It appears that endogenous production of bicarbonate within duodenal epithelial cells is less important than in gastric mucosa since acetazolamide does not inhibit duodenal alkali secretion[10]. Basal secretion is electrogenic and stimulated by prostaglandins[17] whereas other stimulants of secretion appear to activate an electroneutral transport process which is probably chloride–bicarbonate exchange (Figure 7.3). Confirmation that alkalinization occurs in the proximal duodenum has taken place in guinea-pig[40], rat[50], cat[53] and more recently in man[54].

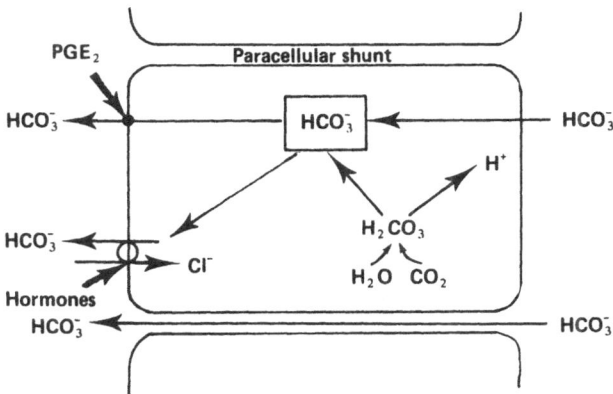

Figure 7.3 Mechanisms of duodenal bicarbonate transport

CONTROL AND REGULATION OF SECRETION

Gastric bicarbonate

Compared with the vast amount of data on gastric acid secretion, knowledge of the control of bicarbonate secretion is very limited. The response of gastric bicarbonate secretion to a wide variety of hormones and neurotransmitters has been obtained from *in vitro* experiments[12,55]. Unfortunately, it cannot be established from these that a particular response is of physiological significance. Nonetheless using such techniques it has been found that gastric alkalinization is stimulated by the cholinergic agonist, carbachol[55], and this suggests at least the presence of cholinergic receptors on the epithelium. The cyclic nucleotide, cGMP, also stimulates alkalinization[55] and this may be the intracellular mediator of secretion although calcium has also been observed to exert an effect[56]. Conversely, isolated gastric mucosal bicarbonate secretion may be inhibited by noradrenaline but not by isoprenaline[56] suggesting that an α-adrenergic process may modulate secretion. Other putative neurotransmitters have not been found to affect gastric bicarbonate secretion in the *in vitro* model. Prostaglandins of the E and F series can be shown to stimulate bicarbonate secretion in the stomach[14,15,57,58] and the inhibition of secretion by non-steroidal anti-inflammatory drugs, such as indomethacin, suggests that endogenous prostaglandins may be important in regulating basal secretion[14,15]. Of the gastrointestinal hormones, both cholecystokinin and pancreatic glucagon are stimulants of secretion whereas GIP and PTH are inhibitory[55]. Almost all other neurohumoral agents which have been tested *in vitro* have no effect, and interestingly this includes gastrin, histamine and secretin. It is therefore clear that the secretion of acid and bicarbonate are under independent control. Local factors such as distension or trauma increase bicarbonate secretion although this is presumably owing to increased passive permeation. The presence of luminal acid itself regulates bicarbonate secretion (Figure 7.4)[59]. This was originally demonstrated in elegant experiments by Garner and Hurst[14] in dogs with Heidenhain pouches, where instillation of acid into the main stomach increased bicarbonate secretion by the pouch. In experiments using a paired mucosal chamber with a common serosal side-solution[59] it has been found that acidification of one mucosa increases bicarbonate secretion by another indicating release of some paracrine agent which mediates the response. Further work has suggested that the response to luminal acid may occur via release of prostaglandins[59] although other mechanisms are likely to play a part. Other luminal contents may also affect the secretion of bicarbonate by the stomach, in particular bile. This is frequently present in the luminal contents owing to duodenogastric reflux and experiments have shown that low concentrations of taurocholate[37,60] inhibit gastric bicarbonate secretion.

Evidence indicates that neural regulation of gastric bicarbonate also occurs.

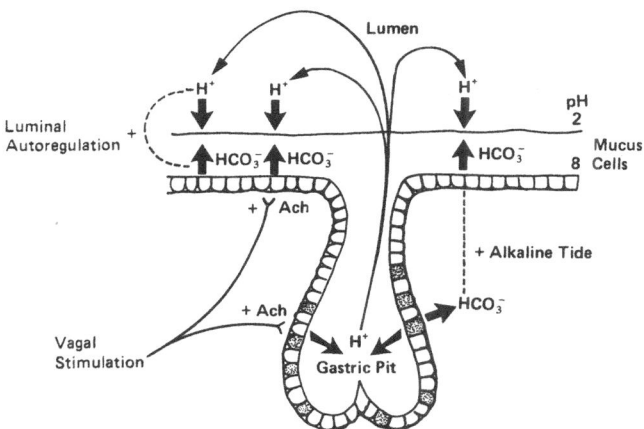

Figure 7.4 Diagram illustrating the interaction between gastric acid and alkali secretion

It has been demonstrated that vagal stimulation increases gastric bicarbonate secretion in cats and that this may involve an axon reflex and possibly Substance P[42]. The vagal stimulation by sham feeding has also been shown to stimulate gastric bicarbonate secretion in man[62], a response that is inhibited by cholinergic antagonists. Endogenous neurones have recently been shown to modify gastric alkali secretion in that electrical field stimulation of isolated mucosa has been shown to increase secretory rate (personal observations).

Duodenal bicarbonate

The response of *in vitro* duodenal mucosa to application of neurohumoral agents differs from that of gastric mucosa and this implies separate control mechanisms. There is no response to carbachol or cGMP but endorphins in low concentrations have been shown to act as stimulants[63,64]. Opiates are present in high concentrations in the mucosa and submucosa of the upper bowel[65,66] and are likely to play a role in the neuroendocrine regulation of duodenal bicarbonate secretion. Cyclic AMP increases secretion and may be an intracellular mediator of the secretory response[12]. Prostaglandins and arachidonic acid increase while indomethacin decreases secretion, and in these respects duodenal alkalinization responds in a way similar to gastric bicarbonate secretion. Of the gastrointestinal hormones, pancreatic glucagon, neurotensin and GIP are stimulants[67,68] but no other hormones affect the output of alkali from isolated duodenal mucosa. Of the local factors, distension may increase bicarbonate secretion owing to passive permeation[69] and acid within the lumen is a potent stimulus to secretion[59,70,71,73]. The effect of acid is independent of damage and is likely to have an important regulatory function.

151

In vivo animal work indicates that vagal stimulation increases bicarbonate secretion by proximal duodenum[72]. This response is abolished by hexamethionium but only inhibited in part by atropine. Experiments using electrical field stimulation indicate that enteric neurones of the lamina propria are capable of stimulating bicarbonate secretion[73] and, in amphibian mucosa, at least, this occurs via release of acetylcholine since it is abolished by atropine[74]. Physical stress in rats inhibits duodenal bicarbonate secretion[75] and this effect is not blocked by atropine and is probably mediated by the sympathetic nervous system. It is possible that there are species differences in the neurohumoral control processes of duodenal alkalinization and this may account for some of the apparent discrepancies observed in animal work. Nonetheless it is clear that neural, hormonal and luminal factors may act in conjunction to adjust bicarbonate output precisely to the prevailing acid load and luminal milieu (Figure 7.4).

HUMAN GASTRODUODENAL BICARBONATE SECRETION

Although the majority of information on gastroduodenal bicabonate secretion has been gained from animal experiments an increasing body of information is being harvested from experiments on the intact human stomach.

Gastric bicarbonate secretion

Patients with achlorhydria have been demonstrated to have alkaline gastric contents[76] but the non-parietal secretion described in this pathological state cannot necessarily be extrapolated to healthy man. Attempts to calculate gastric bicarbonate output in healthy volunteers using a glycine buffer[77] resulted in high calculated outputs which were probably an artefact of the experimental technique. The advent of histamine H_2-receptor antagonists enabled acid secretion to be markedly suppressed and it became possible to measure gastric bicarbonate secretion in healthy subjects. The first reported description of this method was by Rees *et al.*[43] who used an intubation perfusion technique with measurement of pH and pCO_2 in the aspirate, with corrections for salivary contamination and duodenogastric reflux. Such a method is valid because the gastric mucosa has a very low permeability to CO_2 and at a pH of 6 to 7, the luminal pCO_2 is relatively low. Using this method it was possible to demonstrate a basal rate of secretion of 400 μmol/h, a rate which seems to accord with the animal work. Feldman and Barnett have more recently described another technique[44] in which bicarbonate was calculated by the fall in osmolality caused by the interaction of acid and alkali. The method requires some assumptions to be made and requires independent validation[78] since the magnitude of basal secretion using this method seems improbably high (2.6 mM/h). Recently Forssell *et al.* have described a high-volume rapid perfusion technique[45] with continuous computer monitoring of pH and pCO_2 and the basal secretion measurements are more in accordance with those of Rees *et al.*[43].

Human gastric bicarbonate secretion can be stimulated by carbachol and high concentrations of prostaglandins[44,79,80]. In lower, more physiological concentrations, however, prostaglandins do not stimulate secretion but do prevent the inhibition that can otherwise be induced by low concentrations of aspirin or taurocholate[81]. These observations suggest that the inhibitory action of the latter agents is owing to a reduction in mucosal prostaglandin formation and that endogenous prostaglandins play a role in modulating basal secretion, a phenomenon referred to as prostaglandin 'tone'. Luminal acid has been confirmed as a stimulus to bicarbonate secretion in man[82] and clearly this effect may have an important role in the regulation of human gastric bicarbonate secretion and its adjustment to the prevailing pH. Forssell has described an increase in gastric bicarbonate secretion which occurs in response to sham feeding[61] confirming the importance of the vagus nerves in the regulation of secretion. The effect is blocked by benzalkonium which suggests that cholinergic efferents are responsible.

Duodenal Bicarbonate Secretion

A difficulty in demonstrating human duodenal bicarbonate secretion has been to isolate proximal duodenal mucosa from pancreatico-biliary secretions which contain high concentrations of bicarbonate. It had been noted in the past that acid instilled into an isolated, distal duodenal segment was rapidly neutralized with a simultaneous increase in intraduodenal pCO_2 and decrease in osmolality[83]. These early findings indicated that duodenal bicarbonate secretion played a role in acid disposal in man. Isenberg and his colleagues have recently developed a technique that allows measurement of proximal duodenal alkalinization in healthy human volunteers[54]. A 4-cm segment of proximal duodenum is isolated between two occluding balloons and the lumen perfused with markers. Mean basal secretion has been calculated as 140 μmol/cm/h and this rate is increased in a dose-dependent manner following instillation of different concentrations of acid. A prostaglandin analogue, misoprostil, has been shown to stimulate secretion[84] while indomethacin inhibits[85], suggesting that prostaglandins play a role in modulating secretion in man as well as in experimental animals. Much work remains to be done to determine the significance of human duodenal bicarbonate secretion in health and in peptic ulcer disease but these early results confirm that some of the observations from animal experiments are relevant to human physiology.

IMPORTANCE OF THE MUCUS–BICARBONATE BARRIER

The preceding sections illustrate that impressive evidence now exists for active bicarbonate secretion from gastric and duodenal epithelia *in vivo* and for the presence of a pH gradient across the mucus-gel layer. It is unlikely however that mucosal defences can be explained solely on this model and other factors are likely to play a part (Figure 7.5). The mucus–bicarbonate barrier is only able to provide an explanation for defence against luminal acid and yet other noxious agents such as alcohol and bile are frequently present within the lumen for which other protective mechanisms must come into play. Furthermore, experiments indicate that the pH gradient cannot be sustained when intra-luminal pH falls below 1.5[28,29,30], a circumstance which frequently occurs *in vivo*. A number of other protective mechanisms can be observed in the experimental situation. Mucus itself may exert a protective action by virtue of its physical and chemical properties and is capable of anti-oxidant behaviour protecting the mucosa from free radicals[86]. Mucus gel may retard the diffusion of hydrogen ions and unidirectional movement of H^+ towards the lumen is favoured by its linkage with active Na^+ transport by epithelium[87] (see Chapter 6). Furthermore, the phospholipid layer on the epithelial surface has hydrophobic qualities which are enhanced by prostaglandins and are likely to provide a second-line defence against noxious agents[88]. When the defensive layer has been breached, epithelial restitution is likely to be the limiting factor determining mucosal recovery since cells are capable of rapidly migrating to fill small defects[89,90] (see Chapter 8). Changes in mucosal blood flow may also play a part in the normal defence mechanisms of stomach and duodenum[91] (see Chapter 10). All of these processes are capable of being affected by prostaglandins[92] and it is likely that endogenous prostaglandin metabolism is important in modulating changes in the defensive state of the mucosa *in vivo* (see Chapter 9). The current concept therefore is that mucosal protection is a

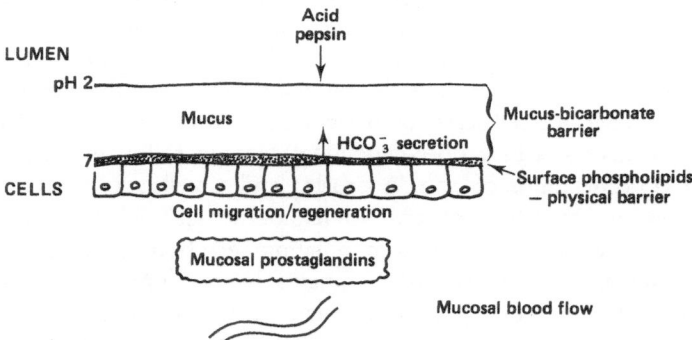

Figure 7.5 Components of gastroduodenal mucosal defence

154

multi-tiered process with the mucus–bicarbonate barrier forming the first-line defence against acid and that different mechanisms may have relatively more importance with different noxious agents. There is no doubt that when the mucus–bicarbonate barrier is breached experimentally, other factors can still maintain mucosal integrity and then assume greater importance. The precise relative importance of these mechanisms *in vivo* and in disease states remain to be determined.

GASTRODUODENAL BICARBONATE SECRETION IN DISEASE

The role of secreted bicarbonate in sustaining the protective mucus–bicarbonate barrier has naturally led to an interest in its involvement in mucosal disease. Experiments have demonstrated the inhibition of bicarbonate secretion[38] and the disruption of the pH gradient[94] by non-steroidal anti-inflammatory drugs. In man, aspirin and indomethacin[96] have been shown to inhibit gastric bicarbonate secretion and indomethacin has also been shown to inhibit duodenal bicarbonate secretion[85]. It is tempting to ascribe the known damaging effects of this group of drugs on gastroduodenal mucosa to these actions. Furthermore prostaglandins, known to stimulate gastroduodenal bicarbonate secretion, have been observed to protect the mucosa from a wide variety of necrotizing agents[95]. Ethanol has been demonstrated to inhibit gastric bicarbonate secretion and it has been suggested that this may play a part in the pathogenesis of alcoholic gastritis. Similarly, the inhibitory effect of noradrenaline on gastric bicarbonate secretion has led to speculation on the role of such an action in the pathogenesis of stress-induced ulcers. Certainly in rats, physical stress reduces duodenal bicarbonate secretion and combined with histamine administration results in ulcer formation. This suggests that a reduction in bicarbonate output produced by stress impairs the ability of mucosa to withstand an acid load[75].

At present, there is very scanty information on gastroduodenal bicarbonate secretion and the integrity of the mucus–bicarbonate barrier in patients with peptic ulcer. Gastric bicarbonate secretion is, not surprisingly, unimpaired in patients with duodenal ulcer[97] and to date, no studies have examined gastric bicarbonate secretion in patients with gastric ulcer or gastritis. Isenberg and his colleagues have measured bicarbonate secretion from the proximal duodenum in patients with duodenal ulcer[98]. The basal rate is similar to healthy controls but there is a poor response to instilled luminal acid. Since a previous study has shown failure of duodenal acidification to release local prostaglandins in duodenal ulcer patients[99], the absent bicarbonate response may be linked to abnormal prostaglandin metabolism in duodenal ulcer disease. Clearly this finding is likely to be of importance and may play a role in the pathogenesis of duodenal ulcer and its recurrent behaviour.

155

THERAPEUTIC MANIPULATION OF GASTRODUODENAL BICARBONATE SECRETION

In developing medical treatment for peptic ulcer, a great deal of effort has been devoted to agents which reduce acid secretion and this has culminated in the highly successful histamine H_2-receptor antagonists and more recently in the H^+-K^+-ATPase ('proton pump') inhibitor, omeprazole. Nonetheless, many patients with duodenal ulcer and most patients with gastric ulcer do not have abnormally high acid output. Although reducing the acid output in these patients may be effective, recent attention has been paid to the therapeutic manipulation of mucosal defences, notably the mucus–bicarbonate barrier, in an attempt to restore the physiological balance between aggressive and protective factors. Of the agents currently available to treat peptic ulcer disease, it is known that cimetidine, pirenzepine, omeprazole and carbenoxolone[100,101] do not affect gastric or duodenal bicarbonate secretion. A number of synthetic prostaglandin analogues have recently become available of which most may be expected, on the basis of animal experiments, to be stimulants of gastroduodenal bicarbonate secretion. However, only misoprostil (16,16-dimethyl-prostaglandin E_2)[42] and 11,16,16-trimethyl-prostaglandin E_2[44] have been demonstrated to exert this effect in man. Of course the prostaglandins are likely to have a number of other actions including effects on mucosal blood flow[102], epithelial cell-membrane properties and mucus gel secretion and thickness which may be equally therapeutically valuable. Unfortunately, analysis of clinical trial data suggests that the ulcer-healing actions of most prostaglandin analogues are related to inhibition of acid production rather than to actions on protective mechanisms[103]. This is not perhaps surprising since defective endogenous prostaglandin production has not been consistently demonstrated in peptic ulcer disease[104]. Nonetheless exogenous prostaglandins do prevent the detrimental actions of non-steroidal anti-inflammatory drugs on the stomach as assessed by both faecal occult bleeding[105] and endoscopy[106] and may have greater potential value in preventing mucosal damage by these drugs or healing peptic ulcers associated with such drugs.

In addition to prostaglandins, a number of currently available ulcer-healing drugs do appear to act on mucosal defence mechanisms (Figure 7.6). Sucralfate is a basic aluminium salt of sucrose sulphate which was originally introduced because of its ability to adhere selectively to ulcerated tissue to form a barrier. It has more recently been found to stimulate prostaglandin E_2 synthesis and release by gastroduodenal mucosa[106] and also to significantly increase gastric, and to a lesser extent, duodenal bicarbonate secretion[107]. Bismuth, the ingredient of tripotassium dicitrato bismuthate, may also stimulate gastroduodenal bicarbonate secretion *in vitro*[108] and this may play a role in its therapeutic action which has long remained unexplained. Aluminium ions have been shown

156

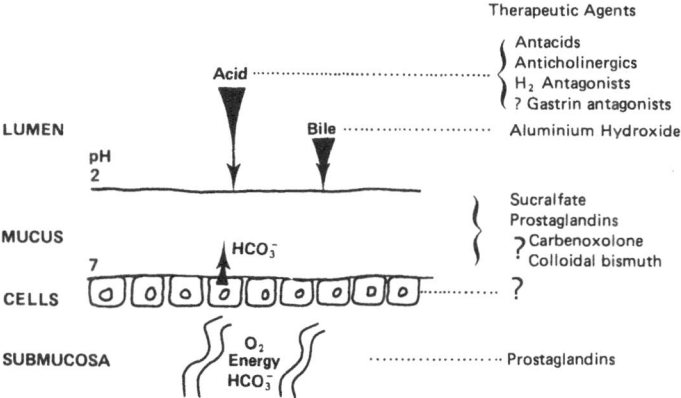

Figure 7.6   Possible mechanisms of action of current ulcer healing agents

to stimulate both gastric and duodenal alkali secretion *in vitro*[109]. This may be an important observation since it can be shown that low doses of antacids containing aluminium are capable of healing ulcers and this may be more owing to stimulation of endogenous bicarbonate secretion than provision of buffering capacity. Carbenoxolone has been shown to increase mucus biosynthesis and the thickness of mucus gel[110] which may be of protective benefit although it does not stimulate bicarbonate secretion[101] and is unlikely to substantially affect the pH gradient. The effect of other drugs on mucosal defences has not been adequately examined. It appears that therapeutic manipulation of gastroduodenal bicarbonate secretion is possible and the ulcer-healing action of current anti-ulcer drugs may in part be mediated by this effect. In future, drugs may be specifically developed for their actions on the 'mucus–bicarbonate' barrier although this will require a better understanding of the regulation of mucus and bicarbonate production.

REFERENCES

1. Schierbeck, N.P. (1892). Ueber Kohlensäure im Ventrikel. *Skand. Archiv. für Physiol.*, **3**, 437–74
2. Pavlov, J.P. (1898). *Die Arbeit der Verdauungsdrüsen.* (Wiesbaden: J. F. Bergman Verlag)
3. Teorell, T. (1939). On the permeability of the stomach mucosa for acids and some other substances. *J. Gen. Physiol.*, **23**, 263–74
4. Thjodleifsson, B. and Wormsley, K.G. (1977). Back diffusion–fact or fiction. *Digestion*, **15**, 53–72
5. Hollander, H.F. (1954). The two-component mucous barrier. *Arch. Intern. Med.*, **94**, 107–20
6. Heatley, N.G. (1959). Mucosubstance as a barrier to diffusion. *Gastroenterology*, **37**, 313–17
7. Davenport, H.W., Warner, H.A. and Code, C.F. (1964). Functional significance of gastric mucosal barrier to sodium. *Gastroenterology*, **47**, 142–52

8. Makhlouf, G.M. (1981). Electrolyte composition of gastric secretion. In Johnson, L.R., Christensen, J., Grossman, M.I. et al. (eds) Physiology of the Gastrointestinal Tract, pp. 551–66. (New York: Raven Press)
9. Flemström, G. and Sachs, G. (1975). Properties of isolated antral mucosa. I. General characteristics. Am. J. Physiol., 228, 1188–98
10. Flemström, G. (1977). Active alkalinization by amphibian gastric fundic mucosa in vitro. Am. J. Physiol., 233, E1–E12
11. Flemström, G. (1981). Gastric secretion of bicarbonate. In Johnson, L.R., Christensen, J., Grossman, M.I. et al. (eds) Physiology of the Gastrointestinal Tract, pp. 603–16. (New York: Raven Press)
12. Flemström, G. and Garner, A. (1982). Gastroduodenal HCO_3^- transport: characteristics and proposed role in acidity regulation and mucosal protection. Am. J. Physiol., 242, G183–G193
13. Garner, A. (1977). Effects of acetylsalicylate on alkalinzation, acid secretion and electrogenic properties in the isolated gastric mucosa. Acta Physiol. Scand., 99, 281–91
14. Garner, A. and Hurst, B.C. (1981). Alkaline secretion by the canine Heidenhain pouch in response to exogenous acid, some gastrointestinal hormones and prostaglandins. In Gati, T., Szollar, L.G. and Ungvary, G. (eds) Advances in Physiological Sciences. Nutrition, Digestion and Metabolism, 12, 215–19. (Oxford: Pergamon)
15. Garner, A., Flemström, G. and Heylings, J.R. (1979). Effects of anti-inflammatory agents and prostaglandins on acid and bicarbonate secretions in the amphibian-isolated gastric mucosa. Gastroenterology, 77, 457–61
16. Garner, A., Hurst, B.C., Heylings, J.R. and Flemström, G. (1981). Role of gastroduodenal HCO_3^- transport in acid disposal and mucosal protection. In Case, R.M., Garner, A., Turnberg, L.A. and Young, J.A. (eds) Electrolyte and Water Transport Across Gastrointestinal Epithelia, pp. 239–52. (New York: Raven Press)
17. Flemström, G. (1980). Stimulation of HCO_3^- transport in isolated proximal bullfrog duodenum by prostaglandins. Am. J. Physiol., 239, G198–G204
18. Rees, W.D.W. and Turnberg, L.A. (1982). Mechanisms of gastric mucosal protection: a role for the 'mucus–bicarbonate' barrier. Clin. Sci., 62, 343–8
19. Allen, A. and Garner, A. (1980). Mucus and bicarbonate secretion in the stomach and their possible role in mucosal protection. Gut, 21, 249–62
20. Flemström, G. and Turnberg, L.A. (1984). Gastroduodenal defence mechanisms. Clin. Gastroenterol., 13(2), 324–57
21. Allen, A., Pain, R.H. and Robson T.R. (1976). Model for the structure of the gastric mucus gel. Nature (London), 264, 88–9
22. Allen, A. (1978). Structure of gastrointestinal mucus glycoproteins and the viscous and gel-forming properties of mucus. Br. Med. Bull., 34, 28–33
23. Pearson, J., Allen, A. and Venables, C. (1980). Gastric mucus: isolation and polymeric structure of the undegraded glycoprotein; its breakdown by pepsin. Gastroenterology, 78, 709–15
23a. Bickel, M. and Kauffman, G.L. (1981). Gastric mucus gel thickness: effect of distension, 16,16-dimethyl prostaglandin E_2 and carbenoxolone. Gastroenterology, 80, 770–5
24. McQueen, S., Hutton, D., Allen, A. and Garner, A. (1983). Gastric and duodenal surface mucus gel thickness in the rat: effects of prostaglandins and damaging agents. Am. J. Physiol., 245, G388–G393
25. Kerss, S., Allen, A. and Garner, A. (1982). A simple method for measuring thickness of the mucus gel layer adherent to rat, frog and human gastric mucosa: influence of feeding, prostaglandin, N-acetylcysteine and other agents. Clin. Sci., 63, 187–95
26. Williams, S.E. and Turnberg, L.A. (1980). Retardation of acid diffusion by pig gastric mucus: a potential role in mucosal protection. Gastroenterology, 79, 299–304
27. Pfeiffer, C.J. (1981). Experimental analysis of hydrogen ion diffusion in gastrointestinal mucus glycoprotein. Am. J. Physiol., 240, G176–G182
28. Ross, I.N., Bahari, H.M.M. and Turnberg, L.A. (1981). The pH gradient across mucus adherent to rat fundic mucosa in vivo and the effect of potential damaging agents. Gastroenterology, 81, 713–18

29. Bahari, H.M.M., Ross, I.N. and Turnberg, L.A. (1982). Demonstration of a pH gradient across the mucus layer on the surface of human gastric mucosa *in vitro. Gut,* **23,** 513–16
30. Ross, I.N. and Turnberg, L.A. (1983). Studies of the 'mucus–bicarbonate' barrier on rat fundic mucosa – the effects of luminal pH and a stable prostaglandin analogue. *Gut,* **24,** 1030–3
31. Takeuchi, K., Magee, D., Critchlow, J. *et al.* (1983). Studies of the pH gradient and thickness of frog gastric mucus gel. *Gastroenterology,* **84,** 331–40
32. Allen, A., Hutton, D., McQueen, S. and Garner, A. (1983). Dimensions of gastroduodenal surface pH gradients exceed those of adherent mucus gel layers. *Gastroenterology,* **85,** 463–76
33. Garner, A. and Heylings, J.R. (1979). Stimulation of alkaline secretion in amphibian-isolated gastric mucosa by 16,16-dimethyl PGE_2 and $PGF_{2\alpha}$: a proposed explanation for some of the cytoprotective actions of prostaglandins. *Gastroenterology,* **76,** 497–503
34. Johansson, C. and Kollberg, B. (1979). Stimulation by intragastrically administered E_2 prostaglandins of human gastric mucus output. *Eur. J. Clin. Invest.,* **9,** 229–32
35. Quigley, E.M.M. and Turnberg, L.A. (1985). Neutral microclimate lines human gastroduodenal mucosa *in vivo. Gut,* **26**(10), A1117
36. Quigley, E.M.M. and Turnberg, L.A. (1986). Can the mucus–bicarbonate barrier withstand low intraluminal pH? – Studies in health and gastroduodenal mucosal disease. *Gut,* **2 7**(10), A1284
37. Rees, W.D.W., Garner, A., Turnberg, L.A. and Gibbons, L.C. (1982). Studies of acid and alkali secretion by rabbit gastric fundus *in vitro*: effect of low concentrations of sodium taurocholate. *Gastroenterology,* **83,** 435–40
38. Rees, W.D.W., Gibbons, L.C. and Turnberg, L.A. (1983). Effects of non-steroidal anti-inflammatory drugs and prostaglandins on alkali secretion by rabbit gastric, fundus *in vitro. Gut,* **24,** 784–9
39. Garner, A. and Flemström, G. (1978). Gastric HCO_3^- secretion in the guinea pig. *Am. J. Physiol.,* **234,** E535–E545
40. Flemström, G. and Garner, A. (1980). Stimulation of gastric acid and bicarbonate secretions by calcium in guinea pig stomach and amphibian isolated mucosa. *Acta Physiol. Scand.,* **110,** 421–8
41. Smeeton, L., Hurst, B., Allen, A. and Garner, A. (1983). Gastric and duodenal HCO_3^- transport *in vivo*: influence of prostaglandins. *Am. J. Physiol.,* **245,** *(Gastrointest. Liver Physiol.,* **8**), G751–G759
42. Fändriks, L. and Delbro, D. (1983). Neural stimulation of gastric bicarbonate secretion in the cat. An involvement of vagal axon-reflexes and substance P? *Acta Physiol. Scand.,* **118,** 301–4
43. Rees, W.D.W., Botham, D. and Turnberg, L.A. (1982). A demonstration of bicarbonate production by the normal human stomach *in vivo. Dig. Dis. Sci.,* **27,** 961–6
44. Feldman, M. and Barnett, C. (1983). Gastric bicarbonate secretion in humans. Effects of pentagastrin, bethanechol, and 11,16,16-trimethyl prostaglandin E_2. *J. Clin. Invest.,* **72,** 295–303
45. Forssell, H., Preshaw, R. and Olbe, L. (1983). Gastric secretion of bicarbonate in man determined with a perfusion technique. In Allen, A., Flemström, G., Garner, A. *et al.* (eds) *Mechanisms of Mucosal Protection in the Upper Gastrointestinal Tract,* pp. 125–7. (New York: Raven Press)
46. Flemström, G. (1980). Cl^- dependence of HCO_3^- transport in frog gastric mucosa. *Uppsala J. Med. Sci.,* **85,** 303–10
47. Flemström, G. and Nylander, O. (1981). Secretion of bicarbonate by guinea-pig duodenum *in vivo. Prostaglandins,* **21**(suppl.), 47–52
48. Flemström, G., Garner, A., Nylander, O. *et al.* (1982). Surface epithelial HCO_3^- transport by mammalian duodenum *in vivo. Am. J. Physiol.,* **243,** G348–G358
49. Flemström, G. (1980). Stimulation of HCO_3^- transport in isolated proximal bullfrog duodenum by prostaglandins. *Am. J. Physiol.,* **239** *(Gastrointest. Liver Physiol.,* **2**), G198–G203
50. Isenberg, J.I., Flemström, G. and Johansson, C. (1983). Mucosal bicarbonate secretion is

significantly greater in the proximal versus distal duodenum in the *in vivo* rat. In Allen, A., Flemström, G., Garner, A. *et al.* (eds) *Mechanisms of Mucosal Protection in the Upper Gastrointestinal Tract*, pp. 175–80. (New York: Raven Press)

51. Simson, J.N.L., Merhav, A. and Silen, W. (1981). Alkaline secretion by amphibian duodenum. I. General characteristics. *Am. J. Physiol.*, **240**, G401–G408
52. Flemström, G., Garner, A. and Hurst, B.C. (1983). Influence of luminal chloride on duodenal epithelial bicarbonate secretion in the cat. *J. Physiol.*, **342**, 14P–15P (Abstract)
53. Case, R.M., Garner, A. and Uddin, K.K. (1983). Simultaneous determination of duodenal and pancreatic bicarbonate transport: differential effects of secretin and prostaglandin E_2 in the cat *in vivo*. *J. Physiol.*, **340**, 36P–37P (Abstract)
54. Isenberg, J.I., Hogan, D.L., Koss, M.A. and Selling, J.A. (1986). Human duodenal mucosal bicarbonate secretion. Evidence for basal secretion, stimulation by hydrochloric acid and a synthetic prostaglandin E_1 analogue. *Gastroenterology*, **21**, 370–8
55. Flemström, G., Heylings, J.R. and Garner, A. (1982). Gastric and duodenal HCO_3^- transport *in vitro*: effects of hormones and local transmitters. *Am. J. Physiol.*, **242**, G100–G110
56. Flemström, G. (1978). Effect of catecholamines, Ca^{2+} and gastrin in gastric HCO_3^- secretion. *Acta Physiol. Scand.* (Special supplement Gastric Ion Transport), 81–90
57. Bolton, J.P. and Cohen, M.M. (1978). Stimulation of non-parietal secretion in canine Heidenhain pouches by 16,16-dimethyl prostaglandin E_2. *Digestion*, **17**, 291–9
58. Kauffman, G.L., Reeve, J.J. and Grossman, M.I. (1980). Gastric bicarbonate secretion: effect of topical and intravenous 16,16-dimethyl prostaglandin E_2. *Am. J. Physiol.*, **239**, G44–G48
59. Heylings, J.R., Garner, A. and Flemström, G. (1984). Regulation of gastroduodenal HCO_3^- transport by luminal acid in the frog *in vitro*. *Am. J. Physiol.*, **246**, G235–G242
60. Rees, W.D.W., Garner, A., Vivian, K.H.B. and Turnberg, L.A. (1981). Effect of sodium taurocholate on secretion by amphibian gastric mucosa *in vitro*. *Am. J. Physiol.*, **240**, G245–G249
61. Forssell, H., Stenquist, B. and Olbe, L. (1985). Vagal stimulation of human gastric bicarbonate secretion. *Gastroenterology*, **89**, 581–6
62. Flemström, G., Sedstedt, G. and Nylander, O. (1986). Beta-endorphin and enkephalins stimulate duodenal mucosal alkaline secretion in the rat *in vivo*. *Gastroenterology*, **90**(2), 368–72
63. Rees, W.D.W., Gibbons, L.C. and Turnberg, L.A. (1986). Influence of opiates on alkali secretion by amphibian gastric and duodenal mucosa *in vitro*. *Gastroenterology*, **90**(2), 323–7
65. Polak, J.M., Bloom, S.R., Sullivan, S.N., Facer, P. and Pearse, A.G.E. (1977). Enkephalin-like immunoreactivity in the human gastrointestinal tract. *Lancet*, **i**, 972–4
66. Ito, S., Takai, K., Shibata, A., Matsubara, Y. and Yanaihara, N. (1979). Met-enkephalin-immunoreactive and gastrin immunoreactive cells in human and canine gastric antrum. *Gen. Comp. Endocrinol*, **38**, 238–45
67. Flemström, G. (1982). Properties of hormone and prostaglandin stimulated duodenal HCO_3^- transport. In Case, R.M., Garner, A., Turnberg, L.A. and Young, J.A. (eds) *Electrolyte and Water Transport across Gastrointestinal Epithelia*, pp. 85–94. (New York: Raven Press)
68. Flemström, G. and Garner, A. (1980). Stimulation of HCO_3^- transport by gastric inhibitory peptide on proximal duodenum of the bullfrog. *Acta Physiol. Scand.*, **109**, 231–2
69. Garner, A., Flemström, G., Heylings, J.R., Hurst, B.C., Hampson, S.E. and Hughes, C.L. (1984). Factors regulating HCO_3^- transport by duodenal epithelia. In Allen, A., Garner, A., Flemström, G. and Turnberg, L.A. (eds) *Mechanisms of Mucosal Protection in the Upper Gastrointestinal Tract*, pp. 153–8. (New York: Raven Press)
70. Heylings, J.R. (1983). A technique for studying the influence of luminal acid on frog gastric and duodenal HCO_3^- transport *in vitro*. *J. Physiol.*, **342**, 4–5
71. Isenberg, J.I., Smedfors, B. and Johansson, C. (1985). Effect of graded doses of intraluminal H^+, prostaglandin E_2 and inhibition of endogenous prostaglandin synthesis on the proximal duodenal bicarbonate secretion in unanaesthetised rat. *Gastroenterology*, **88**, 303–7

72. Flemström, G., Nylander, O., Fandriks, L., Jönsson, C. and Delbro, D. (1985). Regulation of bicarbonate secretion by gastroduodenal mucosa. *Gastroenterol Clin. Biol.*, **9**(12), 16–19

73. Crampton, J., Gibbons, L.C. and Rees, W.D.W. (1985). Effect of electrical field stimulation on bicarbonate secretion by isolated amphibian duodenum. *Gut*, **26**(10), A1110

74. Crampton, J., Gibbons, L.C. and Rees, W.D.W. (1986). Evidence for cholinergic modulation of duodenal bicarbonate secretion. *Gut*, **27**(10), A1254

75. Takeuchi, K., Furukawa, O. and Okabe, S. (1986). Induction of duodenal ulcers in rats under water-immersion stress conditions. Influence of stress on gastric acid and duodenal alkaline secretion. *Gastroenterology*, **91**, 554–63

76. Andre, C., Bruhiere, J., Vague, M. and Lambert, R. (1973). Bicarbonate secretion in the human stomach. *Acta Hepato-Gastroenterol*, **20**, 62–9

77. Okosdinossian, I.T. and El Munshid, H.A. (1977). Composition of the alkaline component of human gastric juice: effect of swallowed saliva and duodenogastric reflux. *Scand. J. Gastroenterol*, **12**, 945–50

78. Flemström, G. (1985). Measurement of gastric bicarbonate secretion. *Gastroenterology*, **88**(6), 2000–1

79. Feldman, M. and Schiller, L.S. (1982). Effect of bethanechol (urecholine) on gastric acid and non-parietal secretion in normal subjects and duodenal ulcer patients. *Gastroenterology*, **83**, 262–6

80. Johansson, C., Aly, A., Nilsson, E. and Flemström, G. (1983). Stimulation of gastric bicarbonate secretion by E_2 prostaglandins in man. In Samuelsson, B., Paoletti, R. and Ramwell, P. (eds) *Advances in Prostaglandin, Thromboxane, and Leukotriene Research*, **12**, 395–401. (New York: Raven Press)

81. Rees, W.D.W., Gibbons, L.C., Warhurst, G. and Turnberg, L.A. (1983). Studies of bicarbonate secretion by the normal human stomach *in vivo* — effect of aspirin, sodium taurocholate and prostaglandin E_2. In Allen, A., Flemström, G., Garner, A. *et al.* (eds) *Mechanisms of Mucosal Protection in the Upper Gastrointestinal Tract*, pp. 119–123. (New York: Raven Press)

82. Crampton, J., Gibbons, L.C. and Rees, W.D.W. (1986). Effect of acid on bicarbonate secretion by the stomach in man: evidence for an autoregulatory reflex. *Gut*, **27**(5), A592

83. Winship, D.H. and Robinson, J.E. (1974). Acid loss in human duodenum. Volume change, osmolal loss and CO_2 production in response to acid loads. *Gastroenterology*, **66**, 181–8

84. Selling, J.A., Hogan, D.L., Koss, M.A. and Isenberg, J.I. (1985). Human proximal versus distal duodenal bicarbonate secretion: effect of endogenous prostaglandin synthesis. *Gastroenterology*, **8**(5), 1580 (Abstract)

85. Cross, C.E., Halliwell, B. and Allen, A. (1984). Antioxidant protection: a function of tracheobronchial and gastrointestinal mucus. *Lancet*, **i**, 1328

86. Smith, G.W., Tasman-Jones, C., Wiggins, P.M. and Lee, S.P. (1985). Pig gastric mucus: a one-way barrier for H^+. *Gastroenterology*, **89**, 1313–18

87. Hills, B.A., Butler, B.D. and Lichtenberger, L.M. (1983). Gastric mucosal barrier: hydrophobic lining to the lumen of the stomach. *Am. J. Physiol.*, **244** (*Gastrointest. Liver Physiol.*, 7), G561–G568

88. Svanes, K., Ito, S., Takeuchi, K. and Silen, W. (1982). Restitution of the surface epithelium of the *in vitro* frog gastric mucosa after damage with hyperosmolar sodium chloride. *Gastroenterology*, **83**, 1409–26

89. Wallace, J.L. and Whittle, B.J.R. (1986). Role of mucus in the repair of gastric epithelial damage in the rat. *Gastroenterology*, **91**, 603–11

90. Leung, F.W., Itoh, M., Hirabayashi, K. and Guth, P.H. (1985). Role of blood flow in gastric and duodenal mucosal injury in the rat. *Gastroenterology*, **88**, 281–9

91. Miller, T.A. (1983). Protective effects of prostaglandins against gastric mucosal damage: current knowledge and proposed mechanisms. *Am. J. Physiol.*, **245** (*Gastrointest. Liver Physiol.*, **8**), G601–G623

92. Flemström, G. and Kivilaakso, E. (1983). Demonstration of a pH gradient at the luminal surface of rat duodenum *in vivo* and its dependence on mucosal alkaline secretion. *Gastroenterology*, **84**, 787–94

93. Robert, A. (1981). Prostaglandins and the gastrointestinal tract. In Johnson L.R., Christensen, J., Grossman, M.I., *et al.* (eds) *Physiology of the Gastrointestinal Tract*, pp. 1407–34. (New York: Raven Press)

94. Crampton, J.R., Gibbons, L.C. and Rees, W.D.W. (1985). Comparison of the effects of indomethacin and fenbufen on gastric secretion of bicarbonate in man. *Gastroenterology*, **90**(5), 1382

95. Feldman, M. and Barnett, C.C. (1985). Gastric bicarbonate secretion in patients with duodenal ulcer. *Gastroenterology*, **88**, 1205–8

96. Isenberg, J.I., Selling, J.A., Hogan, D.L., Thomas, F.J. and Koss, M.A. (1986). Duodenal ulcer patients have impaired proximal duodenal mucosal bicarbonate secretion. *Gastroenterology*, **90**(5), 1472

97. Flemström, G. and Mattsson, H. (1986). Effect of omeprazole on gastric and duodenal bicarbonate secretion. *Scand. J. Gastroenterol*, **21**, (Suppl. 118), 65–7

98. Rees, W.D.W., Garner, A., Heylings, J.R. and Flemström, G. (1981). Effect of carbenoxolone on alkaline secretion by isolated amphibian gastric and duodenal mucosa. *Eur. J. Clin. Invest.*, **11**, 481–6

99. Guth, P.H. (1980). Gastric mucosal blood flow and resistance to injury. In Holtermuller, K.H. and Malagelada, J.R. (eds) *Advances in Ulcer Disease*, pp. 101–9. (Amsterdam: Excerpta Medica)

100. Lauritsen, K., Laursen, L.S., Havelund, T., Bytzer, P., Svendsen, L.B. and Rask-Madsen, J. (1986). Enprostil and ranitidine in duodenal ulcer healing: double-blind comparative trial. *Br. Med. J.*, **292**, 864–6

101. Hawkey, C.J. and Rampton, D.S. (1985). Prostaglandins and the gastrointestinal mucosa: are they important in its function, disease or treatment? *Gastroenterology*, **89**, 1162–88

102. Cohen, M.M., Clark, L., Armstrong, L. and D'Souza, J. (1985). Reduction of aspirin-induced faecal blood loss and low-dose misoprostil tablets in man. *Dig. Dis. Sci.*, **30**(7), 605–11

103. Crampton, J.R., Gibbons, L.C. and Rees, W.D.W. (1986). Sucralfate produces a dose-dependent increase in PGE$_2$ synthesis by mammalian gastric and duodenal mucosa. *Gut*, **27**(5), A606

104. Crampton, J.R., Gibbons, L.C. and Rees, W.D.W. (1985). Effect of sucralfate on isolated amphibian gastroduodenal bicarbonate secretion. *Gut*, **26**(10), A1119

105. Crampton, J.R., Gibbons, L.C. and Rees, W.D.W. (1986). Effect of certain ulcer healing agents on amphibian gastroduodenal bicarbonate secretion. *Scand. J. Gastroenterol.*, **21**, 113–16

106. Crampton, J.R., Gibbons, L.C. and Rees, W.D.W. (1985). Effect of aluminium on bicarbonate secretion by isolated amphibian gastroduodenal mucosa. *Gut*, **26**, A1150

107. Domschke, W., Domschke, S. and Hagel, J. (1977). Gastric epithelial cell turnover, mucus production and healing of ulcers with carbenoxolone. *Gut*, **18**, 817–20

8
Rapid epithelial restitution of the superficially-damaged gastric mucosa

E. R. LACY

Studies begun in the 1950s and 1960s[1-5] elucidated some of the mechanisms by which extremely steep ionic gradients could be maintained across the gastric mucosa. The concept of the 'gastric mucosal barrier' was developed during this time from physiological experiments which showed that luminally-applied agents such as bile acids, various alcohols, hypertonic solutions and salicylates increased gastric mucosal permeability but also often resulted in frank bleeding into the gastric lumen[6-8]. Under these conditions which broke the barrier, there was a rapid back diffusion of hydrogen ions from the gastric lumen into the tissue and a concomitant loss of tissue sodium ions. From these studies, a feed forward loop was hypothesized which suggested that acid back diffusion not only resulted in tissue damage but indirectly stimulated parietal cells to secrete more acid into the lumen which initiated additional cycles of this loop[9]. While there is substantial experimental evidence to verify each component of this model, the cause and effect relationship between breaks in the gastric mucosal barrier and the development of gastric erosions is not understood[6]. Until recently there has not been sufficient data from which to postulate a mechanism by which this feed forward cycle (acid back diffusion, tissue damage, parietal cell stimulation, acid secretion) could be terminated. This in turn has put emphasis on the prophylactic aspects of gastric mucosal defence while little attention has been focused on the reparative aspects of the damaged barrier.

It therefore appeared logical to define the morphological and physiological limits of the gastric mucosal barrier and the conditions (or agents) which would compromise this barrier. The scientific literature is now replete with physiological data concerning the strengths, times, and doses of various agents which increase gastric mucosal permeability or, in the current scientific vernacular, 'break the gastric mucosal barrier'[6]. It was within this context that the concept of prostaglandin-mediated 'cytoprotection' was enthusiastically received[10-13]. The phenomenon of gastric 'cytoprotection' was originally defined from gross observations of rat gastric mucosae exposed to various necrotizing agents (which were commonly termed 'barrier breakers') with and without prior treatment with a prostaglandin[12]. Pretreatment with an extremely low dose of one of a number of different prostaglandins (PGs) or prostaglandin analogs reduced or eliminated macroscopic haemorrhagic lesions present in stomachs receiving only the necrotizing agent (e.g. absolute ethanol). It was assumed that the absence of macroscopic lesions in the PG pretreatment group was synonymous with an undamaged mucosa and the gastric mucosal barrier had under these circumstances not been broken[10-13]. Further extensions of these assumptions concluded that the epithelial cells themselves had been protected by the PG pretreatment[10-13]. Both gross observations and histological analysis have repeatedly confirmed Robert and colleagues' observations[10-12] that PG pretreatment does indeed protect the gastric mucosa from grossly visible haemorrhagic lesions. Contrary to general belief, however, microscopic analysis showed that the gastric mucosal barrier was not preserved since the superficial epithelium had been extensively damaged[14-20]. However, quantitative light microscopical analysis of PG-pretreated mucosa subjected to absolute ethanol challenge showed that the depth to which the damage extended into the tissue was reduced when compared to the mucosa of rats challenged with absolute ethanol only[14]. These findings showed that while PG did not completely protect the mucosa from damage as originally assumed, these fatty-acid derivatives protected against gross haemorrhagic lesions as well as lessening the severity of the damage in regions of the stomach that grossly appeared normal[14].

The studies described above confirmed observations first made in the 1940s concerning the nature of luminally-induced gastric damage[21]. Histologically, there appear to be two different types of damage that result from exposure of the gastric mucosa to full-strength necrotizing agents such as absolute ethanol[22]. Linear haemorrhagic lesions are focal regions where there is extensive damage deep into the parenchyma with associated accumulations of red blood cells (haemostasis and haemorrhage), extracellular haemoglobin, and platelets[23-30]. The superficial as well as the glandular epithelium in these areas is also damaged. This grossly-visible type of lesion is repaired in a lengthy process of cellular mitosis and rebuilding of the connective tissue matrix and vasculature[24-26,28,31,32]. The term 'healing' is appropriate in this case because of the fully-developed inflammatory response and the stages of subsequent tissue repair.

The other type of damage is limited to the superficial mucosa and does not exhibit macroscopic haemorrhage[21,27,29,30,33–42]. Histologically, there is minimal extravasation of erythrocytes or haemolysis, although endothelial cell damage is present. This type of damage can be found in grossly normal-appearing regions of the ethanol-challenged stomach (between haemorrhagic lesions) or throughout the surface of stomachs pretreated with PG and subsequently challenged with a necrotic agent[22]. Recently, it has been shown that damage to the interfoveolar and upper gastric pit epithelium is rapidly repaired by active migration of mucous cells which line the deeper walls of the gastric pits[30,37,39,41]. This process occurs in the *in vitro* amphibian[41] and guinea pig[39] gastric mucosa within hours and in the *in vivo* rat stomach within minutes[30,37]. The term 'rapid epithelial restitution' has been used to describe this phenomenon because of its independence from a circulatory (inflammatory) response, as evidenced from the *in vitro* studies, the speed at which the mucosal surface is re-epithelialized, and the fact that it is a process of cell migration and not cell replication (mitosis)[40]. The process of rapid epithelial restitution of the damaged mucosal surface occurs in an orderly sequence of events which are described below.

STAGES IN RAPID EPITHELIAL RESTITUTION

1. Epithelial necrosis

Figures 8.1 to 8.3 show a normal rat gastric mucosa and the cytological damage induced *in vivo* by an exposure to absolute ethanol for less than one minute which produces superficial damage only. Within 30 sec after exposure to the ethanol, the interfoveolar and upper gastric pit cells are severely damaged (Figure 8.3). The apical plasma membrane of these mucous cells is broken to varying degrees and much of the intracellular contents have leaked out (Figure 8.4). Many of the membranes around the mucous granules rupture, spilling their contents into the cell and the gastric lumen. Surprisingly, however, in ethanol-, aspirin- and salicylate-treated gastric mucosa the zonula occludentes (tight junctions) between adjacent cells remain intact and appear ultrastructurally 'normal' by transmission electron microscopy (Figure 8.4). This is contrary to the damage by luminal hypertonic urea in which there are characteristic blebs within the strands of the tight junctional complex, as observed in mouse stomachs[43]. After ethanol exposure (Figure 8.3), more of the basolateral plasma membrane than its apical counterpart remains intact, thus allowing visualization of the cell outline. The cytoplasmic matrix is largely extracted and the organelles appear severely damaged to the point of being unrecognizable. However, the nucleus remains visible but the chromatin is clumped. In the

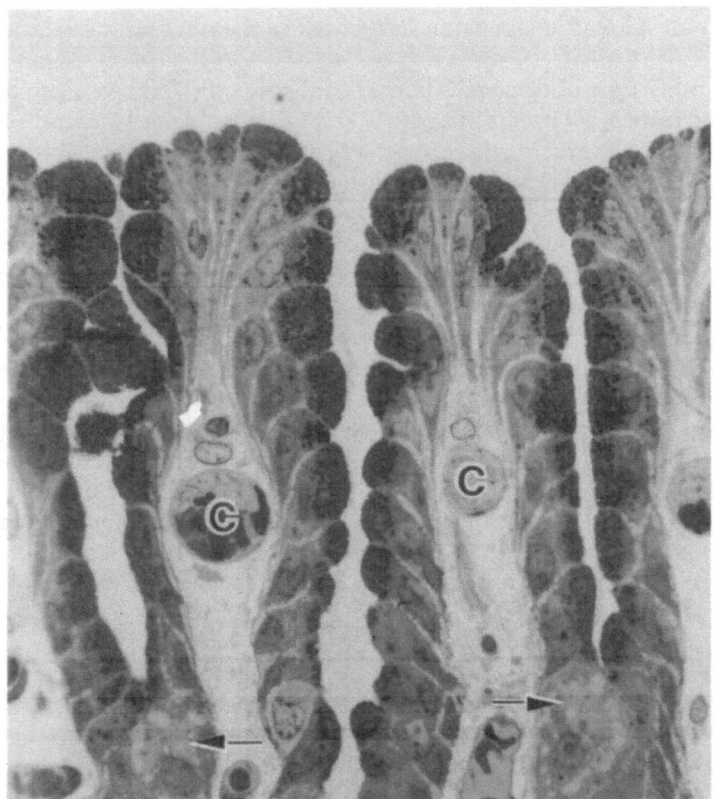

Figure 8.1 Photomicrograph of normal superficial mucosa of the rat. The gastric pits and the interfoveolar regions are lined by mucous cells. Arrows indicate parietal cells demarcating the upper border of the gastric glands. C, capillaries. × 780

gastric pits the expelled contents of apposing mucous cells form a necrotic mass which occludes the gastric pit opening (Figure 8.3).

2. Exfoliation

The process of exfoliation of the necrotic epithelium begins as early as 30 sec after ethanol exposure *in vivo* as the interfoveolar and upper gastric pit cells lift off the underlying basal lamina. As Figure 8.3 shows, however, the necrotic epithelium at this time is still attached to the viable-appearing cells deeper in the gastric pits. At least morphologically, the damage does not appear to be graded in its severity from the lumen towards the gastric glands. Figure 8.3 illustrates the deepest penetration of the ethanol-induced damage as deter-

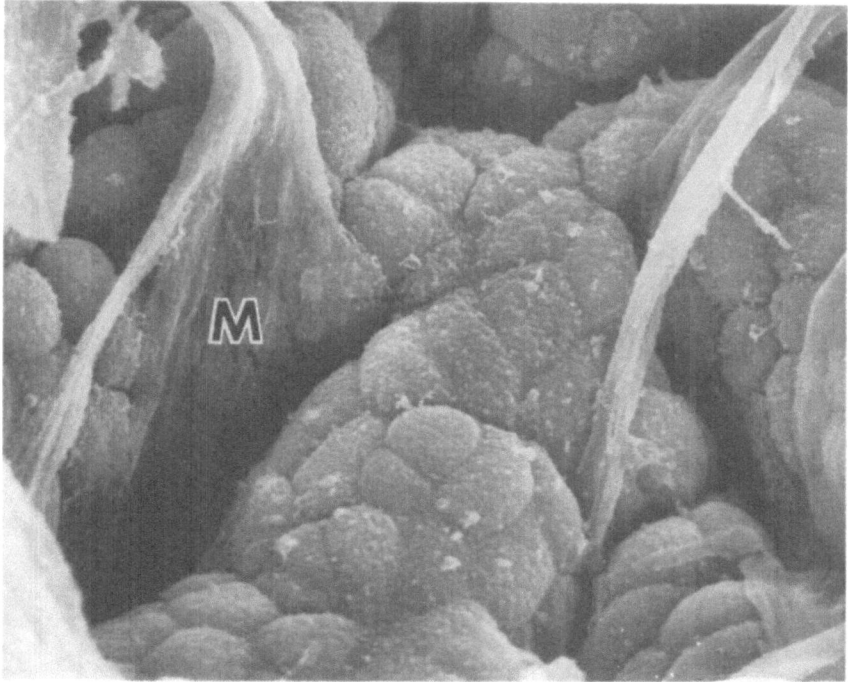

Figure 8.2 Scanning electron micrograph of normal rat gastric mucosa showing interfoveolar and upper gastric pit mucous cells. Mucus (M) extends from gastric pits into the lumen. × 1740

mined by light microscopy. By three minutes after ethanol exposure, the necrotic cells have broken away from the underlying viable cells (Figure 8.5). In the *in vitro* frog preparation, a thick, fluffy layer of dead cells and mucus (detached from the mucosa) develops approximately 30 min after exposure to hypertonic sodium chloride[41]. The close proximity of epithelial cells lining the upper portion of adjacent gastric pits, their outward exfoliation from the basal lamina, and the intermingling of their mucus and cytoplasmic contents account for the formation of a single mucoid necrotic epithelial layer over the damaged mucosa (Figure 8.3). Transmission electron microscopy has shown that the newly formed space between the necrotic epithelial sheet and the underlying basal lamina is filled with a homogeneously, finely-textured substance similar to that in the adjacent capillaries, suggesting its vascular origin. Furthermore, fibrin has consistently been observed in this region[27,30]. Subsequent analysis has verified that this material consists in part of plasma albumin[44,45]. In addition, there were remnants of plasma membrane from the exfoliated mucous cells as well as recognizable cells themselves which occasionally remain attached

167

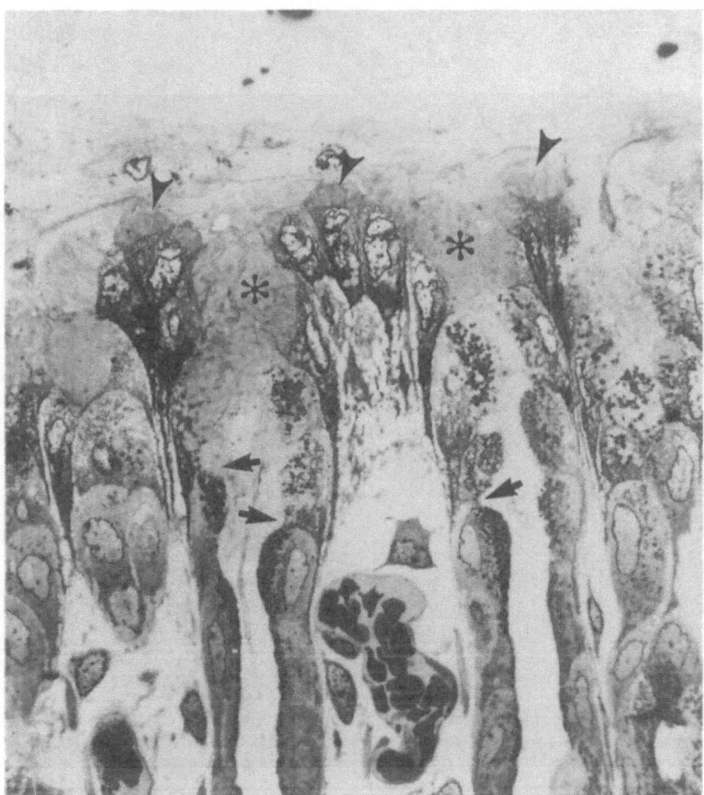

Figure 8.3 Photomicrograph of rat superficial gastric mucosa after exposure to absolute ethanol for 30 sec. The interfoveolar and upper gastric pit epithelial cells are necrotic. Arrowheads indicate superficial epithelial cells which have cellular contents spilling into gastric lumen. Contents from ruptured cells in each gastric pit coalesce to form a plug (asterisks) which is in lateral continuity with the necrotic superficial mucous cells. Arrows indicate the depth of damage. Mucous cells below arrows appear morphologically intact. × 780

to the basal lamina as the necrotic epithelial sheet lifted off. The juxtaposition of this exfoliated mucoid layer between the gastric lumen and the damaged surface appears to facilitate rapid epithelial restitution of the mucosal surface, as will be discussed below.

3. Re-epithelialization by cellular migration

Physiological studies of gastric mucosae mounted in Ussing-type chambers or gastric pouches and subsequently exposed to luminal 'barrier breakers'

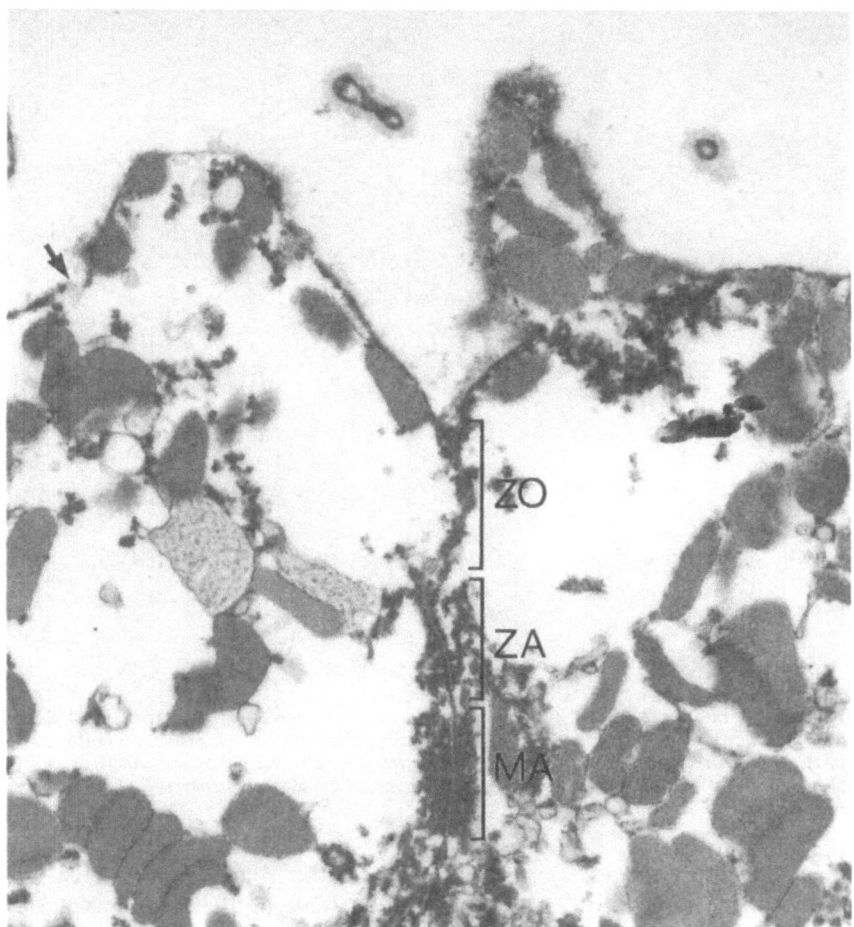

Figure 8.4 Transmission electron micrograph of junctional region of two adjacent necrotic cells which have exfoliated into the gastric lumen. Note the varying thickness of the apical plasma membrane which has some accumulations of a densely-stained fuzzy material as well as discrete breaks (arrow). The junctional complex remains intact: ZO = zonula occludens (tight junction), ZA = zonula adherens (intermediate junction), MA = macula adherens (desmosome). The cytoplasm is extracted except for numerous uniformly dense bodies with segments of membrane around them. × 18,650

have shown a significant reduction in the transmucosal potential difference[17,39,41,46-49]. Electrical signs of mucosal recovery were noted as early as 10 min after the initial insult[17,39], suggesting an extremely rapid process of repair. This is followed by a continued return of the potential difference

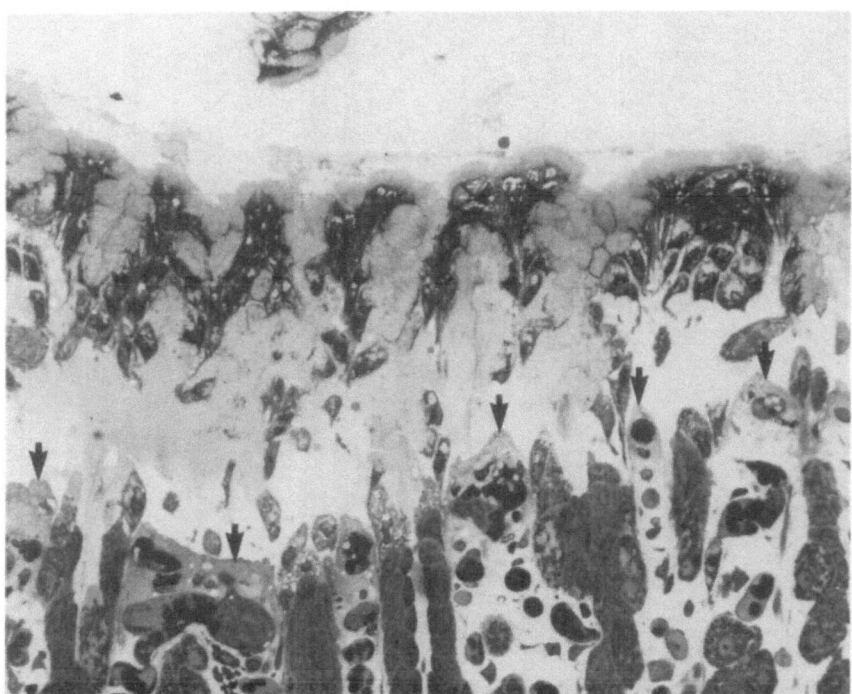

Figure 8.5 Photomicrograph of rat gastric mucosa 3 min after exposure to luminal ethanol (absolute). The interfoveolar and upper gastric pit epithelium has exfoliated into the gastric lumen. Adjacent necrotic tissue has fused to form a single mucoid mass which covers the damaged mucosal surface. Arrows indicate the denuded basal lamina between adjacent gastric pits. × 320

towards control values, as monitored 30 min to several hours later. This recovery was verified by histological analyses showing that a notable amount of the damaged surface was re-covered with flattened epithelial cells migrating from deeper within the gastric pits[27,30,37,39–42]. This short time course for repair obviated cell replacement by mitosis as the mechanism for renewal of the epithelial surface. Further evidence for the speed of this process in the rat came from morphometric analysis which showed that 15 min after the superficial epithelium had been destroyed (98% of the gastric surface area), almost one-half of the damaged surface had been re-populated with migrating cells. By one hour later, nearly 95% of the mucosal surface was re-epithelialized[37]. Sixty to ninety minutes post-insult in the frog, there was evidence of cell migration which continued for two to four hours[41].

The cells responsible for epithelial restitution were the viable mucous neck cells positioned along the gastric pits. The intervening basal lamina was initially

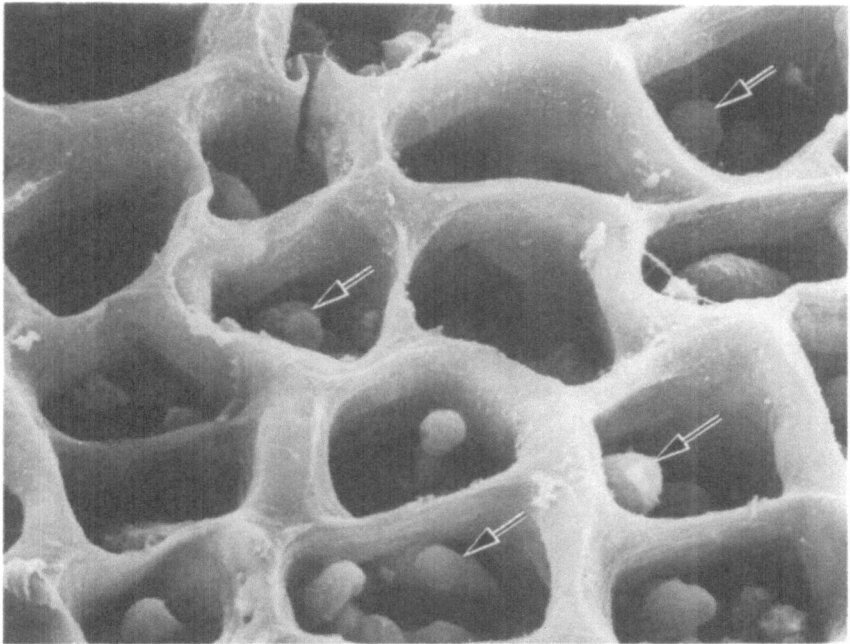

Figure 8.6 Scanning electron micrograph of rat gastric mucosa 3 min after ethanol exposure showing superficial basal lamina denuded of epithelial cells. The overlying necrotic mucoid layer (Figure 8.5) has been physically removed to obtain this view. Viable mucous cells remain deep in the gastric pit (arrows). × 900

devoid of epithelial cells which had exfoliated into the gastric lumen (Figures 8.5 and 8.6). As early as three minutes after ethanol administration in the rat, the first morphological signs of restitution were observed. A few low cuboidal mucous cells in the gastric pits rapidly changed their morphology and extended large, flat extensions of their free surface, called lamellipodia, over the denuded basal lamina as shown in Figures 8.7 to 8.9. Parietal cells were never observed to have lamellipodia or to actively migrate, although they were occasionally pulled onto the surface by the migrating epithelial sheet[30,37]. In addition, migrating cells projected some long cylindrical filopodia from their free surface.

The lamellipodia were most consistently devoid of mucous granules and mitochondria but did contain microfilaments and occasionally endoplasmic reticulum (Figure 8.9). These filaments are most likely actin and associated proteins which are characteristically present in the leading edge of migrating cells in culture[50,51]. Further evidence comes from studies of rat and frog restituting mucosae in which the potent microfilament disrupting drug, cytochalasin (B or D), inhibits gastric mucous cell migration[37,42]. Transmission

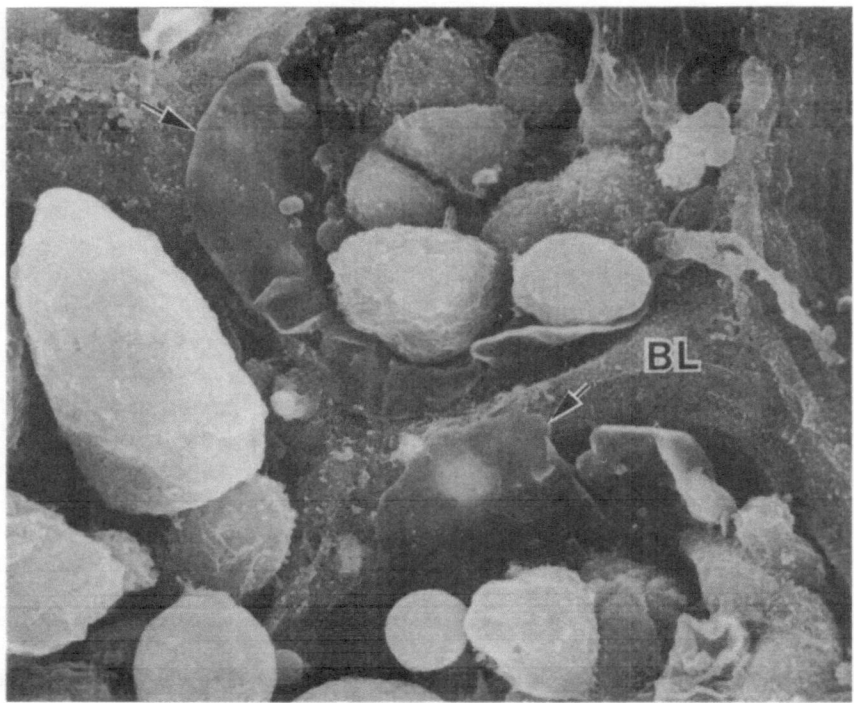

Figure 8.7 Scanning electron micrograph of rat gastric mucosa approximately 15 min after exposure to ethanol. The viable epithelial cells in the gastric pits shown in Figure 8.6 have extended lamellipodia (arrows) and are migrating across the basal lamina (BL). × 2500

electron microscopy has shown that application of cytochalasin D to the damaged rat mucosa inhibits the formation of lamellipodia (thus restitution) and causes large membrane-bound vacuoles to form within the mucous cells at the edge of the viable epithelium[37]. Microtubule-disrupting drugs such as nocodozole did not affect the morphological sequence of the restituting epithelium in the rat[37]. In the bullfrog, however, Svanes and colleagues found that colchicine added to the nutrient solution (blood side) of damaged mucosal preparations in the Ussing chamber caused a rapid stimulation of H^+ secretion and an inhibition in the normal post-injury rise in potential difference and resistance[41]. The histology of the frog mucosal preparations did not differ from controls in which the mucous cells extended lamellipodia and migrated as described above[41].

Indirect evidence has suggested that the presence of a relatively intact basal lamina is necessary for the migration of these epithelial cells during restitution[52]. Ultrastructural studies showed that hydrochloric acid in the gastric lumen after

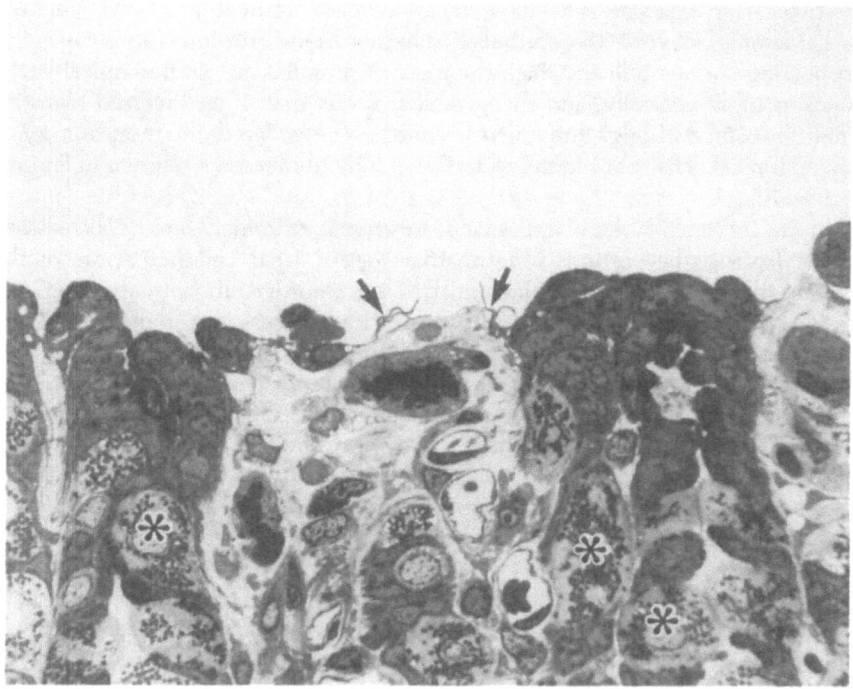

Figure 8.8 Photomicrograph of rat gastric mucosa approximately 15 min after ethanol exposure. Migrating mucous cells have extended lamellipodia (arrows). Asterisks indicate parietal cells. Note the hemostasis in the superficial capillaries which are filled with platelets and erythrocytes. × 780

the initial ethanol insult resulted in dissolution of the exposed basal lamina with swelling and solubilization of the underlying collagen fibrils[30,53]. Under these conditions, the viable epithelial cells in the gastric pits were unable to migrate and re-cover the denuded basal lamina[53]. Furthermore, we have noted that after ethanol exposure there are occasional patches where the lamina propria was directly exposed to the lumen because the basal lamina had been destroyed. Electron micrographs showed lamellipodia did not readily cover this exposed area of the connective tissue matrix.

As lamellipodia meet, they form intercellular junctions in the process of re-epithelializing the mucosal surface. Tight junctions between newly-occluded lamellipodia were observed as early as 30 min after damage[37]. Svanes and co-workers[41] showed that tight junction formation of restituting bullfrog mucosa was dependent upon the presence of Ca^{2+} in the bathing medium[42]. At present, we are unable to define any further conditions which dictate the mechanism or location of tight-junction formation in this newly-forming epithelium.

173

Once the adjacent cells have made contact, formed junctions, and the basal lamina covered, the epithelial cells then transform into more typically-appearing surface cells in which the mucous granules are located apically, the nucleus more centrally, and the overall shape is that of an inverted teardrop (Figure 8.10). Although the mucosal surface is re-covered, the morphology of the epithelial cells is not identical to the uninjured mucosa as shown in Figures 8.1 and 8.10.

In the rat, the process of epithelial restitution is extremely rapid. Calculations made from tissue sections indicate that these gastric cells are some of the fastest migrating cells (1–6 μm/min)[21,37] yet recorded. In both the frog and guinea pig *in vitro* studies[39,41], the restitution process was morphologically similar to that described for the rat[30,37] but also substantially slower. The stripped guinea-pig mucosal preparation in Ussing chambers[39] subjected to hypertonic NaCl showed an initial drop in the potential difference which started to recover after 30 min and was back to normal after two hours. The concomitant morphological studies showed that by 30 min, the guinea-pig gastric mucosal epithelium had significantly restituted[39]. Likewise, studies of *ex vivo* rat stomachs[17,30] showed a rise in potential difference 10 min after the mucosa was subjected to 40% ethanol. At 60 min later, the potential difference had returned to about one-half the control value while morphologically there was considerable epithelial restitution. The failure of the potential difference to return to control levels probably reflects the observation that haemorrhagic lesions (which heal much slower) were produced by the ethanol and subsequent HCl exposure. As pointed out on p. 164, deep vasocongestion (particularly with subsequent acid exposure) causes severe damage that is not rapidly restituted as opposed to damage confined to the superficial mucosa.

The study of rapid epithelial restitution is comparatively young and conditions which alter the process are just beginning to be understood. Some factors which are necessary for optimal restitution include an intact basal lamina, presence of free calcium, and a functional microfilament network in the lamellipodia. There have been reports of accelerated epithelial restitution in mucosa pretreated with prostaglandins before an ethanol challenge[28,54]. Although these studies implicate prostaglandins as having a direct effect on the speed of the migrating epithelial cells, there is a caveat to this conclusion. It has been shown histologically that prostaglandin pretreatment of rat gastric mucosa results in significantly shallower damage to the gastric mucosa than the untreated controls[14]. It seems reasonable to expect that if the epithelial cells of both groups (prostaglandin pretreated and the untreated controls) migrate at the same speed, then the cells positioned nearer to each other (the prostaglandin pretreated group) will meet, form junctions, and re-establish the epithelium faster than the cells which were initially farther apart. Studies to

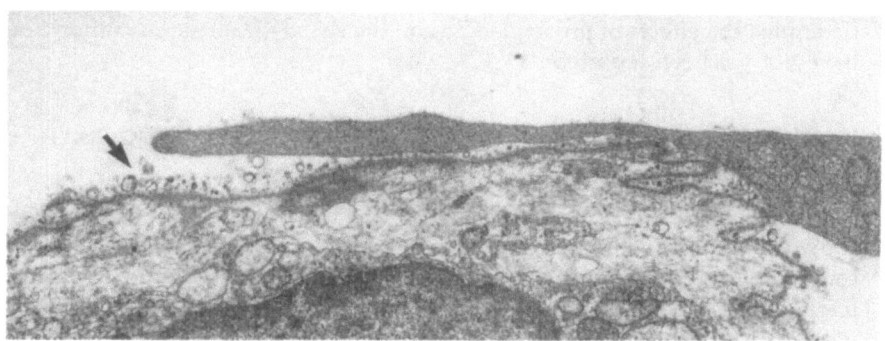

Figure 8.9 Transmission electron micrograph showing the leading edge of a lamellipodium (note the more distal position of the mitochondria located at the far right of the micrograph) extending over the basal lamina which has some necrotic debris still attached (arrow). × 8820

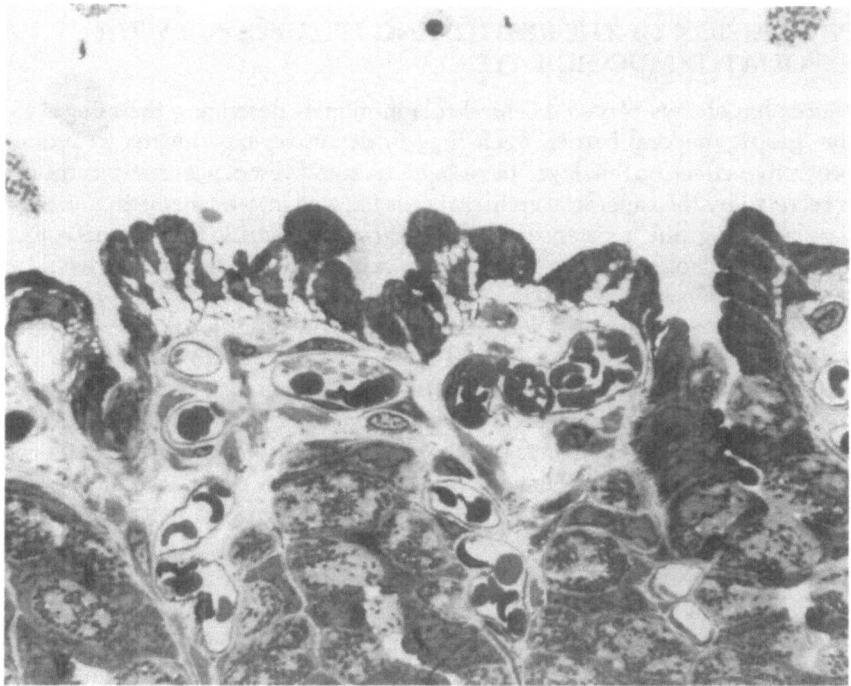

Figure 8.10 Photomicrograph of superficial rat gastric epithelium approximately 60 min after ethanol exposure. The surface is now re-epithelialized with irregularly-shaped mucous cells which have formed intercellular junctions. × 780

determine the effects of prostaglandins on the speed of cellular migration itself have not yet been reported.

RAPID EPITHELIAL RESTITUTION AND REPEATED MUCOSAL CHALLENGE

Studies utilizing physiological parameters to access mucosal integrity have shown that repeated doses of necrotizing agents such as ethanol and aspirin cause a progressive mucosal resistance to subsequent damage[55-60]. These findings are contrary to histological and ultrastructural reports of rat stomachs which were exposed to repeated doses of concentrated ethanol. These latter studies showed severely-damaged mucosae after each ethanol challenge[47,61]. At present, there is only speculation to explain the divergent results from these two groups of data. It seems clear that simultaneous physiological and morphological studies on the same mucosa are necessary to understand the various factors involved in repeated damage and repair processes.

PROTECTION OF THE RESTITUTING EPITHELIUM BY THE EXFOLIATED MUCOID LAYER

Mucus has always played a central role in models describing the integrity of the 'gastric mucosal barrier' even though definitive experiments to prove a protective effect of this layer have been elusive[62]. Evidence that bicarbonate is secreted by the superficial epithelial cells fits well into a scheme that includes data showing the existence of a pH gradient across the normal mucus layer[63-66]. Teleologically in this scheme, acid in the gastric lumen would be retarded by the alkaline sink next to the epithelial cells.

Recent morphological evidence challenges the traditional role of gastric mucus since observations of normal rat gastric mucosa do not show a continuous protective mucus sheet over the superficial epithelial cells[67]. Rat gastric mucus appears as ropes and strands which emanate from mucous cells in the gastric pits, isthmus and glands but not typically from the interfoveolar mucous cells[67], as illustrated in Figure 8.2. Increasing evidence suggests that one of the primary functions of gastric mucus may be in the protection it affords to the rapidly restituting epithelium[52]. As explained above, damage to the superficial mucosa results in exfoliation of the superficial epithelium as a single sheet cemented together by the expelled mucus. This layer consists of recognizable necrotic epithelial cells, some blood components, and extracellular mucus. It has been called a mucus cap[67], a gelatinous layer[61], or a mucoid layer[52]. To test the hypothesis that this layer was protective, rat stomachs which had previously been subjected to a superficially-damaging exposure of ethanol were allowed to restitute and were re-challenged with a rapid exposure (30 sec)

176

to absolute ethanol[61]. Animals in which the mucoid layer had been physically removed before the second ethanol challenge had extensive damage to the superficial mucosa. Those rats in which the mucoid layer was not removed had no additional damage to the restituted mucosa[61]. These findings were subsequently corroborated by studies showing that the mucolytic agents, pepsin and N-acetylcysteine, applied to the mucoid layer before application of hydrochloric acid, inhibited the restitution process[45]. It appears likely from the microscopic studies of rat gastric mucosa that the exfoliated mucous cells (and contents) may protect the underlying mucosa under more normal, physiological situations encountered during the ingestion of drugs such as aspirin as well as a variety of noxious foods and drink.

These studies present an alternative view to the classical role that mucus plays in gastric mucosal protection. In the present scheme, mucus (and the associated cellular debris plus plasma components) forms a formidable barrier to luminal contents *after* superficial damage and has little if any protective role *before* the insult.

PLASMA SHEDDING

Concomitant with epithelial exfoliation after superficial injury, there is an outpouring of alkaline fluid into the lumen[19,61]. Davenport[8,9] called this phenomenon 'plasma shedding' which probably represents no more than a gastric version of the initial (inflammatory) response to injury: increased capillary permeability, observed in numerous other tissues. The vascular origin of this alkaline fluid is corroborated by the increased amounts of labelled albumin found in gastric juice after damage[9,44,45]. This response to superficial injury would appear to dilute noxious agents in the gastric lumen, preventing their rapid penetration into the mucosa, but also would provide an optimal alkaline environment with abundant plasma nutrients for epithelial restitution[27,61,68,69].

FUTURE PROSPECTS

Rapid epithelial restitution offers a new avenue into the study of the etiology of gastric erosions. It can no longer be assumed that breaks in the gastric mucosal barrier initiate a series of deleterious consequences that irreversibly lead to pathological conditions. It can now be hypothetized that gastritis and gastric erosions may in fact be due to an initial failure of the mucosa to rapidly restitute and not to rupture of the gastric mucosal barrier. It appears paramount for future studies to define the limits and the cellular basis for this restitution process. Pertinent problems include defining the biochemical dynamics of such extraordinarily rapid changes in cell shape during migration, the role of the basal lamina and its interaction with the lamellipodia, the *de novo* formation of tight junctions, and the role of mucus and bicarbonate in restitution. Pathological conditions which alter restitution would further our understanding of the process. Based on morphological and physiological similarities with laboratory animals, there is reason to believe that restitution also occurs in humans. Unfortunately, we have no data to confirm this hypothesis.

ACKNOWLEDGEMENTS

The excellent technical assistance of Ms K. Cowart and Ms M. Hinson is gratefully acknowledged. This work was supported in part by a grant from the National Institutes of Health AM06345.

References

1. Davenport, H.W. (1964). Gastric mucosal injury by fatty and acetylsalicylic acids. *Gastroenterology*, **46**, 245–53
2. Davenport, H.W., Warner, H.A. and Code, C.F. (1964). Functional significance of gastric mucosal barrier to sodium. *Gastroenterology*, **47**, 142–52
3. Code, C.F., Scholer, J.F. and Orvis, A.L. (1955). Barrier offered by gastric mucosa to absorption of sodium. *Am. J. Physiol.*, **183**, 604
4. Davenport, H.W. (1965). Damage to the gastric mucosa: effects of salicylate and stimulation. *Gastroenterology*, **49**, 189–96
5. Davenport, H.W. (1967). Ethanol damage to canine oxyntic glandular mucosa. *Soc. Exp. Biol. Med.*, **126**, 657–62
6. Fromm, D. (1981). Gastric mucosal barrier: In Johnson, L.R. (ed.) *Physiology of the Gastrointestinal Tract*, pp. 733–48. (New York: Raven Press)
7. Davenport, H.W. (1970). Backdiffusion of acid through the gastric mucosa and its physiological consequences. In Glass, G.B.J. (ed.) *Progress in Gastroenterology*, p. 48. (New York: Grune and Stratton)
8. Davenport, H.W. (1974). Plasma protein shedding by the canine oxyntic glandular mucosa induced by topical application of snake venom and ethanol. *Gastroenterology*, **67**, 264–70
9. Davenport, H.W. (1966). Fluid produced by the gastric mucosa during damage by acetic and salicylic acids. *Gastroenterology*, **50**, 487–99
10. Robert, A. (1975). Antisecretory, anti-ulcer, cytoprotective and diarrheogenic properties of prostaglandins. *Adv. Prostaglandin Thromboxane Res.*, **2**, 507–20
11. Robert, A. (1979). Cytoprotection by prostaglandins. *Gastroenterology*, **77**, 761–7
12. Robert, A., Nezamis, J.E., Lancaster, C. and Hanchar, A.J. (1979). Cytoprotection by prostaglandins in rats. Prevention of gastric necrosis produced by alcohol, HCl, NaOH, hypertonic NaCl and thermal injury. *Gastroenterology*, **77**, 433–43
13. Miller, T.A. (1983). Protective effects of prostaglandins against gastric mucosal damage: current knowledge and proposed mechanisms. *Am. J. Physiol.*, **245**, G601–23
14. Lacy, E.R. and Ito, S. (1982). Microscopic analysis of ethanol damage to rat gastric mucosa after treatment with a prostaglandin. *Gastroenterology*, **83**, 619–25
15. Lacy, E.R. and Ito, S. (1984). Ethanol-induced insult to the superficial rat gastric epithelium: a study of damage and rapid repair. In Allen, A., Flemström, G., Garner, A., Silen W. and Turnberg, L.A. (eds) *Mechanisms of Mucosal Protection in the Upper Gastrointestinal Tract*, pp. 49–56. (New York: Raven Press)
16. Guth, P.H., Paulsen, G. and Nagata, H. (1984). Histologic and microcirculatory changes in alcohol-induced gastric lesions in the rat: effect of prostaglandin cytoprotection. *Gastroenterology*, **87**, 1083–90

17. Wallace, J.L., Morris, G.P., Krausse, E.J. and Greaves, S.E. (1982). Reduction by cyto-protective agents of ethanol-induced damage to the rat gastric mucosa: a correlated morphological and physiological study. *Can. J. Physiol. Pharmacol.*, **60**, 1688–99
18. Ohno, T., Ohtsuki, H. and Okabe, S. (1985). Effect of 16,16-dimethyl prostaglandin E$_2$ on ethanol-induced and aspirin-induced gastric damage in the rat. Scanning electron micro-scopic study. *Gastroenterology*, **88**, 353–61
19. Tarnawski, A., Hollander, D., Stachura, J., Krause, W.J. and Gergely, H. (1985). Prostaglandin protection of the gastric mucosa against alcohol injury – a dynamic time-related process. *Gastroenterology*, **88**, 334–52
20. Whittle, B.J.R. and Steel, G. (1985). Evaluation of the protection of rat gastric mucosa by a prostaglandin analogue using cellular enzyme markers and histologic techniques. *Gastroenterology*, **88**, 315–27
21. Grant, R. (1945). Rate of replacement of the surface epithelial cells of the gastric mucosa. *Anat. Rec.*, **91**, 175–85
22. Lacy, E.R. (1985). Prostaglandins and histological changes in the gastric mucosa. *Dig. Dis. Sci.*, **30**, 83S–94S
23. Duchateau, A., Thiefin, G., Zeithoun, P. and Barzaghi, F. (1983). Hémolyse intra-muqueuse dans la lésion nécrotique gastrique par alcool absolu chez le rat. *Gastroenterol. Clin. Biol.*, **7**, 150–7
24. Lev, R., Kawashima, K. and Glass G.B.J. (1976). Morphological features and healing of stress ulcers induced by alcohol and restraint. *Arch. Pathol. Lab. Med.*, **100**, 554–8
25. Helander, H.F. (1983). Morphological studies on the margin of gastric corpus wounds in the rat. *J. Submicrosc. Cytol.*, **15**, 627–43
26. Blom, H. and Helander, H.F. (1981). Quantitative ultrastructural studies on parietal cell regeneration in experimental ulcers in rat gastric mucosa. *Gastroenterology*, **80**, 334–43
27. Ito, S. and Lacy, E.R. (1985). Morphology of rat gastric mucosal damage, defense, and restitution in the presence of luminal ethanol. *Gastroenterology*, **88**, 250–60
28. Ito, S. and Lacy E.R. (1984). Characteristics of ethanol induced lesions in rat gastric mucosa. In Allen, A., Flemström, G., Garner, A., Silen, W. and Turnberg, L.A. (eds) *Mechanisms of Mucosal Protection in the Upper Gastrointestinal Tract*, pp. 57–63. (New York: Raven Press)
29. Lacy, E.R. (1986). Effects of absolute ethanol, misoprostol, cimetidine, and phosphate buffer on the morphology of rat gastric mucosae. *Dig. Dis. Sci.*, **31**, 101S–7S
30. Morris, G.P. and Wallace, J.L. (1981). The roles of ethanol and of acid in the production of gastric mucosal erosions in rats. *Virchow's Arch. (Cell Pathol.)*, **38**, 23–38
31. Townsend, S.F. (1961). Regeneration of the gastric mucosa in rats. *Am. J. Anat.*, **109**, 133–47
32. Helpap, B., Hattori, T. and Gedigk, P. (1981). Repair of gastric ulcer. A cell kinetic study. *Virchow's Arch. (Pathol. Anat.)*, **392**, 159–70
33. Yeomans, N.D. (1976). Electron microscopic study of the repair of aspirin-induced gastric lesions. *Dig. Dis. Sci.*, **21**, 533–41
34. Hingson, D.J. and Ito, S. (1971). Effect of aspirin and related compounds on the fine structure of mouse gastric mucosa. *Gastroenterology*, **61**, 156–77
35. Yeomans, N.D., St. John D.J.B. and de Boer, W.G.R.M. (1973). Regeneration of gastric mucosa after aspirin-induced injury in the rat. *Dig. Dis. Sci.*, **18**, 773–80
36. Ferguson, A.R. (1928). A cytological study of the regeneration of gastric glands following the experimental removal of large areas of mucosa. *Am. J. Anat.*, **42**, 403–41
37. Lacy, E.R. and Ito, S. (1984). Rapid epithelial restitution of the rat gastric mucosa after ethanol injury. *Lab. Invest.*, **51**(5), 573–83
38. Dinoso, V.P., Ming, S. and McNiff, J. (1976). Ultrastructural changes of the canine gastric mucosa after topical application of graded concentrations of ethanol. *Am. J. Dig. Dis.*, **21**, 626–32
39. Rutten, M.J. and Ito, S. (1983). Morphology and electrophysiology of guinea pig gastric mucosal repair *in vitro*. *Am. J. Physiol.*, **244**, G171–82
40. Ito, S., Lacy, E.R., Rutten, M.J., Critchlow, J. and Silen, W. (1984). Rapid repair of injured gastric mucosa. *Scand. J. Gastroenterol.*, (Suppl. 101), 87–95

179

41. Svanes, K., Ito, S., Takeuchi, K. and Silen, W. (1982). Restitution of the surface epithelium of *in vitro* frog gastric mucosa after damage with hyperosmolar sodium chloride: morphologic and physiologic characteristics. *Gastroenterology*, **82**, 1409–26
42. Critchlow, J., Magee, D., Ito, S., Takeuchi, K. and Silen, W. (1985). Requirements for restitution of the surface epithelium of frog stomach after mucosal injury. *Gastroenterology*, **88**, 237–49
43. Eastwood, G.L. and Kirchner, J.P. (1974). Changes in the fine structure of mouse gastric epithelium produced by ethanol and urea. *Gastroenterology*, **67**, 71–84
44. Szabo, S., Trier, J.S., Brown, A. and Schnoor, J. (1985). Early vascular injury and increased vascular permeability in gastric mucosal injury caused by ethanol in the rat. *Gastroenterology*, **88**, 228–36
45. Wallace, J.L. and Whittle, B.J.R. (1986). Role of mucus in the repair of gastric epithelial damage in the rat. Inhibition of epithelial recovery by mucolytic agents. *Gastroenterology*, **91**, 603–11
46. Svanes, K., Critchlow, J., Takeuchi, K., Magee, D., Ito, S. and Silen, W. (1984). Factors influencing reconstitution of frog gastric mucosa: role of prostaglandins. In Allen, A., Flemström, G., Garner, A., Silen, W. and Turnberg, L.A. (eds) *Mechanisms of Mucosal Protection in the Upper Gastrointestinal Tract*, pp. 33–9. (New York: Raven Press)
47. Dinoso, V.P., Chey, W.Y., Siplet, H. and Lorder, S.H. (1970). Effects of ethanol on the gastric mucosa of the Heidenhain pouch of dogs. *Dig. Dis. Sci.*, **15**, 809–19
48. Biggerstaff, R.J. and Leitch, G.J. (1977). Effects of ethanol on electrical parameters of the *in vivo* rat stomach. *Dig. Dis. Sci.*, **22**, 1064–8
49. Shanbour, L.L. (1980). Effects of alcohol on acid secretion and ion transport in the gastric mucosa. Alcohol and the gastrointestinal tract. *INSERM*, **95**, 390–404
50. Dipasquale, A. (1975). Locomotion of epithelial cells: factors involved in extension of the leading edge. *Exp. Cell Res.*, **95**, 425–39.
51. Allen, R.D. (1981). Cell motility. *J. Cell Biol.*, **91** (suppl.), 148S–55S
52. Lacy, E.R. (1987). Gastric mucosal defense after superficial injury. *Clin. Invest. Med.*, **10**, 189–200
53. Lacy, E.R., Rutten, M.J. and Ito, S. (1983). The role of the basal lamina in gastric mucosa reepithelization after surface cell destruction. *Anat. Rec.*, **205**, 104a
54. Wallace, J.L. and Whittle, B.J.R. (1985). Acceleration of recovery of gastric epithelial integrity by 16,16-dimethyl prostaglandin E_2. *Br. J. Pharmac.*, **86**, 837–42
55. Miller, T.A. and Henagan, J.M. (1984). Indomethacin decreases resistance of gastric barrier to disruption by alcohol. *Dig. Dis. Sci.*, **29**, 141–9
56. Lev, R., Siegel, H.I. and Glass, G.B.J. (1972). Effects of salicylates on the canine stomach: a morphological and histochemical study. *Gastroenterology*, **62**, 970–80
57. Ivey, K.J., Tarnawski, A., Stachura, J., Werner, H., Mach, T. and Burks, M. (1980). The induction of gastric mucosal tolerance to alcohol by chronic administration. *J. Lab. Clin. Med.*, **96**, 922–32
58. Deregnaucourt, J. and Code, C.F. (1979). Increased resistance of the gastric mucosal barrier to barrier breakers in the rat. *Gastroenterology*, **77**, 309–12
59. Bolton, J.P. and Cohen, M.M. (1977). Effect of repeated aspirin administration on the gastric mucosal barrier and cell turnover. *J. Surg. Res.*, **23**, 251–6
60. St. John, D.J.B., Yeomans, N.D., McDermott, F.T. and de Boer, W.G.R.M. (1973). Adaptation of the gastric mucosa to repeated administration of aspirin in the rat. *Dig. Dis. Sci.*, **18**, 881–6
61. Lacy, E.R. (1985). Gastric mucosal resistance to a repeated ethanol insult. *Scand. J. Gastroenterol.*, **20** (Suppl. 110), 63–72
62. Allen, A. (1981). Structure and function of gastrointestinal mucus. In Johnson, L.R. (ed.) *Physiology of the Gastrointestinal Tract*, pp. 617–39. (Raven Press: New York)
63. Kivilaakso, E. and Flemström, G. (1984). Surface pH gradient in gastroduodenal mucosa. *Scand. J. Gastroenterol.*, **19** (Suppl. 105), 50–2
64. Ross, I.N., Bahari, H.M.M. and Turnberg, L.A. (1981). The pH gradient across mucus adherent to rat fundic mucosa *in vivo* and the effect of potential damaging agents. *Gastroenterology*, **81**, 713–8

65. Takeuchi, K.M., Magee, J., Critchlow, J., Matthews, J. and Silen, W. (1983). Studies of the pH gradient and thickness of frog gastric mucus gel. *Gastroenterology*, **84**, 331–40
66. Williams, S.E. and Turnberg, L.A. (1980). Retardation of acid diffusion by pig gastric mucus: a potential role in mucosal protection. *Gastroenterology*, **79**, 299–304
67. Morris, G.P., Harding, R.K. and Wallace, J.L. (1984). A functional model for extracellular gastric mucus in the rat. *Virchow's Arch. (Cell Pathol.)*, **46**, 239–51
68. Takeuchi, K. and Okabe, S. (1983). Role of luminal alkalinization in repair process of ethanol-induced mucosal damage in rat stomach. *Dig. Dis. Sci.*, **28**, 993–1000
69. Svanes, K., Takeuchi, K., Ito, S. and Silen, W. (1983). Effect of luminal pH and nutrient bicarbonate concentration on restitution after gastric surface cell injury. *Surgery*, **94**, 494–500

9
Prostanoids and related mediators in gastric damage and disease

B. J. R. WHITTLE and J. L. WALLACE

INTRODUCTION

Endogenous metabolites of arachidonic acid, formed via the cyclo-oxygenase and lipoxygenase enzymic pathways (Figure 9.1) have been implicated as local mediators or modulators of gastric mucosal function and disease. Prostaglandins of the E and I series, PGE_2 and prostacyclin respectively, are formed by gastric mucosal tissue[1]. These prostanoids can inhibit gastric acid secretion, stimulate gastric bicarbonate and mucus secretion, can induce vasodilation in the mucosal microcirculation and prevent the vascular stasis induced by damaging agents and can affect sodium and chloride ionic flux[2-6]. These prostanoids and their synthetic analogues protect the gastric mucosa from damage, an action which may be brought about by their effects on several of the above parameters[1-6].

Since prostanoids exert such potent actions on gastric function and integrity, it is not surprising that alterations in local prostaglandin formation have been implicated as a mechanism underlying gastric damage and disease. The depletion of endogenous prostanoids by non-steroid anti-inflammatory agents, which directly inhibit the cyclo-oxygenase enzyme, is a likely mechanism contributing to the gastric mucosal damage induced by these drugs, both in experimental models and in their clinical use. Local alterations in prostanoid turnover have also been implicated in the pathogenesis of peptic ulcer disease.

Other arachidonate metabolites (or eicosanoids) may be involved in the

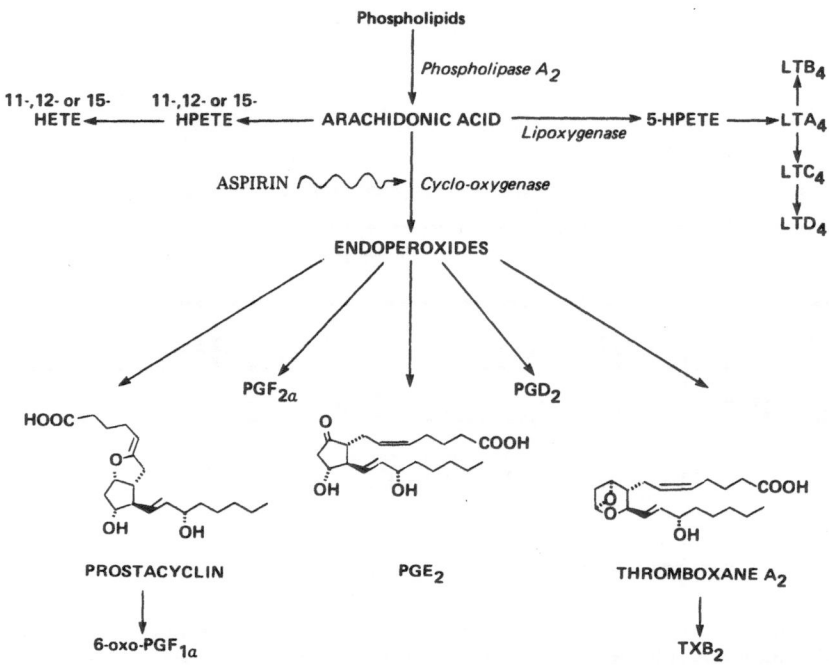

Figure 9.1 Metabolism of arachidonic acid by the cyclo-oxygenase and lipoxygenase pathways

pathogenesis of gastric damage. The cyclo-oxygenase product, thromboxane A_2 has been demonstrated to exert pro-ulcerogenic actions[7]. Likewise, products of the lipoxygenase pathway including the leukotrienes may exert deleterious actions on the gastric mucosa[1]. In addition, the endogenous release of the related phospholipid, platelet-activating factor (PAF) may underlie the gastrointestinal damage and ulceration associated with such diseases as septic shock[8]. Thus, several endogenous lipid mediators have a potential role in the aetiology of gastric damage and disease.

PROSTANOID DEPLETION AND GASTRIC INTEGRITY

Effects of cyclo-oxygenase inhibitors on mucosal prostanoid metabolism

Early studies demonstrated that indomethacin at ulcerogenic doses, reduced the level of prostaglandins in homogenates of rat gastric mucosa, bioassayed as PGE_2 and the levels of both PGE_2 and $PGF_{2\alpha}$ in the stomach, determined by radioimmunoassay[9,10]. The clinically-used compounds indomethacin, aspirin, naproxen, flurbiprofen or ketoprofen all caused a dose-related inhibition of

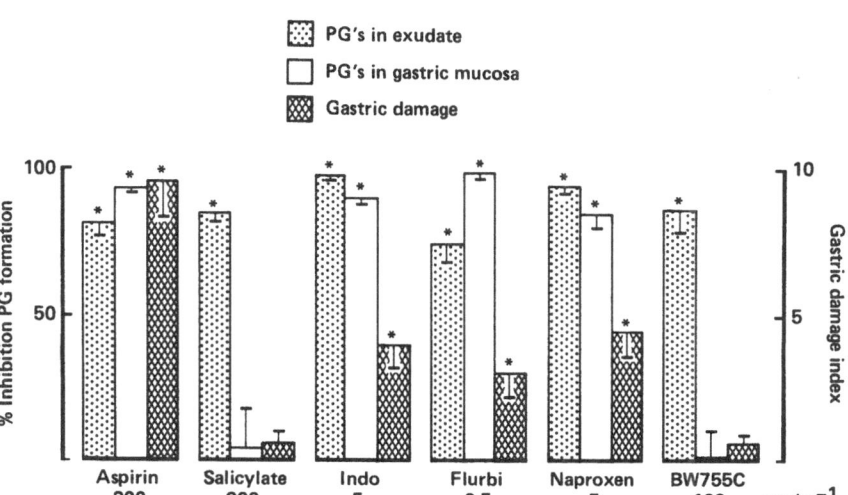

Figure 9.2 Gastric damage and the inhibition of prostaglandin formation in the rat gastric mucosa and inflammatory exudate by non-steroid anti-inflammatory drugs. The compounds (Indo = indomethacin, Flurbi = fluribiprofen) were administered three times over 24 h, and prostacyclin formation in gastric mucosal strips *ex vivo* (□) and PGE_2 levels in carrageenin-induced inflammatory exudate in an implanted sponge (▩) was determined by bioassay. Gastric mucosal damage (▩) was assessed macroscopically in terms of a damage score. Results are shown as mean ± S.E. of 5–12 experiments, where * represents $p < 0.01$. Data are adapted from Whittle *et al.*[11]

gastric mucosal prostaglandin generation[11] determined *ex vivo* following either parenteral and oral administration (Figure 9.2). Using similar techniques, others have confirmed that intragastric or intravenous administration of aspirin inhibits both PGE_2 and prostacyclin generation by the rat, cat and dog gastric mucosa *ex vivo*[12–14].

In other studies, intravenous administration of indomethacin reduced the levels of PGE_2 in mucosal interstitial fluid, sampled from implanted hollow dialysis tubes in the dog stomach[15]. Studies in the pig with a 10-day intragastric treatment with several anti-inflammatory drugs including aspirin, indomethacin, sulindac and diclofenac caused a significant fall in the mucosal 'levels' of both PGE_2 and the prostacyclin breakdown product, 6-keto-$PGF_{1\alpha}$, determined by RIA following a rapid freezing procedure[16].

The effects of aspirin following oral ingestion on human gastric mucosal cyclo-oxygenase activity using the vortex generation technique have also been reported by several groups[17,18]. A similar degree of inhibition of PGE_2 formation in biopsies of fundic, antral and duodenal mucosa following administration of aspirin over 24 h was achieved in either healthy volunteers or duodenal ulcer patients[17].

Table 9.1 Inhibition of cyclo-oxygenase in homogenates of rat gastric mucosa and ileum by anti-inflammatory agents

| | IC_{50} (μM) | |
	Gastric mucosa	Ileum
Indomethacin	3.9	5.8
Flurbiprofen	0.5	0.4
Naproxen	3.9	6.3
Ketoprofen	5.5	7.3
Meclofenamate	11.3	–
Paracetamol*	1325	> 1000
BW 755C*	380	265
NDGA*	150	–

Results are shown as the IC_{50} values (concentration causing 50% inhibition of prostacyclin formation, determined by bioassay procedures) following 10-min pre-incubation *in vitro* with tissue homogenate;* represents biphasic dose–response curves with stimulation of prostacyclin formation at lower concentrations. Data are adapted from Boughton-Smith and Whittle[19].

Studies *in vitro* using several non-steroid anti-inflammatory drugs showed that these compounds were potent inhibitors of prostanoid formation from endogenous precursor in rat gastric mucosa and ileum (Table 9.1) as determined by bioassay or radioimmunoassay (RIA)[19]; the effective concentrations were comparable to those inhibiting cyclo-oxygenase activity in other tissue preparations. Concentrations of indomethacin similar to these have also been reported to inhibit prostaglandin biosynthesis *in vitro* in homogenates and microsomal preparations of human gastric mucosa[20,21].

Relationship between endogenous prostanoids and gastric damage

When administered in divided doses over 24 h, indomethacin, flurbiprofen and naproxen all induced a comparable degree of gastric erosion formation which paralleled the inhibition of mucosal prostacyclin production[11]. In contrast, sodium salicyclate or the experimental agent BW 755C did not inhibit mucosal cyclo-oxygenase nor cause macroscopic damage, supporting the association between these two events (Figure 9.2). Others have likewise shown that BW 755C or sodium salicylate does not inhibit prostaglandin generation in fundic mucosal tissue from rat or dog[13,22]. In the cat, bolus intravenous injection of aspirin inhibited mucosal PGE_2 and 6-oxo-$PGF_{1\alpha}$ generation and induced the formation of deep-penetrating ulcers in the antrum during histamine-stimulated acid secretion, whereas equimolar doses of sodium salicylate did not have such actions[14]. These findings are given support from the clinical studies that show that sodium salicylate produced far less gastro-intestinal irritation than did aspirin, as determined by faecal blood loss[23].

The analgesic antipyretic agent, paracetamol, which is not considered a major gastric irritant, only inhibited prostaglandin formation in rat gastric mucosal homogenates *in vitro* at high concentrations[19] and had little action on prostaglandin formation after administration in the rat gastric mucosa *ex vivo*[24]. Furthermore paracetamol caused only a small reduction in mucosal PGE_2 synthesis in human fundic and antral mucosal biopsies following oral ingestion[17].

In the pig, an overall association between the inhibition of gastric prostaglandin formation and the potential to induce gastric lesions on chronic administration was found with seven out of eight anti-inflammatory agents tested[16].

Non-steroid anti-inflammatory drugs are well-recognized to cause local irritant actions on the gastric mucosa. This 'barrier-breaking' activity does not appear to be related to the inhibition of endogenous prostaglandin biosynthesis[1,13] and results from a direct action, initially exerted on the surface epithelial cells. Both local irritancy and the inhibition of prostaglandin biosynthesis are of importance when considering the gastric toxicity of non-steroid anti-inflammatory agents, especially since both processes interact synergistically to produce more extensive gastric injury than either activity alone[25]. Indeed, experimental studies indicate that either mechanism alone may cause only limited damage to the gastric mucosa[26]. Such synergy must be taken into account when assessing the correlation between cyclo-oxygenase inhibition and the potential of these agents to induce damage. Indeed, such an interactive situation is likely to occur in the therapeutic administration of the aspirin-like drugs.

Although neither sodium salicylate nor BW 755C reduced gastric mucosal cyclo-oxygenase following oral or parenteral administration, both agents substantially reduced the prostanoid levels in experimental inflammatory exudates in the rat (Figure 9.2). Such tissue-selective inhibition of pro-inflammatory prostanoids, while sparing protective prostanoid biosynthesis in the gastric and intestinal mucosa, would form the basis of a biochemical approach to the development of anti-inflammatory agents devoid of gastro-intestinal toxicity.

Role of endogenous prostanoids in maintaining mucosal integrity

The gastric damage that follows challenge with low concentrations of topical irritants such as acidified bile salts or ethanol is greatly augmented by concurrent administration of cyclo-oxygenase inhibitors[26]. Intravenous or subcutaneous administration of such agents in doses inhibiting mucosal cyclo-oxygenase by greater than 60% significantly potentiated mucosal damage by topical irritants such as acidified taurocholate or ethanol in the rat or dog[27,28]. These findings give support for a role of endogenous prostanoids in the maintenance of mucosal integrity. Although cyclo-oxygenase products do not appear to regulate mucosal 'barrier' function, their actions on the mucosal

187

microcirculation and other potentially protective processes appear to be of physiological importance. Significant suppression of endogenous prostanoid biosynthesis thus greatly augments the susceptibility of the mucosal tissue to damage by normally-weak irritants.

In studies on chronic mild stress in rats, the gastric mucosa was found to be more resistant to injury by ethanol than in non-stressed rats[29]. The findings suggested that this protection resulted from stimulation of endogenous prostanoid biosynthesis[29]. Stimulation of endogenous prostaglandin formation has also been implicated as one mechanism by which topical application of weak irritants to the mucosal surface can protect against subsequent challenge by more concentrated irritants[30,31]. Such processes may again reflect prostaglandin-mediated physiological defence mechanisms of the gastric mucosa against damage.

Role of prostanoids in the pathogenesis of peptic ulcer disease

Alterations in endogenous prostaglandin turnover, resulting from changes in substrate availability, or the activity of cyclo-oxygenase or isomerase and synthase enzymes, as well as effects on metabolism, degradation and elimination of endogenous prostanoids may have importance not only in drug-induced gastric damage, but also in the pathogenesis of peptic ulcer disease. Early studies on levels of prostaglandins, notably PGE_2, in plasma and gastric juice from peptic ulcer patients may be of limited value since these prostanoids are rapidly and extensively metabolized during their passage through the gastric mucosa and determination of the levels of prostaglandin metabolites in gastric juice would be more appropriate.

In a study where the *ex vivo* generation of PGE_2 in biopsies of human gastric mucosa was determined using bioassay techniques, no difference was found in the maximal generation of PGE_2 in oxyntic, antral and duodenal mucosa from healthy volunteers or from patients with duodenal ulcer[17]. It is possible that the technique of vortex generation of prostaglandins in gastric tissue *ex vivo* is insufficiently sensitive to reflect any subtle changes in endogenous turnover of mucosal prostaglandins *in vivo*. A reduction in antral and corpus mucosal prostaglandin E_2 levels determined by RIA was seen in gastric ulcer patients compared to normal volunteers, and was associated with atrophic gastritis[32].

In non-proliferative culture of human gastric mucosa, PGE_2 and 6-keto-$PGF_{1\alpha}$ production, determined by RIA, was significantly lower in antral tissue of patients with active duodenal ulcer disease than in that of control patients[33]. However, there was no difference between production of the prostanoids in duodenal mucosa from either group. In patients treated with cimetidine for four weeks and presumably with healed duodenal ulcers, antral prostanoid production was comparable to that from control subjects[33]. In other studies on incubated human duodenal biopsy material, mucosal tissue taken from the proximity of the ulcer site produced less 6-keto-PGF$_{1\alpha}$ determined by RIA than healthy tissue from non-ulcerated subjects[34].

It is difficult to establish the cause or effect of the prostaglandin depletion in such circumstances of peptic ulceration. However, the evidence does favour the concept that a reduction in prostaglandin synthesis in gastric mucosa, while not solely initiating damage, may well exacerbate the development of such lesions or make the tissue more susceptible to damage by other pathological events.

ACTIONS AND ROLE OF THROMBOXANE A$_2$

Although depletion of prostanoids of the E and I series may have a deleterious effect on the gastric mucosa, not all eicosanoids exert protective actions. Thus, the cyclo-oxygenase product, thromboxane A$_2$ (TXA$_2$), derived predominantly from platelets, is a potent vasoconstrictor in many vascular beds[35]. It is highly labile, with a half-life of less than 30 sec under physiological conditions, and therefore to study its pharmacological actions, it must be generated locally. When its precursor, arachidonic acid was infused into canine gastric arterial circulation, so as to incubate with blood flowing to a chambered segment of fundic mucosa *in situ*, dose-related vasoconstriction in gastric circulation was observed[36,37]. This response was abolished by indomethacin and reflects the biotransformation of archidonic acid by blood-borne platelets to TXA$_2$, which was detected by RIA as the breakdown product, TXB$_2$[38]. Furthermore, the specific thromboxane synthetase inhibitor, 1-benzylimidazole, abolished this vasoconstriction, reversing it to a vasodilator response[7]. Under conditions where canine gastric mucosa was concurrently exposed to low concentrations of acidified bile salts, TXA$_2$ biosynthesized in blood from arachidonic acid *in vivo*, induced extensive damage and necrosis in the gastric tissue[7].

Since TXA$_2$ is so highly labile, further studies have been conducted with the chemically-stable epoxy-methano endoperoxide analogue, U-46619, which acts as a thromboxane mimetic. In the canine gastric circulation, local intra-arterial administration of U-46619 induced dose-related vasoconstriction, as seen with TXA$_2$[36]. In the presence of topically-applied acidified bile salts, intra-arterial infusion of U-46619 induced extensive haemorrhagic necrosis of the gastric mucosa[28]. Thus, these thromboxanes reduced the ability of mucosa to withstand challenge from normally-mild irritants. This action may be related to their vasoconstrictor properties, although direct cytolytic actions on the mucosal cells cannot be entirely excluded.

To investigate further the actions of the thromboxane mimetic on gastric microcirculation, the *in vivo* microscopy technique described by Guth and colleagues[39] was used to study gastric submucosal arteriolar and venular responses in the pentobarbital-anaesthetized rat. Topical application of U-46619 to the exposed submucosal vascular bed reduced vessel diameter in both arterioles and venules, reaching plateau responses within 2 min of application[40]. At the highest concentration of U-46619 studied (1 μM), the reduction in vessel diameter was comparable for both arterioles and venules. Intense focal vasoconstriction in the venules was clearly demonstrated, leading to sluggish blood flow and stasis within the vessels[40].

These potent microcirculatory and damaging actions of the thromboxanes raise the possibility that local generation of TXA$_2$, perhaps following platelet activation in the microcirculation or as a result of local trauma or general shock may be involved in the pathogenesis of gastric ulcerogenesis. Studies with selective thromboxane synthase inhibitors in experimental models give some support to this concept[41,42]. Thus, OKY-1581 reduced bile-salt induced gastric necrosis, although it failed to inhibit that induced by ethanol[41]. Further, 1-benzylimidazole substantially inhibited gastric damage induced by acid-ethanol[42]. However, 1-benzylimidazole also inhibited indomethacin-induced erosions[42]. Since the dose of indomethacin used would inhibit cyclo-oxygenase, and therefore itself would reduce TXA$_2$ formation, the mechanisms of its protective action are not fully clear. However, the involvement of TXA$_2$ in gastric damage resulting from local ischaemia and other microcirculatory disorders requires further consideration.

In studies on human mucosal tissue, biopsy material taken from the proximity of the ulcer site produced less 6-keto-PGF$_{1\alpha}$ than from tissue from healthy control subjects[34]. As the PGE$_2$ and TXA$_2$ levels were not altered, a general reduction in cyclo-oxygenase activity was unlikely. Such a selective reduction of prostanoid formation could reflect the contribution of different mucosal cells and their different sensitivity to inhibition. This change in the profile of arachidonate metabolites, which would lead to an imbalance between local levels of the cytotoxic thromboxane and the protective prostanoid, prostacyclin, could contribute to the pathogenesis of peptic ulceration.

Platelet adhesion, aggregation and subsequent plug formation play a major role in the control of cutaneous and vascular haemostasis. Since TXA$_2$ is a potent inducer of platelet aggregation, it has been implicated as a mediator in the process of haemostasis. Thus, inhibition of thromboxane synthesis can reduce platelet aggregation and prolong cutaneous bleeding time in man. Using a standard incision in the gastric mucosa of rat, dog and rabbit to initiate bleeding, the role of TXA$_2$ in the termination of gastric haemorrhage was determined and compared to that in the mesenteric artery[43]. Direct inhibition of platelet aggregation following intravenous infusion of prostacyclin or by administration of the thromboxane synthetase inhibitor, 1-benzylimidazole, prolonged mesenteric bleeding yet did not alter that from the gastric mucosa.

In contrast to the mesenteric artery, heparin significantly prolonged gastric bleeding[43]. These findings suggest that TXA_2 biosynthesis and platelet aggregation play a minimal role in the initial haemostatic events in the gastric mucosa and that the arrest of gastric haemorrhage is brought about by processes primarily involving the coagulation system.

Local or systemic administration of non-steroid anti-inflammatory drugs, in doses sufficient to inhibit cyclo-oxygenase did not prolong gastric bleeding[43]. Thus, interference with TXA_2 formation or platelet aggregation plays little part in the bleeding associated with the gastric irritancy associated with these agents.

ACTIONS AND ROLE OF LIPOXYGENASE PRODUCTS

At present, little is known concerning the role of the endogenous arachidonate metabolites formed by the lipoxygenase enzymes (Figure 9.1) in the gastric mucosa. The hydroperoxy intermediates such as 5-, 12- or 15-HPETE (hydroperoxyeicosatetraenoic acid) in common with other lipid peroxides may exert tissue-destructive actions. The local accumulation of such products, or the free radicals that they subsequently can form, could therefore be involved in the pathogenesis of gastric damage.

Leukotriene B_4 (LTB_4) is a potent chemotactic agent and has been proposed as a pro-inflammatory mediator of chronic inflammation[44]. Its role in inflammatory diseases of the upper gastrointestinal tract, including gastritis or in the inflammatory zone of the ulcer crater has yet to be explored. Leukotriene C_4 (LTC_4) identified as one constitutent of SRS-A (Slow Reacting Substance of Anaphylaxis) can affect vascular smooth muscle tone and its permeability to plasma[45,46]. Using *in vivo* microscopy techniques in the rat, locally-applied LTC_4 has been demonstrated to be a potent vasoconstrictor in the gastric microcirculation, especially in the submucosal venules[40]. Such findings thus identify this arachidonate product as a further endogenous mediator with pro-ulcerogenic potential. The predominant venular constriction led to vaso-congestion and stasis in the microcirculation, which represent histological characteristics of several forms of gastric damage including that induced by local application of ethanol[39,47,48]. Indeed, recent studies have identified the release of LTC_4 from the rat gastric mucosa following ethanol challenge[49,50].

The involvement of lipoxygenase products in gastric damage has been explored by the use of lipoxygenase inhibitors. Although BW 755C is classed as a dual inhibitor of both cyclo-oxygenase and lipoxygenase pathways in most tissues, it fails to inhibit prostanoid formation in the gastric mucosa, as discussed above. Hence BW 755C is a useful pharmacological probe to study lipoxygenase inhibition in this tissue. In anti-inflammatory doses, BW 755C inhibited gastric mucosal damage induced by acidified ethanol, as determined

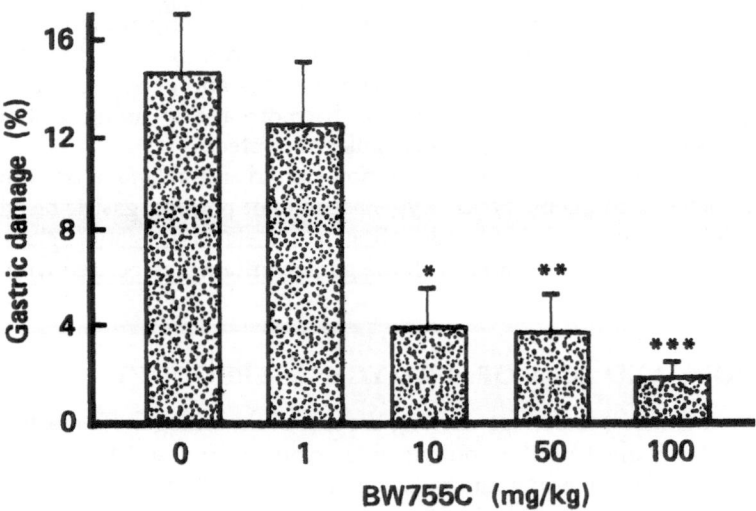

Figure 9.3 Inhibition by BW 755C of gastric mucosal damage induced by the oral admin-istration for 1 h of acidified ethanol (40% ethanol in 100 mM HCl). BW 755C was orally-administered, 1 h prior to challenge. Results are shown as macroscopic damage, expressed as a percentage of the total mucosal area, mean ± S.E. for 4–9 rats in each group, where * represents $p < 0.05$, ** $p < 0.01$, ***$p < 0.001$. Results are taken from Wallace and Whittle[51]

by both macroscopic and histological measurement (Figure 9.3). The ability of BW 755C to prevent such gastric damage may therefore reflect the inhibition of the biosynthesis of pro-ulcerogenic lipoxygenase products[51]. The less-specific lipoxygenase inhibitor NDGA has also been demonstrated to reduce ethanol-induced gastric necrosis[49]. Measurement of the biosynthesis of lipoxy-genase products including LTC_4 and LTB_4 in gastric and duodenal tissue from patients with peptic ulcer disease will provide interesting data on the profile of arachidonate metabolites and their role in peptic ulceration.

ACTIONS AND ROLE OF PAF-ACETHER

A further lipid mediator which has potent actions on the gastrointestinal tract is platelet-activating factor[52] also known as PAF, PAF-acether, or AGEPC. Although PAF is not a metabolite of arachidonic acid, its immediate precursor, lyso-PAF is released from membrane-bound phospholipids by the action of phospholipase A_2, the enzyme which releases arachidonic acid. Lyso-PAF, which has very limited biological activity, is metabolized into PAF by the acetyl CoA transferase, which is subsequently broken down back to lyso-PAF

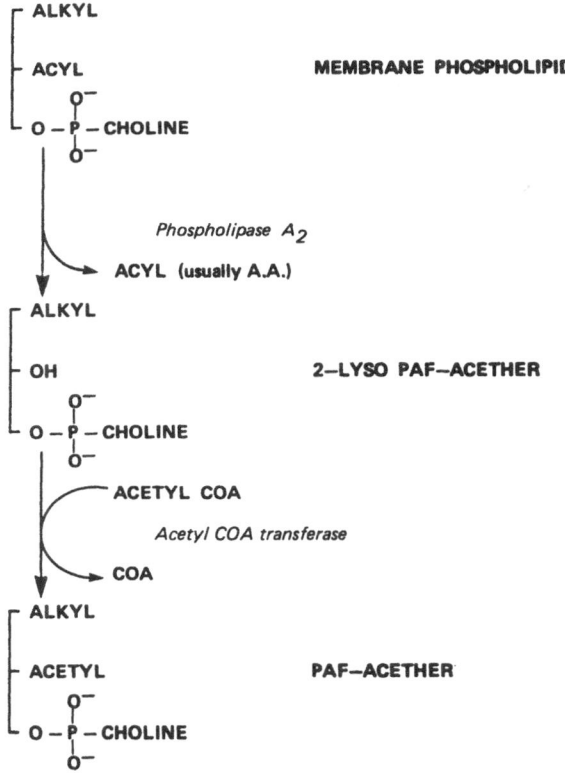

Figure 9.4 Formation of PAF from membrane phospholipids following activation of phospholipase A_2

by the enzyme acyl hydrolase (Figure 9.4). PAF is a low molecular weight phospholipid characterized by an ether linkage at the 1'-position (usually with a fatty acid chain of 16 or 18 carbons) and an acetyl group at the 2'-position of a phosphatidylcholine[53] giving the structure of 1-O-alkyl-2-O-acetyl-*sn*-glyceryl-3-phosphocholine (Figure 9.4). The cellular sources of PAF can include neutrophils, macrophages, monocytes, basophils, endothelial cells, mast cells and platelets, all of which have been shown to release PAF *in vitro*[52,54].

PAF has been implicated as a mediator of allergic and inflammatory processes[54] and its potent pro-inflammatory actions make it a possible candidate as an endogenous mediator of gastrointestinal damage[55,56]. Indeed, in recent studies, PAF has been identified as the most potent endogenous pro-ulcerogenic agent for the stomach as yet known[8].

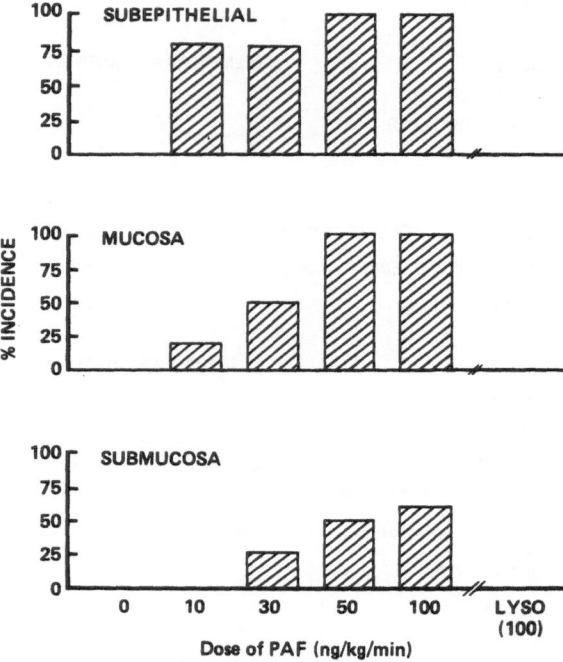

Figure 9.5 Histological assessment of the gastric mucosal damage induced by intravenous infusion of PAF and lyso-PAF. Results show the incidence of tissue disruption in the subepithelial, mucosal and submucosal regions, characterized as vasocongestion and necrosis

Role of PAF in gastro-intestinal damage

Intravenous infusion of PAF at low doses resulted in extensive gastric mucosal congestion and necrosis in the rat, cat or dog. The damage induced by PAF was dose-related and also involved the duodenum, jejunum, ileum and caecum[56]. The distal colon, however, did not appear to be susceptible to PAF-induced damage. As the dose of PAF was increased, the vascular congestion increased progressively in terms of severity and the depth of tissue involved (Figure 9.5). It is noteworthy that lyso-PAF, the precursor-breakdown product of PAF, did not produce such vasocongestion or damage.

The finding that picomole doses of PAF caused subepithelial vasocongestion suggested that this compound might predispose the gastric mucosa to ulceration when given at extremely low doses[57]. Thus, using an *ex vivo* gastric chamber preparation, the rat gastric mucosa was challenged with a relatively low concentration of ethanol (20%) or sodium taurocholate (2 mM). These mild irritants caused only minimal gastric damage when applied topically to the gastric mucosa during an intravenous infusion of the vehicle. However, chal-

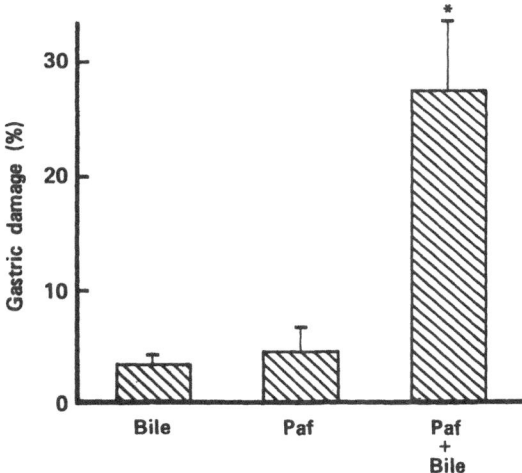

Figure 9.6 Potentiation of gastric mucosal damage induced by topical application of acidified sodium taurocholate (2 mM in 50 mM HCl) to the rat chambered stomach *in situ* by a 5-min intravenous infusion of PAF (100 ng kg^{-1}min^{-1}). Results are shown as damage, expressed as the percentage of total area of mucosa, mean ± S.E. of 4–6 experiments, where * represents $p < 0.02$. Data are adapted from Wallace and Whittle[57]

lenge with these agents during a 5-min infusion of PAF, caused a dose-related increase in the gastric damage (Figure 9.6). A significant increase in ethanol-induced mucosal damage was observed with a dose of PAF as low as 1 ng/kg/min (2 pmoles/kg/min)[57].

The mechanism of the ulcerogenic action of PAF is not clearly understood. The systemic hypotension induced by PAF[58] would contribute to an increase in mucosal susceptibility to injury. However, there are several lines of evidence suggesting that this is not the sole mechanism. Other equally-hypotensive agents (isoprenaline, prostacyclin or nitroprusside) did not share the potent ulcerogenic or pro-ulcerogenic actions of PAF[8]. Furthermore, non-hypotensive doses of PAF significantly augmented 20% ethanol-induced gastric damage[57].

The histological observations suggest that mucosal vascular stasis is the primary effect of PAF infusion which would lead to ulceration. Such stasis could be precipitated by a direct vasoconstrictor effect of PAF. However, using *in vivo* microscopy techniques to study the actions of PAF on rat gastric submucosal vessels, no such vasoconstriction action could be demonstrated in the arterioles or venules, the vessels that regulate mucosal blood flow[59]. Direct observation did however indicate a sluggish blood flow in these microvessels. Furthermore, a profound reduction in blood flow and subsequent stasis in the mucosal capillaries was also noted. Since infusion of PAF results in marked haemoconcentration[60], the increased viscosity of blood under such conditions would contribute to the sluggish mucosal blood flow observed *in vivo*.

PAF-induced aggregation of neutrophils or platelets might also contribute to gastrointestinal mucosal vasocongestion by blocking the microcirculation, especially under conditions of increased blood viscosity. While there is histological evidence supporting a role for neutrophil aggregation[56], a contribution of platelet aggregation in the ulcerogenic action of PAF in the rat is unlikely, since PAF does not aggregate rat platelets. Furthermore, the ulcerogenic actions of PAF were observed in rats made thrombocytopenic by prior administration of anti-platelet serum[8].

Prostaglandins, particularly of the E series, markedly reduce the gastric damage and ulceration induced by a variety of ulcerogens[1-6]. However, neither PGE_2 nor its 16,16-dimethyl analogue significantly reduced PAF-induced gastric damage[61]. These studies thus demonstrate that the protective properties of such prostanoids observed in most models of experimental ulceration do not extend to this form of damage. The presence of high concentrations of acid in the stomach are not necessary for PAF-induced ulcerogenesis, since pretreatment with anti-secretory doses of cimetidine did not reduce this mucosal damage.

Role of mediators in PAF-induced damage

It is possible that the actions of PAF in the gastrointestinal tract are exerted via other mediators. However, histamine, noradrenaline and the cyclo-oxygenase products of arachidonic acid do not appear to play major roles as mediators of PAF-induced gastric damage. Such damage was not prevented by pretreatment with antagonists of histamine H_1-receptors (mepyramine), histamine H_2-receptors (cimetidine) or α-adrenergic (phentolamine) receptors[8], as shown in Figure 9.7. Furthermore, inhibitors of cyclo-oxygenase (indomethacin, acetylsalicylic acid) or thromboxane synthetase (1-benzylimidazole), failed to reduce the extent of gastric damage[62] as shown in Figure 9.8. However, pretreatment with the glucocorticoid anti-inflammatory agents, dexamethasone or prednisolone, or with the dual lipoxygenase/cyclo-oxygenase inhibitor, BW 755C, did produce a significant reduction of PAF-induced gastric damage (Figure 9.8). These latter agents also significantly reduced the extent of haemoconcentration induced by PAF administration[62]. Such observations could reflect a contribution of lipoxygenase products of arachidonic acid to PAF-induced gastric damage.

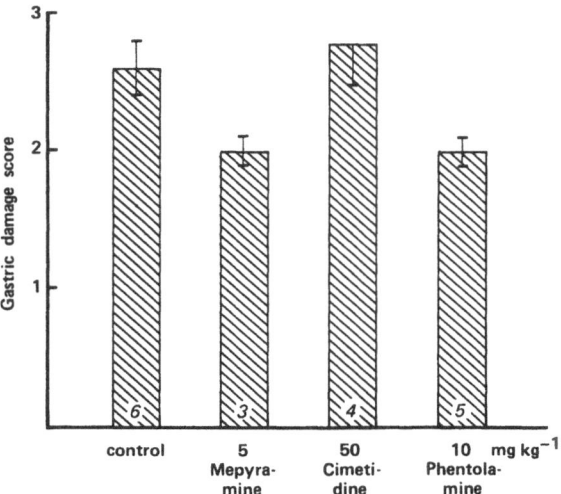

Figure 9.7 Failure of the histamine H_1- and H_2-receptor antagonists, mepyramine and cimetidine, respectively, or the α-adrenergic receptor antagonist, phentolamine to inhibit the gastric mucosal damage induced by a 20-min infusion of PAF ($50\,\text{ng kg}^{-1}\text{min}^{-1}$). Results, shown as the macroscopically-determined gastric damage score, are the mean $\pm$ S.E. of (n) experiments. Data are adapted from Rosam, Wallace, and Whittle[8]

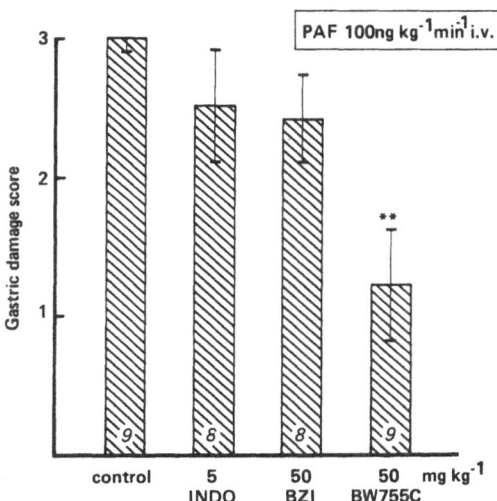

Figure 9.8 Effect of the cyclo-oxygenase inhibitor, indomethacin (INDO), the thromboxane synthatase inhibitor, 1-benzylimidazole (BZI), and the dual cyclo-oxygenase/lipoxygenase inhibitor, BW 755C on gastric mucosal damage induced by intravenous infusion of PAF ($100\,\text{ng kg}^{-1}\text{min}^{-1}$). Results, shown as the gastric damage score, are the mean $\pm$ S.E. of (n) experiments, where ** represents $p < 0.01$. Data are adapted from Wallace and Whittle[62]

197

Role of PAF in septic shock

Septic shock is a major risk factor for gastrointestinal ulceration[63]. Septic or endotoxin shock is additionally characterized by systemic hypotension, pulmonary hypertension, endothelial disruption and increased vascular permeability, all of which can be reproduced in animals by infusion of PAF[64]. It has been demonstrated that PAF is released into the blood following endotoxin administration in the rat[60]. The concentration of PAF in the blood reached 4.7 nm, 10 mins after endotoxin administration, comparable to that achieved following an intravenous injection of 300 pmoles/kg of PAF. As discussed above, PAF can exert pro-ulcerogenic actions in doses as low as 2 pmoles/kg in the rat. Thus, appropriate concentrations of PAF can be achieved in the blood following endotoxin administration to induce gastrointestinal damage. It is thus possible that the endogenous release of PAF contributes to the gastrointestinal damage associated with endotoxaemia and related diseases. Others have also suggested that PAF in combination with endotoxin may contribute to necrotizing enterocolitis[55].

Pretreatment with corticosteroids can inhibit the gastrointestinal damage following experimental septic shock[65], and corticosteroid therapy is known to be beneficial to patients in septic shock[66]. Such actions in endotoxin shock may be related to the ability of corticosteroids to inhibit phospholipase A_2[67], a primary enzyme in the biosynthesis of PAF[68].

Recently, several groups have demonstrated that specific PAF antagonists can ameliorate the hypotensive actions and reduce the mortality which follows endotoxin administration in rats[69,70]. Since chemically-dissimilar PAF antagonists could produce similar protective actions, this gives good support to the involvement of endogenously-released PAF in the pathology of septic shock.

The ability of the PAF antagonist, CV-3988, to reduce gastrointestinal damage following endotoxin shock in the rat has also been studied[71]. Intravenous infusion of lipopolysaccharide from *Salmonella typhosa* induced pronounced hypotension. Upon macroscopic examination 30 min later, the stomach and small bowel were found to have extensive regions of hyperaemia and haemorrhage. In the stomach, this damage was usually found in the corpus region[71]. The jejunum and terminal ileum were the most severely affected regions of the small intestine, while the distal colon was devoid of damage. This profile and distribution of damage in the gastrointestinal tract is comparable to that observed following intravenous infusion of PAF. Pre-treatment with CV-3988, in a dose that could inhibit PAF-induced gastric damage, abolished the prolonged hypotensive action of endotoxin and significantly reduced the damage to the small intestine and stomach (Table 9.2). More recently, these findings have been extended by the use of two further structurally-dissimilar

Table 9.2 Effects of the PAF-antagonists, CV-3988, on gastrointestinal damage induced by endotoxin

Treatment	n	Damage score	
		Small intestine	Stomach
Endotoxin	11	2.8 ± 0.1	2.8 ± 0.1
Endotoxin + CV-3988	9	$0.6 \pm 0.3^*$	0.8 ± 0.2

Lipopolysaccharide from *Salmonella typhosa* was infused intravenously (1.25 mg/kg) for 10 min. Rats were pretreated, 10 min prior to endotoxin, with CV-3988 infused intravenously (1 mg kg^{-1}min^{-1} for 10 min). The macroscopically-visible signs of gastric and small intestinal damage were scored on a 0 (normal) to 3 (extensive damage) scale. Results, shown as mean $\pm$ SE of (n) animals, where * represents $p < 0.001$, are taken from Wallace and Whittle[71].

PAF antagonists, BN-52021 and RO-193704 which also prevented endotoxin-induced gastric and intestinal damage[72].

These findings thus support the involvement of endogenously-released PAF as a mediator of gastrointestinal damage associated with septic shock[73]. It is not yet known whether the release of PAF from circulating or entrapped blood cells under other circumstances such as haemorrhagic shock would also lead to gastric damage. It is conceivable that in conditions characterized by infiltration of inflammatory cells, or in the sequence of events following local tissue damage, the release of PAF directly into the mucosal tissue may occur. Thus, both systemic and local release of PAF could serve to either initiate or further amplify gastric ulceration under pathological conditions. The clinical usefulness of specific PAF-antagonists for such conditions remains to be explored.

CONCLUSIONS

Identification of the potent protective actions of PGE$_2$ and prostacyclin on the gastric mucosa, coupled with the characterization of the endogenous formation of these prostanoids by the mucosa, has provided one mechanism to explain the ability of the mucosa to resist the continual challenge by acid, pepsin, bile salts and ingested irritants. Interference with endogenous prostaglandin formation by non-steroid anti-inflammatory agents may therefore contribute to the damage which they induce. A reduction in gastric mucosal prostanoid formation could also be a predisposing factor in the natural history of development of peptic ulceration. The influence of other factors, including diet and cigarette smoking[74], on prostanoid formation and turnover may well be an important aspect in understanding the nature of peptic ulcer disease.

The involvement of the aggressive actions of TXA$_2$, lipoxygenase products including LTC$_4$ and the related lipid mediator, PAF, in gastric damage must await further clarification. However, the identification and characterization of such products as candidates for endogenous pro-ulcerogenic mediators should provide new pharmacological approaches to investigate the pathogenesis of gastric ulceration. This should in turn lead to the development of novel selective agents for the effective therapeutic intervention in peptic ulcer disease.

References

1. Whittle, B.J.R. and Vane, J.R. (1987). Prostanoids as regulators of gastrointestinal function. In Johnson, L.R. (ed.) *Physiology of the Gastro-intestinal Tract*, 2nd Edn pp. 143–80 (New York, Raven Press)
2. Robert, A. (1976). Antisecretory, antiulcer, cytoprotective and diarrheogenic properties of prostaglandins. In B. Samuelsson and J.R. Vane (eds) *Advances in Prostaglandin and Thromboxane Research*, **2**, pp. 507–20 (Raven Press: New York)
3. Allen, A. and Garner, A. (1980). Mucus and bicarbonate secretion in the stomach and their possible role in mucosal protection. *Gut*, **21**, 249–62
4. Miller, T.A. (1983). Protective effects of prostaglandins against gastric mucosal damage: Current knowledge and proposed mechanisms. *Am. J. Physiol.*, **245**, G601–G623
5. Hawkey, C.J. and Rampton, D.S. (1985). Prostaglandins and the gastrointestinal mucosa: are they important in its function, disease, or treatment? *Gastroenterology*, **89**, 1162–88
6. Robert, A., Nezamis, J.E., Lancaster, C. and Hanchar, A.J. (1979). Cytoprotection by prostaglandins in rats – prevention of gastric necrosis produced by alcohol, HCl, NaOH, hypertonic NaCl and thermal injury. *Gastroenterology*, **77**, 433–43
7. Whittle, B.J.R., Kauffman, G.L. and Moncada, S. (1981). Vasoconstriction and thromboxane A_2 induces ulceration of the gastric mucosa. *Nature (London)*, **292**, 472–74
8. Rosam, A-C., Wallace, J.L. and Whittle, B.J.R. (1986). Potent ulcerogenic actions of platelet-activating factor on the stomach. *Nature (London)*, **319**, 54–6
9. Fitzpatrick, F.A. and Wynalda, M.A. (1976). *In vivo* suppression of prostaglandin biosynthesis by non-steroidal anti-inflammatory agents. *Prostaglandins*, **12**, 1037–51
10. Main, I.H.M. and Whittle, B.J.R. (1975). Investigation of the vasodilator and antisecretory role of prostaglandins in the rat gastric mucosa by use of non-steroidal anti-inflammatory drugs. *Br. J. Pharmacol.*, **53**, 217–24
11. Whittle, B.J.R., Higgs, G.A., Eakins, K.E., Moncada, S. and Vane. J.R. (1980). Selective inhibition of prostaglandin production in inflammatory exudates and gastric mucosa. *Nature (London)*, **284**, 271–3
12. Konturek, S.J., Piastucki, I., Brzozowski, T., Radecki, T., Dembinskia-Kiec, A., Zmuda, A. and Gryglewski, R. (1981). Role of prostaglandins in the formation of aspirin-induced gastric ulcers. *Gastroenterology*, **80**, 4–9
13. Ligumsky, M., Grossman, M.I. and Kauffman, G.L. Jr, (1982). Endogenous gastric mucosal prostaglandins: their role in mucosal integrity. *Am. J. Physiol.*, **242**, G337–G341
14. Whittle, B.J.R., Hansen, D. and Salmon, J.A. (1985). Gastric ulcer formation and cyclo-oxygenase inhibition in cat antrum follows parenteral administration of aspirin but not salicylate. *Eur. J. Pharmacol.*, **115**, 153–7
15. Bunnett, N.W., Walsh, J.H., Debas, H.T., Kauffman, G.L. and Golanska, E.M. (1983). Measurement of prostaglandin E_2 in the interstitial fluid from dog stomach after feeding and indomethacin. *Gastroenterology*, **85**, 1391–8
16. Rainsford, K.D. and Willis, C. (1982). Relationship of gastric mucosal damage induced in pigs by anti-inflammatory drugs to their effects on prostaglandin production. *Dig. Dis. Sci.*, **27**, 624–35
17. Konturek, S.J., Obtulowicz, W., Sito, E., Oleksy, J., Wilkon, S. and Kiec-Dembinska, A. (1981). Distribution of prostaglandins in gastric and duodenal mucosa of healthy subjects and duodenal ulcer patients: Effects of aspirin and paracetamol. *Gut*, **22**, 283–9
18. Cohen, M.M. and MacDonald, W.C. (1982). Mechanism of aspirin injury to the human gastroduodenal mucosa. *Prost. Leuk. Med.*, **9**, 241–55
19. Boughton-Smith, N.K. and Whittle, B.J.R. (1983). Stimulation and inhibition of prostacyclin formation in the gastric mucosa and ileum *in vitro* by anti-inflammatory agents. *Br. J. Pharmac.*, **78**, 172–80

20. Bennett, A., Stamford, I.F. and Unger, W.G. (1973). Prostaglandin E_2 and gastric acid secretion in man. *J. Physiol.*, **229**, 349–60
21. Peskar, B.M. (1977). On the synthesis of prostaglandins by human gastric mucosa and its modification by drugs. *Biochem. Biophys. Acta*, **487**, 307–14
22. Peskar, B.M., Weiler, H. and Peskar, B.A. (1982). Effects of BW 755C on prostaglandin synthesis in the rat stomach. *Biochem. Pharmacol.*, **31**, 1652–3
23. Leonards, J.R. and Levy, G. (1973). Gastrointestinal blood loss from aspirin and sodium salicylate tablets in man. *Clin. Pharmacol. Ther.*, **14**, 62–6
24. Van Kolfscholten, A.A., Dembinska-Kiec, A. and Basista, M. (1981). Interaction between aspirin and paracetamol on the production of prostaglandins in the rat gastric mucosa. *J. Pharm. Pharmacol.*, **33**, 462–3
25. Whittle, B.J.R. (1983). The potentiation of taurocholate-induced rat gastric erosions following parenteral administration of cyclo-oxygenase inhibitors. *Br. J. Pharmac.*, **80**, 545–51
26. Whittle, B.J.R. (1977). Mechanisms underlying gastric mucosal damage induced by indomethacin and bile salts, and the actions of prostaglandins. *Br. J. Pharmacol.*, **60**, 455–60
27. Lewi, H.J. and Carter, D.C. (1980). Intravenous prostaglandin synthetase inhibitors potentiate the effect of topical taurocholate on transmucosal ion flux. In Fielding, L.R. (ed.) *Gastrointestinal Mucosal Blood Flow*, pp. 192–201 (Churchill Livingstone: London)
28. Whittle, B.J.R. and Moncada, S. (1983). Ulceration induced by an endoperoxide analogue and by indomethacin in the canine stomach. In Samuelsson, B., Paoletti, R. and Ramwell, P. (eds.) *Advances in Prostaglandin, Thromboxane and Leukotriene Research*, **12**, pp. 373–8 (Raven Press: New York)
29. Wallace, J.L. and Cohen, M.M. (1984). Gastric mucosal protection with chronic mild restraint: role of endogenous prostaglandins. *Am. J. Physiol.*, **247**, G127–132
30. Konturek, S.J., Brzozowski, T., Piastucki, I., Radecki, T., Dembinski, A. and Dembinska, A. (1982). Role of locally generated prostaglandins in adaptive gastric cytoprotection. *Dig. Dis. Sci.*, **27**, 967–71
31. Robert, A., Nezamis, J.E., Lancaster, C., Davis, J.P., Field, S.O. and Hanchar, A.J. (1983). Mild irritants prevent gastric necrosis through 'adaptive cytoprotection' mediated by prostaglandins. *Am. J. Physiol.*, **245**, G113–G121
32. Wright, J.P., Young, G.O., Klaft, L.J., Weers, L.A., Price, S.K. and Marks, I.N. (1982). Gastric mucosal prostaglandin E levels in patients with gastric ulcer disease and carcinoma. *Gastroenterology*, **82**, 263–67
33. Rachmilewitz, D., Branski, D., Sharon, P. and Karmeli, F. (1984). Possible role of endogenous prostanoids in the pathogenesis of peptic ulcer. In Allen, A., Flemström, G., Garner, A., Silen, W. and Turnberg, L.A. (eds.) *Mechanisms of mucosal protection in the upper gastrointestinal tract*, pp. 329–33 (Raven Press: New York)
34. Hillier, K., Smith, C.L., Jewell, R., Arthur, M.J.P. and Ross, G. (1985). Duodenal mucosa synthesis of prostaglandins in duodenal ulcer disease. *Gut*, **26**, 237–40
35. Whittle, B.J.R. and Moncada, S. (1983). The pharmacological interactions between prostacyclin and thromboxanes. *Br. Med. Bull.*, **39**, 232–8
36. Kauffman, G.L. and Whittle, B.J.R. (1982). Gastric vascular actions of prostanoids and the dual effect of arachidonic acid. *Am. J. Physiol.*, **242**, G582–587
37. Walus, K.M., Gustaw, P. and Konturek, S.J. (1980). Differential effects of prostaglandins and arachidonic acid on gastric circulation and oxygen consumption. *Prostaglandins*, **20**, 1089–102
38. Kauffman, G.L., Whittle, B.J.R. and Salmon, J.A. (1982). Gastric venous prostaglandin concentrations during basal and stimulated acid secretion in the dog. *Proc. Soc. Exptl. Med.*, **169**, 233–8
39. Guth, P.H., Paulson, G. and Nagata, H. (1984). Histologic and microcirculatory changes in alcohol-induced gastric lesions in the rat: Effect of prostaglandin cytoprotection. *Gastroenterology*, **87**, 1083–90
40. Whittle, B.J.R., Oren-Wolman, N. and Guth, P.H. (1985). Gastric vasoconstrictor actions of leukotriene C_4, $PGF_{2\alpha}$ and thromboxane mimetic U-46619 on rat submucosal microcirculation *in vivo*. *Am. J. Physiol.*, **248**, G580–G586

41. Konturek, S.J., Brzozowski, T., Prastuki, I., Radecki, T. and Dembinska-Kiec, A. (1963). Role of prostaglandins and thromboxane biosynthesis in gastric necrosis produced by taurocholate and ethanol. *Dig. Dis. Sci.*, **28**, 154–60

42. Whittle, B.J.R. (1984). Cellular mediators in gastric damage: actions of thromboxane A$_2$ and its inhibitors. In Allen, A., Garner, A., Flemström, G., Silen, W. and Turnberg, L.A. (eds) *Mechanisms of Mucosal Protection in the Upper Gastrointestinal Tract*, pp. 295–301 (Raven Press: New York)

43. Whittle, B.J.R., Kauffman, G.L. and Moncada, S. (1986). Hemostatic mechanisms, independent of platelet aggregation arrest gastric mucosal bleeding. *Proc. Natl. Acad. Sci. USA*, **83**, 5683–7

44. Palmer, R.M.J., Stepney, R., Higgs, G.A. and Eakins, K.E. (1980). Chemokinetic activity of arachidonic acid lipoxygenase products on leukocytes from different species. *Prostaglandins*, **20**, 411–18

45. Samuelsson, B., Hammarstrom, S., Murphy, R.C. and Borgeat, P. (1980). Leukotrienes and slow reacting substances of anaphylaxis (SRS-A). *Allergy*, **35**, 373–81

46. Piper, P.J. (ed.) (1986). *The Leukotrienes. Their Biological Significance.* (New York: Raven Press)

47. Morris, G.P. and Wallace, J.L. (1981). The roles of ethanol and of acid in the production of gastric mucosal erosions in rats. *Virchow's Arch. (Cell Pathol.)*, **38**, 23–38

48. Lacy, E.R. and Ito, S. (1982). Microscopic analysis of ethanol damage to rat gastric mucosa after treatment with a prostaglandin. *Gastroenterology*, **83**, 619–25

49. Peskar, B.M., Lange, K., Hoppe, U. and Peskar, B.A. (1986). Ethanol stimulates formation of leukotriene C$_4$ in rat gastric mucosa. *Prostaglandins*, **31**, 283–93

50. Boughton-Smith, N.K. and Whittle, B.J.R. (1987). Prostaglandin inhibition of ethanol-induced release of gastric mucosal leukotrienes. *Gastroenterology*, **92**, 1325

51. Wallace, J.L. and Whittle, B.J.R. (1985). Role of prostanoids in the protective actions of BW 755C on the gastric mucosa. *Eur. J. Pharmacol.*, **115**, 45–52

52. Benveniste, J. (1974). PAF – a new mediator of anaphylaxis and immune complex deposition from rabbit and human basophils. *Nature (London)*, **249**, 581–2

53. Demopoulos, C.A., Pinckard, R.N. and Hanahan, D.J. (1979). Platelet-activating factor: evidence for 1-O-alkyl-2-acetyl-sn-glyceryl-3-phosphorylcholine as the active component (a new class of lipid chemical mediators). *J. Biol. Chem.*, **254**, 9355–8

54. Braquet, P., Shen, T.Y., Touqui, L. and Vargaftig, B.B. (1987). Perspectives in platelet activating factor research. *Pharmacol. Rev.*, **39**, 97–145

55. Gonzalez-Crussi, F. and Hsueh, W. (1983). Experimental model of ischemic bowel necrosis. The role of platelet-activating factor and endotoxin. *Am. J. Pathol.*, **112**, 127–35

56. Wallace, J.L. and Whittle, B.J.R. (1986). Profile of gastrointestinal damage induced by platelet-activating factor. *Prostaglandins*, **32**, 137–41

57. Wallace, J.L. and Whittle, B.J.R. (1986). Picomole doses of platelet-activating factor predispose the gastric mucosa to damage by topical irritants. *Prostaglandins*, **31**, 989–98

58. Humphrey, D.M., McMannus, L.M., Satouchi, K., Hanahan, D.J. and Pinckard, R.N. (1982). Vasoactive properties of acetyl glyceryl ether phosphorylcholine and analogues. *Lab. Invest.*, **46**, 422–7

59. Whittle, B.J.R., Morishita, T., Ohya, T., Leung, F.W. and Guth, P.H. (1986). Microvascular actions of platelet-activating factor (PAF) on the rat gastric mucosa and submucosa. *Am. J. Physiol.*, **251**, 772–8

60. Doebber, J.W., Wu, M.S. and Shen, T.Y. (1984). Platelet activating factor intravenous infusion in rats stimulates vascular lysosomal hydrolase secretion independent of blood neutrophils. *Biochem. Biophys. Res. Comm.*, **125**, 980–7

61. Steel, G., Wallace, J.L. and Whittle, B.J.R. (1987). Failure of prostaglandin E$_2$ and its 16,16-dimethyl analogue to prevent the gastric mucosal damage induced by PAF. *Br. J. Pharmac.*, **90**, 365–71

62. Wallace, J.L. and Whittle, B.J.R. (1986). Effects of inhibitors of arachidonic acid metabolism on PAF-induced gastric mucosal necrosis and haemoconcentration. *Br. J. Pharmac.*, **89**, 415–22

63. Shumer, W. (1979). Septic shock. *J. Am. Med. Assoc.*, **242**, 1906–7

64. Bessin, P., Bonnet, J., Apffel, D., Soulard. C., Desgroux, L., Pelas, I. and Benveniste, J. (1983).

Acute circulatory collapse caused by platelet-activating factor (PAF-acether) in dogs. *Eur. J. Pharmacol.*, **86**, 403–13

65. Payne, J.G. and Bowen, J.C. (1981). Hypoxia of the canine gastric mucosa caused by *Escherichia coli* sepsis and prevented by methyl prednisolone therapy. *Gastroenterology*, **80**, 84–9

66. Nicholson, D.P. (1982). Glucocorticoids in the treatment of shock and the adult respiratory distress syndrome. *Clin. Chest Med.*, **3**, 121–32

67. Flower, R.J. and Blackwell, G.J. (1979). Anti-inflammatory steroids induce biosynthesis of a phospholipase A_2 inhibitor which prevents prostaglandin generation. *Nature (London)*, **278**, 456–9

68. Mencia-Huerta, J.M. and Benveniste, J. (1979). Platelet-activating factor and macrophages, I. Evidence for the release from rat and mouse peritoneal macrophages and not from mastocytes. *Eur. J. Immunol.*, **9**, 409–15

69. Doebber, T.W., Wu, M.S., Robbins, J.C., Choy, M., Chang, M.N. and Shen, T.Y. (1985). Platelet activating factor (PAF) involvement in endotoxin-induced hypotension in rats. Studies with PAF-receptor antagonist kadsurenone. *Biochem. Biophys. Res. Comm.*, **127**, 799–808

70. Terashita, Z., Imura, Y., Nishikawa, K. and Sumida, S. (1985). Is platelet activating factor (PAF) a mediator of endotoxin shock? *Eur. J. Pharmacol.*, **109**, 257–61

71. Wallace, J.L. and Whittle, B.J.R. (1986). Prevention of endotoxin-induced gastrointestinal damage by CV-3988, an antagonist of platelet-activating factor. *Eur. J. Pharmac.*, **124**, 209–10

72. Wallace, J.L., Steel, G., Whittle, B.J.R., Lagente, V. and Vargeftig, B. (1987). Evidence for platelet-activating factor (PAF) as a mediator of endotoxin-induced gastro-intestinal damage in the rat: Effects of three PAF antagonists. *Gastroenterology*, **93**, 765–73

73. Whittler, B.J.R., Boughton-Smith, N.K., Hutcheson, I.R., Espluges, J.V. and Wallace, J.L. (1987). Increased intestinal formation of Paf in endotoxin-induced damage in the rat. *Br. J. Pharmacol.*, **92**, 3–4

74. McCready, D.R., Clark, L. and Cohen, M.M. (1985). Cigarette smoking reduces human gastric luminal prostaglandin E_2. *Gut*, **26**, 1192–6

10
Gastric microvasculature and mucosal protection

P. E. O'BRIEN

INTRODUCTION

The hypothesis that ischaemia is a central factor in the pathogenesis of gastric mucosal disease was first proposed by Virchow in 1853. That hypothesis remains unproven today although data have been collected characterizing gastric microcirculation, identifying effects of damaging and protective or therapeutic agents on the microvasculature, and demonstrating associations between alteration of gastric microcirculation and various forms of gastric erosion and ulceration. This review selectively describes the structure and function of the microvasculature as it relates to known methods of gastric mucosal defence, reviews the studies of an association between changes in the microcirculation and changes in the capacity of the mucosa to resist injury and examines links between the microcirculation and acid peptic disease of the stomach.

STRUCTURE OF THE GASTRIC CIRCULATION

The stomach receives blood from the coeliac axis via six principal arteries and a number of secondary arteries. There are extensive anastomoses between these vessels and with vessels originating from the superior mesenteric artery. These anastomoses ensure that, with less than complete vascular isolation of the stomach, sufficient perfusion persists. Experimental partial devascularization of the stomach is frequently not associated with a change in function or with

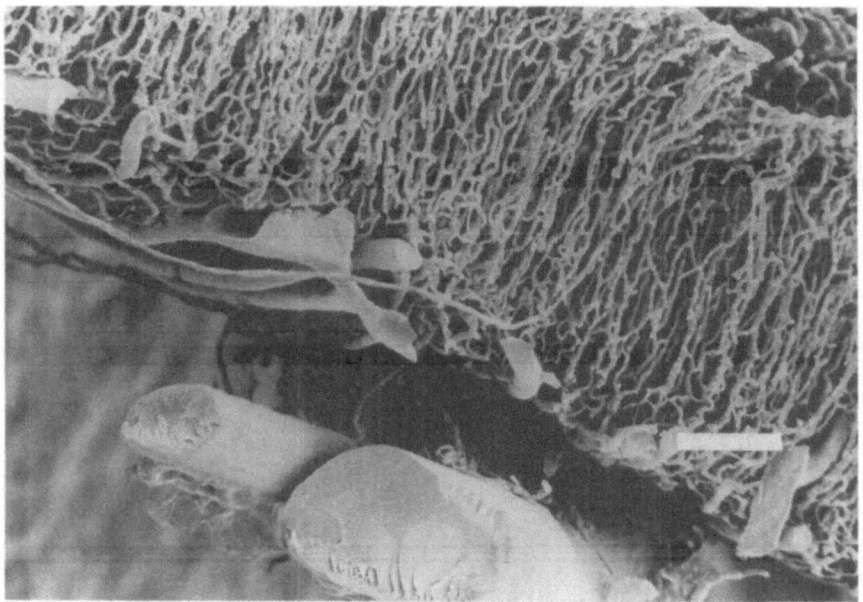

Figure 10.1   A lateral view of a microvascular cast of rat gastric mucosa showing a large artery and vein, smaller submucosal vessels and a capillary network arising from the submucosal arterioles and passing in a generally vertical direction towards the gastric lumen. Calibration bar equals 100 μm

disease[1] although in some models both a decrease in flow and an increase in gastric ulcer formation have been noted[2]. Partial devascularization of the stomach occurs with the operation of highly-selective vagotomy used in the treatment of duodenal ulcer disease. A marked decrease in the rate of perfusion of the lesser curve of the stomach has been noted in these patients soon after the procedure and episodes of necrosis of the lesser curve have been recorded, a complication which is thought to reflect effects on perfusion of the gastric wall[3].

Between 70 and 90% of the blood passing to the stomach is delivered to the mucosa[4,5]. The arrangement of the vessels, at the level of the submucosa and within the mucosa, has been characterized by the examination of micro-vascular casts by scanning electron microscopy[6,7]. At the level of the sub-mucosa, arteries divide into arterioles which then form capillaries passing into the mucosa. Arterioles do not appear to pass beyond the submucosa (Figure 10.1). Within the mucosa, the capillaries pass in a generally vertical direction between the gastric glands towards the lumen of the stomach to form a honeycomb-like network of capillaries immediately deep to the surface epi-thelium (Figure 10.2). These capillaries drain into infrequent venules at this

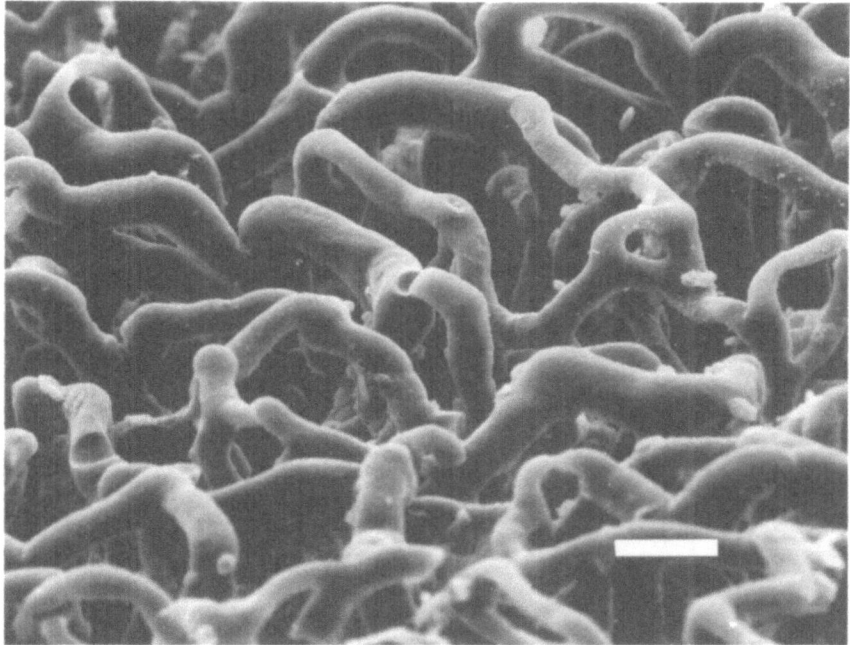

Figure 10.2   Loops of subsurface capillaries forming a honeycomb-like network about the region of the gastric glands. Calibration bar equals 20 μm

level of the mucosa which pass directly through the mucosa to the submucosa without receiving any further tributaries (Figure 10.3). In the rat stomach, each venule drains the capillary blood from approximately 60 gastric glands[8].

Although early studies[9,10] described the presence of arterio-venous (A-V) anastomoses in the gastric mucosa or submucosa, recent studies using microspheres[11,12], microvascular casts[6] and *in vivo* microscopy[13] have failed to demonstrate the presence of any A-V shunts. Given the sensitivities of these various techniques, it appears most unlikely that A-V shunting would account for more than 1% of gastric mucosal blood flow.

The ultrastructure of the mucosal microvessels and the relationship to the gastric mucosal cell reflects an important role in gastric mucosal defence. The capillaries passing between the gastric glands towards the lumen have a close proximity to the parietal and surface epithelial cells[6]. Diffusion distances between capillaries and the serosal surface of parietal cells is commonly less than 0.3 μm and is typically between 0.5 and 1.0μm for surface epithelium. These capillaries show endothelial vesicles and fenestrations. Carbonic anhydrase can be demonstrated in the endothelium in the region of these fen-

207

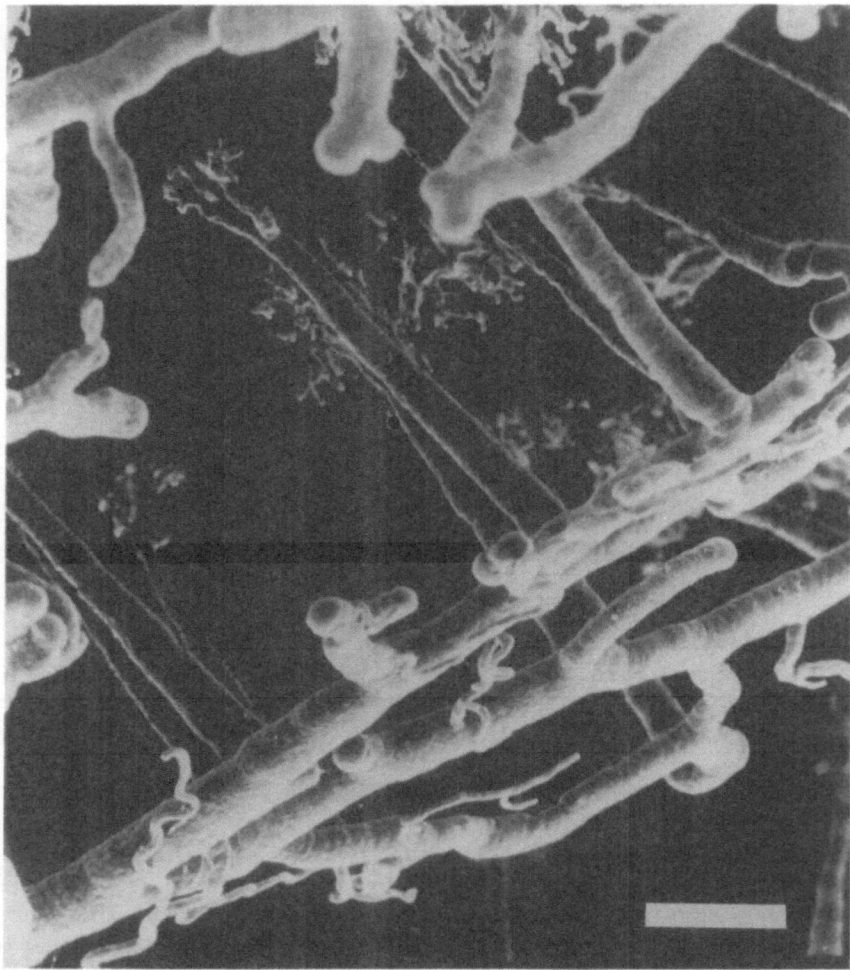

Figure 10.3 A partial venous cast showing submucosal vessels in the foreground and intramucosal venules passing vertically from the gastric lumen. Small tufts of residual capillaries are seen to be filled. Note the absence of capillaries entering into the venule at any point other than the subsurface region. Calibration bar equals 50 μm

estrations[14]. A close proximity between the parietal cells and the capillary endothelium, and the presence of carbonic anhydrase at that site, makes possible the transfer into the microcirculation of HCO_3^- generated by these cells in the process of acid secretion. In contrast, the endothelial cells of the venules contain few vesicles, are not fenestrated and generally separated from gastric epithelial cells by a minimum distance of 10–30 μm.

THE ROLE OF THE MICROVASCULATURE IN GASTRIC MUCOSAL DEFENCE MECHANISMS

The gastric mucosa has a complex array of defence mechanisms to enable it to resist damage by gastric acid[15]. These may be grouped into either barriers to diffusion, including the mucus–bicarbonate barrier[16] and the impermeability of the luminal membrane of gastric epithelial cells[17], or mechanisms for removing back-diffused acid from mucosa, either by neutralization within gastric epithelium or interstitium or by clearance from mucosa into the systemic circulation. If damage to the mucosa does occur, there is a capacity for rapid restitution of minor breaks in epithelial continuity[18] and further, the rapid turnover of gastric epithelium permits more rapid healing of significant lesions.

The microvasculature assists these mechanisms in several important ways. Firstly, the microcirculation through the mucosa permits the maintenance of normal acid–base status by supply of HCO_3^- from the systemic circulation or by local transport of the alkaline tide derived from active acid secretion. Secondly, it provides the metabolic support necessary for these energy dependent defence mechanisms, and thirdly, it provides a pathway for clearance of injurious agents, either intramucosal acid or irritants, from the interstitium of the mucosa.

1. Maintenance of acid–base status

A close proximity exists between parietal cells and the capillary endothelium. Transfer of HCO_3^- into capillaries is enhanced by the CO_2–$H_2CO_3^-$ switch catalysed by endothelial carbonic anhydrase[19]. The alkalinized blood then passes further towards the gastric lumen and at the level of the most superficial capillary network, there is also close proximity with the surface epithelial cells. The actively secreting gastric mucosa is better able to cope with exposure to acid in the gastric lumen than is a non-secreting mucosa[20], presumably owing to the transfer of the 'alkaline tide' of HCO_3^- into the mucosal capillaries. The HCO_3^- is then available for secretion into the mucus layer[21] or for intra-cellular neutralization of back-diffusing H^+.

This protective influence can be seen directly by increasing the HCO_3^- concentration available to isolated gastric mucosa. Conversely a decrease of HCO_3^- concentration or inhibition of carbonic anhydrase decreases the ability of the mucosa[22] to cope with H^+. The degree of gastric ulceration in several *in vitro* and *in vivo* models is inversely related to the HCO_3^- concentration in interstitial fluid[23–25].

The functional importance of the arrangement of gastric microvessels thus becomes evident (Figure 10.4). At times of active acid secretion and therefore lowered luminal pH, the alkaline tide is transferred by capillary network to the surface epithelium thereby increasing its capacity to cope with the acidic

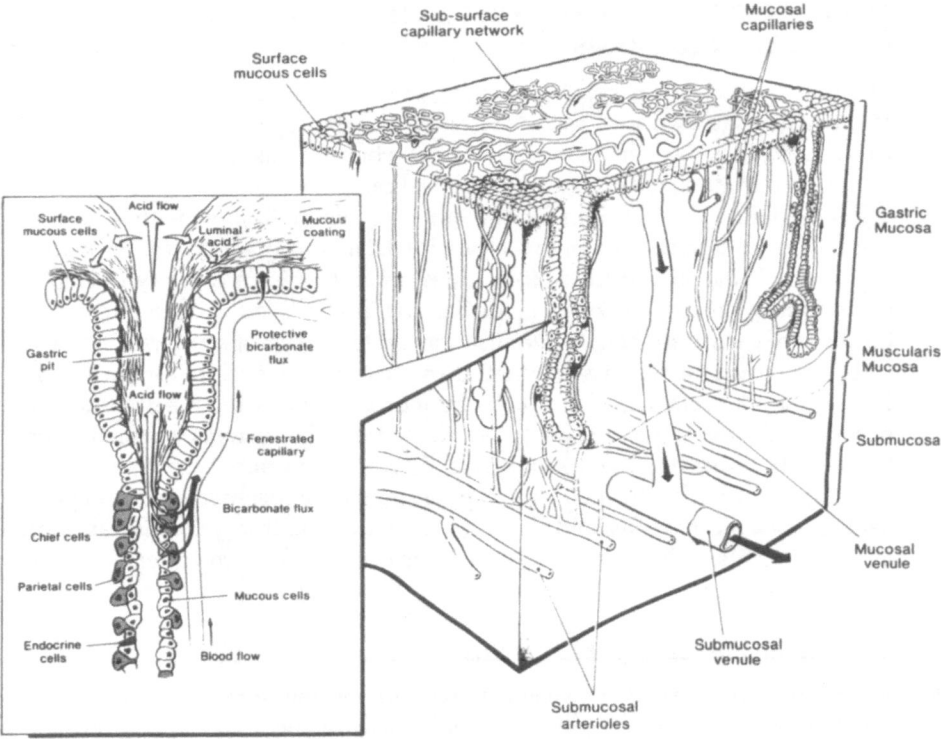

Figure 10.4 A diagram indicating the general organization of microvessels within gastric mucosa. The inset indicates the pathway for transport of interstitial HCO_3^- from the region of parietal cells to surface epithelium (from Ref. 7 with permission)

luminal fluid. The venules draining the capillary network are infrequent, thick walled and placed at a maximal distance from the surrounding gastric glands. Loss of the alkaline tide directly into the venous circulation must therefore be comparatively slight.

When focal areas of ischaemia exist, such as with stress ulceration[26], this arrangement for concomitant reinforcement of gastric mucosal defence at times of active acid secretion is subverted. Regions of the fundus and body which continue to be perfused also continue to secrete H^+ and are thereby protected by the derived alkaline tide. Adjacent areas which are non-secreting owing to ischaemia remain exposed to the acid secreted into the lumen but are relatively deprived of HCO_3^- to assist in defence against this acid.

210

2. Provision of metabolic support

Most, if not all, of the proposed defence mechanisms for the stomach are metabolically active and energy-dependent. The gastric epithelium is largely aerobic and as such is dependent on a constant supply of oxygen for oxidative metabolism, with energy stored in the form of ATP[27]. Reduction of ATP levels is associated with an impairment of the resistance of mucosa to injury[28]. Because of the absence of significant glycogen stores available in gastric mucosa, little anaerobic metabolism is possible and hypoxia is associated with rapid depletion of ATP levels. Haemorrhagic shock reduces the perfusion of superficial microvessels of fundic mucosa[29] and is associated with reduction of the redox potentials of the respiratory chain cytochromes[30]. The changes in microvascular filling, reduction of the respiratory chain cytochromes and reduction of ATP levels seen in association with haemorrhagic shock are more pronounced in the fundic mucosa than in gastric antrum[29–31].

3. Clearance of intra-mucosal irritants

The microcirculation is structured in such a way as to optimally clear acid and other potentially injurious agents from the interstitium of mucosa. The dense network of fenestrated capillaries lies directly beneath the principal absorptive areas of the mucosa and has the potential to transfer H^+ and toxic agents rapidly into thick-walled venules which pass directly out of the mucosa into the systemic circulation. Weak acids such as aspirin and other non-steroidal anti-inflammatory drugs (NSAIDs), and rapidly-diffusable compounds, such as ethanol, are readily absorbed across gastric mucosa and into the systemic circulation. Failure of perfusion of the stomach would be expected to result in increasing accumulation of these agents in gastric epithelial cells with greater cytolytic effects as a consequence[32].

CHANGE IN THE MICROCIRCULATION AS A PART OF GASTRIC MUCOSAL INJURY

In exploring the role of the microvasculature in the pathogenesis of gastric mucosal disease, most studies to date have focused on the microvascular effects of agents known to be injurious to the stomach or the microvascular changes during formation of acute gastric erosions.

Topical applications of injurious agents causes changes in the structure of microvessels and of the flow patterns through them. Scanning electron microscopy of microvascular casts, prepared after exposure of the rat stomach to absolute ethanol, shows gross disruption of the normal structure with large foci of loss of patency of the capillary network, frequently extending almost to the submucosal vessels[33]. Normal filling of the submucosal arterioles and

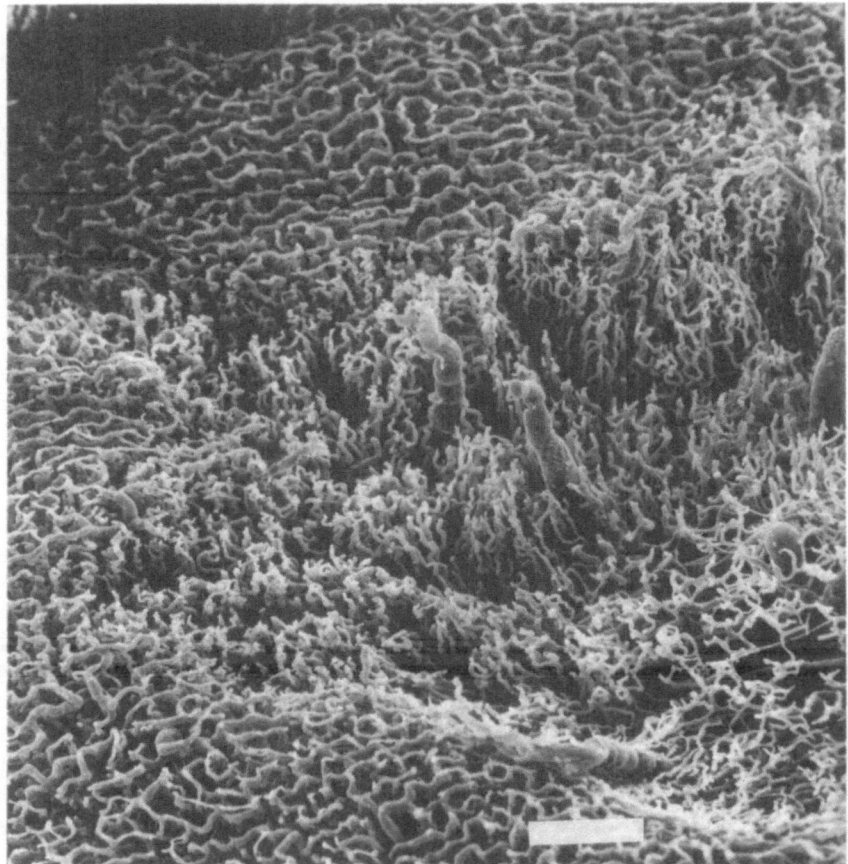

Figure 10.5 An area of a microvascular cast of rat gastric mucosa after exposure to 1 ml of absolute ethanol. There is an area in which there is almost complete lack of filling of the mucosal capillaries with submucosal vessels visible in the background. Note that the venules have filled and indicate the depth of loss of capillary patency. The area in the immediate foreground and at the top show normal subsurface capillary network. Calibration bar equals 200 μm

of the mucosal venules persists indicating that the primary vascular lesion is at the level of the mucosal capillaries. (Figure 10.5).

In vivo microscopy of the rat stomach shows cessation of flow in the superficial capillaries within 1 min of exposure to absolute ethanol and similar changes are observed with exposure to 0.6 M HCl or 0.2 M NaOH[34,35]. Parallel measurement of focal mucosal flow rate using laser Doppler velocimetry (LDV) shows a reduction of 30% of flow rate at 5 min after exposure to the irritant[35].

Notably, however, there is no significant change in LDV measures at 3 min suggesting that vascular change after injury is sequential, with damage to the subsurface capillary network preceding damage to capillaries deeper in the mucosa.

In spite of extensive study, the effects of topical irritants on the rate of gastric mucosal blood flow (GMBF) remain conflicting and the significance of possible changes unclear. Generally, topical aspirin and bile salts increase total GMBF, as measured by aminopyrine clearance[36], radiolabelled microspheres[37] or antipyrine clearance[38]. However, acidified aspirin and bile acids have been associated with a reduction of GMBF using aminopyrine clearance[39]. The techniques of measurement are clearly an important consideration and, for the aminopyrine clearance technique, at least, evidence now indicates that it is probably not a valid method, particularly for damaged mucosa[37,40]. Furthermore, the sequence of microvascular response to irritants may be important. It is possible that an increase of GMBF is a response to mucosal damage following initial vasoconstriction[41]. The route of administration may also be relevant as intravenous aspirin is associated with a decreased GMBF, possibly through an inhibitory effect on endogenous prostaglandin synthesis[42,43].

Further, it is increasingly apparent that, since gastric erosions and ulcers are focal disorders, potentially pathogenic changes in the microvasculature are also likely to be focal. With serial endoscopic examination of acutely-ill patients, Lucas and colleagues observed focal areas of pallor followed by hyperaemia preceding the development of gastric erosions[26]. In experimental models of stress ulceration, focal decrease in GMBF appears to precede the formation of erosions[44,45]. Exposure of gastric mucosa to aspirin also causes areas of focal pallor[37]. McGreevy and Moody[46], using radiolabelled microspheres, were unable to demonstrate any focal reduction of GMBF at the sites of aspirin-induced erosions. However, more recent studies with measurement of focal GMBF using H_2 gas clearance, showed a significant reduction of flow at the sites of pallor[47].

Studies of the sequence of tissue damage indicate that the microvascular changes occur prior to epithelial damage and erosion formation. Increased permeability of the mucosal microvessels to Evans Blue or albumin precedes the development of erosions[33,48]. Monastral Blue B, which labels damaged endothelium, is seen in the mucosal capillaries within 1 min of exposure to 75% or 100% ethanol and precedes the development, at the sites of labelled microvessels, of interstitial oedema and the formation of haemorrhagic erosions[48]. Examination of microvascular casts shows exudation of casting material from damaged microvessels apparently prior to loss of overlying epithelium[33]. Ultrastructural studies of rat stomach after aspirin exposure also shows the mucosal microvessels to be the primary point of damage[49]. Increasingly, particularly for aspirin- and ethanol-induced erosions, the data point to the development of erosions as an example of ischaemic infarction of tissue. (Figure 10.6).

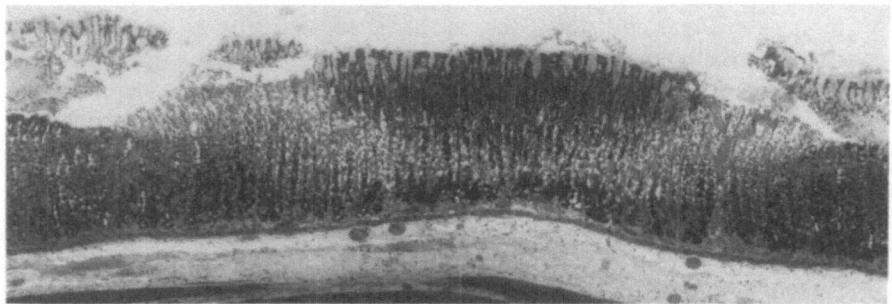

Figure 10.6 A histological section of rat fundic mucosa after exposure to absolute ethanol. There is an area of necrosis extending deep into the mucosa, almost to the level of the submucosa. A central area of epithelium has lifted off the remaining mucosa and is almost separated from the normal tissue by a cleft containing grossly damaged cells

PROTECTION OF GASTRIC MUCOSA AGAINST INJURY – ROLE OF THE MICROVASCULATURE

The recent recognition of the protective effect of prostaglandins (PG) on the gastrointestinal tract has stimulated extensive study of pharmacological means for enhancing gastric mucosal defence. Although other agents appear to provide varying degrees of protection, none has the apparent effectiveness of prostaglandins and some appear to act by stimulating endogenous PG synthesis. Thus the prostaglandins, particularly PGE_2, have become the benchmark for putative protective agents for gastric mucosa. The ability of topical application of prostaglandins to protect the stomach against a variety of necrotizing agents has been termed 'cytoprotection'[50]. The mechanism of this action has been the focus of much study and the subject of several excellent reviews[51–53]. A considerable body of data now exists which tests the hypothesis that effects of prostaglandins on the microvasculature are a central, if not a primary step, in the process of cytoprotection. The following data are important in examining the validity of this hypothesis.

1. Cytoprotection or vasoprotection?

The observations made in the original descriptions of cytoprotection by Robert et al.[50] were, to a large extent, of vascular events. As erosions are not visible to the naked eye, the observations were of bleeding onto the surface, intramucosal haemorrhage, as indicated by petechiae and 'red streaks', and debris from cellular breakdown and degraded mucus. Pretreatment by pro-staglandin prevents these vascular events although histological examination shows that damage to surface epithelium is not prevented[54]. The histological expression of cytoprotection is the absence of 'deep necrotic lesions', segmental areas of damaged mucosa extending almost to the level of the submucosa which separate from the surrounding apparently normal mucosa (Figure 10.6). These areas have the appearance of ischaemic infarcts and correlate well with the areas of loss of patency of the capillary network seen in microvascular casts (Figure 10.4) and with areas of circulatory stasis seen on *in vivo* microscopy[34,35].

2. Cytoprotective prostaglandins are vasoactive

The gastric mucosa generates prostaglandins of the E series, prostacyclin (PGI_2) and prostaglandin $F_{1\alpha}$. PGI_2 is consistently a vasodilator[55]. A number of studies have examined the effect of PGE_2 or its analogues on the rate of GMBF. Considerable variation in the results have been reported, reflecting not only the variability of measuring GMBF, owing to differences of techniques and experimental models, but also whether the dose given was anti-secretory or 'cytoprotective' and whether it was applied topically or given intravenously. In general, PGE_2 has been reported to increase the rate of GMBF in the resting (non-stimulated) gastric mucosa[56-58]. In a number of studies however, anti-secretory doses of PGE_2 are associated with a decrease of GMBF, particularly in the histamine-stimulated stomach[59-62].

Even when administered at 'cytoprotective doses' conflicting data exist. Holm-Rutili[63,64] used the technique of *in vivo* microscopy of rat stomach to measure the velocity of red blood cells and vessel diameters in superficial microvessels of rat gastric mucosa. Topical application of PGE_1 and PGE_2 caused a dose-related increase of red cell velocity of the order of 400–500%, without change in vessel diameter or in the rate of acid secretion. Topical application of 16,16-dimethyl-PGE_2 at a dosage which did not inhibit spon-taneous acid secretion, caused an increase of approximately 50% of red cell velocity in the superficial capillaries. This latter finding contrasts with that of Leung *et al.*[65] who also studied the effect of 'cytoprotective' dosage of 16,16-dimethyl-PGE_2 on the GMBF or rat stomach, using the H_2 gas-clearance technique. They noted a reduction of approximately 15% of GMBF at a dosage of 16,16-dimethyl-PGE_2 which did protect against ethanol damage to the rat stomach. The protective effect was associated with maintenance of the pretreatment level of GMBF. They concluded that the cytoprotective effect of this prostaglandin analogue was achieved by maintaining, rather than increasing, GMBF.

3. Cytoprotective agents maintain the integrity of the microcirculation

It is increasingly evident that focus on the increase of GMBF, as a mode of action of prostaglandins may be inappropriate. The effects of PGE_2 on the rate of GMBF seems to be inconsistent. Furthermore, there is poor correlation between the effects of various prostaglandins on GMBF and their cyto-protective capacity. Prostacyclin is a potent vasodilator and yet is not as effective a cytoprotective agent[50] as PGE_2. $PGF_{2\alpha}$ is both a vasoconstrictor and cytoprotective. Thus we must consider the possibility that prostaglandins mediate their protective effect more by preserving the integrity of the mic-rovasculature and maintaining normal microcirculation than by a primary effect on flow rate.

The structural integrity of the microvasculature has been shown to be preserved by pretreatment with prostaglandin prior to injury. Ethanol injury to rat stomach causes damage to the endothelium of mucosal microvessels[35], stasis within superficial capillary network[34], loss of patency of mucosal micro-vessels[33] and increased permeability of microvessels to albumin[33,34]. Each of these changes can be seen to occur early in the sequence of injury, generally preceding epithelial cell loss. Figure 10.7 shows a microvascular cast of rat gastric mucosa which had been exposed to absolute ethanol after pretreatment with PGE_2. There has been complete protection against loss of patency of deep mucosal capillaries, such as is seen in Figure 10.5. There is however, incomplete filling of the most superficial capillary loops and a few small exudates from superficial capillaries. Pretreatment by PGE_2 or an analogue limits the extent of these microvascular changes in response to ethanol and at the same time protects mucosa against cellular damage. As pretreatment by prostaglandin does not appear to induce a barrier to diffusion of damaging agents such as aspirin or ethanol into mucosa[66,67] the site of action of pro-staglandins is thus likely to be at the level of microvessels.

There are several possible mechanisms for this protective effect on micro-vessels. Firstly, prevention of the increased capillary permeability which results from endothelial damage will have the beneficial effect of avoiding interstitial oedema. Several studies have indicated that this is a potentially important component of gastric mucosal injury in shock[68,69], possibly owing to reduced oxygenation through increased diffusion distance between capillaries and epithelium or owing to impairment of maintenance of acid–base balance from stasis of intersitial fluid. Increased capillary permeability may also lead to increased blood viscosity to an extent sufficient to induce cessation of flow in some capillaries. Secondly, avoidance of plasma skimming may improve the haematocrit of blood in the superficial capillaries and thereby better maintain oxygenation of the epithelium[5]. Studies of gastric microcirculation using microspheres suggest the presence of plasma skimming in the normal micro-

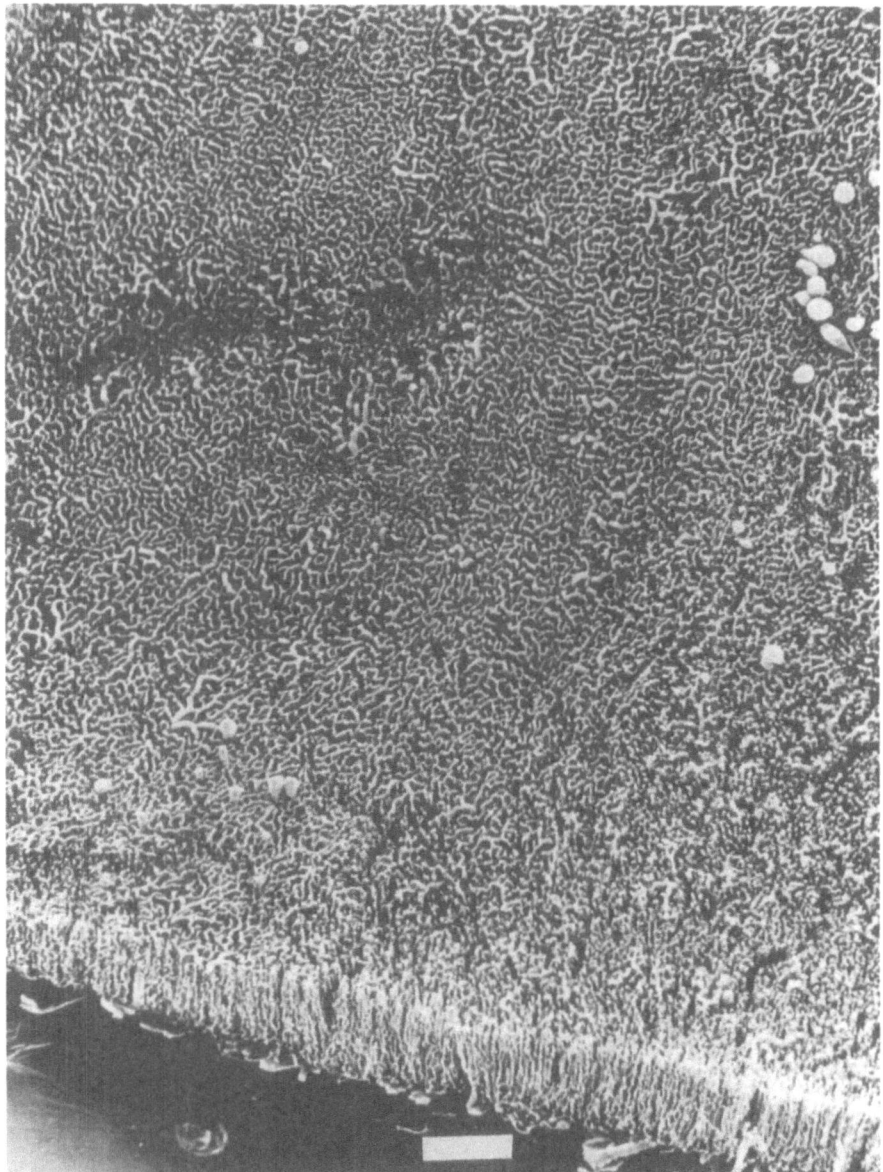

Figure 10.7 A microvascular cast of rat fundic mucosa which had been pretreated with PGE₂ (75 mg/kg intragastrically) followed by exposure to 1 ml of absolute ethanol. The lower right aspect of the cast shows some areas where the subsurface capillary network is incomplete. There are some small spherical exudates in the upper field. The remainder of the cast is, at this magnification, of normal appearance. Calibration bar equals 500 μm

217

circulation[70]. It is not known however, if prostaglandins modify this process. Thirdly, it is possible that prostaglandins may be truly cytoprotective to the endothelial cell. The initial point of injury in the unprotected mucosa appears to be the endothelium of microvessels with secondary stasis possibly as a result of leukocyte, platelet or red-cell thrombus formation[35].

4. Does cytoprotection occur in isolated gastric mucosa?

If cytoprotection could be demonstrated convincingly in an experimental system isolated from the circulation it would be clear that the effects of prostaglandins on the microvasculature were, at best, only a partial contributor to the process. However few studies appear to have pursued this approach. Schiessel et al.[71] found that 16,16-dimethyl-PGE_2 stimulated the bidirectional flux of Cl^- in isolated sheets of amphibian gastric mucosa. As the increased Cl^- flux is linked with the transfer of nutrient HCO_3^- into the cells, these workers considered that this vital step in the protection of the surface epithelium was supported by prostaglandins. Terano and co-workers[72] measured the viability of cell cultures of rat fundic mucosa by radio-labelled chromium-release assay and by dye exclusion and found that 16,16-dimethyl-PGE_2 appeared to protect the cells from damage by aspirin and sodium taurocholate. The relevance of these effects to the observation of protection against gross damage to the intact animal remains unclear.

Of greater importance is the study of Barzilai et al.[73] who described a cytoprotective effect of 16,16-dimethyl-PGE_2 in closed sacs of isolated amphibian gastric mucosa. The sacs were stimulated with histamine and incubated in nutrient solutions of differing buffer content. The protective effect was noted only in sacs incubated with 5 mM of phosphate buffer, gassed with 100% oxygen. The concentration of 16,16-dimethyl-PGE_2 used in these experiments (2.8×10^{-6}M) is sufficient to inhibit basal acid secretion in isolated amphibian gastric mucosa[74] but, as it was unable to inhibit the acid secretory rate of open sheets of histamine-stimulated mucosa, the authors argued that the effect of the prostaglandin analogue was not owing to inhibition of acid secretion and was therefore 'cytoprotective'. It is noteworthy, however, that if they inhibited acid secretion with the histamine H_2-receptor antagonist, metiamide, the cytoprotective effect of 16,16-dimethyl-PGE_2 was not seen.

THE MICROVASCULATURE AND GASTRIC MUCOSAL DISEASE

Although 135 years have passed since Virchow linked chronic peptic ulcer with mucosal ischaemia, there are as yet few studies which convincingly demonstrate that ischaemia is a central factor in the development or persistence of peptic ulcer disease or that failure of revascularization is an important component in failure of healing. In acute ulcerative conditions, particularly stress ulceration, a much more convincing link with mucosal ischaemia is present.

Reduction of the blood supply of the stomach appears to be associated with the development of peptic ulcer. Varhaug et al.[2] induced ischaemia of cat gastric mucosa by extensive devascularization and the blood flow through different regions of the stomach was measured, using radiolabelled microspheres. A marked reduction in mucosal blood flow was detected and one week after devascularization, ulcers were seen to have developed in the midportion of the greater curvature, at the site which had the most pronounced reduction in GMBF. Chronic gastric ulceration can be produced in the rat by ligation of the two major supplying arteries[75]. Extensive ulceration of the glandular stomach occurred over 3–5 days and healed over 1–3 months. The extent of ulceration could be modified, if during the initial 5 days, the rat was fed a buffering liquid diet, suggesting that acid-peptic digestion was occurring in the presence of ischaemia.

Stress ulceration is a form of acid-peptic digestion of gastric mucosa in critically-ill patients. The presence of ischaemia is almost invariable in this clinical setting and in experimental models of stress ulceration[76,77]. Most patients at risk of stress ulcers have had periods of sustained hypotension. Lucas et al.[26] performed sequential gastroscopic examination of severely traumatized patients and found the earliest observable lesion in the development of stress ulcer to be a focal area of mucosal pallor surrounded by a zone of hyperaemia. Histological studies of stomachs which had been resected for control of bleeding stress ulcers shows the presence of a coagulation type of ischaemic necrosis[78]. In a wide range of experimental models of stress ulceration, the induction of ischaemia is a central component[44,79,80]. The focal nature of the microcirculatory change was emphasized by Harjola and Sivula[44]. With the induction of haemorrhagic shock, rabbit gastric mucosa showed sharply demarcated foci of pallor. When blood volume was restored, these areas became hyperaemic and haemorrhagic as erosions developed.

It is evident from this described sequence that the possibility of ischaemia–reperfusion injury owing to the generation of oxygen-derived free radicals should be considered[81]. In support of this possibility, treatment with the hydroxyl radical scavenger, dimethylsulfoxide, has been shown to reduce the number and extent of stress ulcers in rats suffering cold restraint[82]. Further, pretreatment with superoxide dismutase and with allopurinol protects rats against haemorrhagic shock-induced gastric lesions[83]. An early event in reperfusion injury is an increase in vascular permeability, a pathway to injury similar to that seen after exposure of the stomach to toxic agents.

CONCLUSIONS

Adequate blood flow to the stomach is an essential component of normal gastric mucosal defence and reduction in perfusion is associated with the occurrence of mucosal damage. A significant body of data now exists showing that many agents which are toxic to the stomach have a primary, or at least a very early, effect on the gastric microvasculature.

Protection of the gastric mucosa by prostaglandins is partly dependent on maintaining the integrity of the microcirculation although it is not essential that mucosal perfusion is increased. It is likely that prevention of a decreased perfusion induced by damaging agents is sufficient to exert a protective effect.

REFERENCES

1. Jacobson, E.D. (1965). The circulation of the stomach. *Gastroenterology*, **48**, 85–109
2. Varhaug, J.E. and Svanges, K. (1979). Gastric ulceration and changes in acid secretion and increased blood flow after partial gastric devascularisation in cats. *Acta Chir. Scand.*, **145**, 313–19
3. Halvorsen, J.F., Heimann, P., Solhaug, J.H. and Jacobsen, K.B. (1975). Localised vascular necrosis of lesser curve of the stomach complicating highly selective vagotomy. *Br. Med. J.*, **2**, 590–1
4. Delaney, J.P. and Grim, E. (1964). Canine gastric blood flow and its distribution. *Am. J. Physiol.*, **207**, 1195–202
5. Lundgren, O. (1985). Gastric mucosal hemodynamics. *Gastroenterol. Clin. Biol.*, **9**, 26–9
6. Gannon, B.J., Browning, J. and O'Brien, P. (1982). The microvascular architecture of the glandular mucosa of the rat stomach. *J. Anat.*, **135**, 667–83
7. Gannon, B., Browning, J., O'Brien, P., Rogers, P. (1984). Mucosal microvascular architecture of the fundus and body of human stomach. *Gastroenterology*, **86**, 866–75
8. Holm-Rutili, L. and Obrink, K.J. (1985). Rat gastric mucosal microcirculation *in vivo*. *Am. J. Physiol*, **248**, G741–G746
9. Barlow, T.E., Bentley, F.H. and Walder, D.N. (1951). Arteries, veins and arteriovenous anastomoses in the human stomach. *Surg. Gynecol. Obstet.*, **93**, 657–71
10. Nylander, G. and Olerud, S. (1961). The vascular pattern of the gastric mucosa of the rat following vagotomy. *Surg. Gynecol. Obst.*, **112**, 475–80
11. Delaney, J.P. and Grim, E. (1964). Canine gastric blood flow and its distribution. *Am. J. Physiol.*, **207**, 1195–202
12. Archibald, L.H., Moody, F.G. and Simons, M. (1975). Measurement of gastric blood flow with radioactive microspheres. *J. Appl. Physiol.*, **38**, 1051–6
13. Guth, P.H. and Smith, E. (1975). Neural control of gastric mucosal blood flow in the rat. *Gastroenterology*, **69**, 935–40
14. Lonnerholm, G. (1983). Carbonic anhydrase in the monkey stomach and intestine. *Acta Physiol. Scand.*, **117**, 273–9
15. O'Brien, P.E. (1983). The nature of gastric mucosal defence against acid. In Carter, D.C. (ed.) *Peptic Ulcer*, pp. 28–43. (London: Churchill Livingstone)
16. Allen, A. and Garner, A. (1980). Mucus and bicarbonate secretion in the stomach and their possible role in mucosal protection. *Gut*, **21**, 249–62
17. Spenney, J.G., Shoemaker, R.L. and Sachs, G. (1974). Microelectrode studies of fundic gastric mucosa: cellular coupling and shunt conductance. *J. Membrane Biol.*, **19**, 105–28
18. Silen, W. and Ito, S. (1985). Mechanisms for rapid re-epithelialization of the gastric mucosal surface. *Annu. Rev. Physiol.*, **47**, 217–29
19. Lutjen-Drecoll, E., Eichhorn, M. and Barany, E.H. (1985). Carbonic anhydrase in epithelia

and fenestrated juxtaepithelial capillaries of *Macaca fascicularis. Acta Physiol. Scand.*, **124**, 295–307

20. O'Brien, P.E. and Silen, W. (1976). Influence of acid secretory state on the gastric mucosal tolerance to back diffusion of H^+. *Gastroenterology*, **71**, 760–5

21. Flemström, G. (1977). Active alkalinization by amphibian gastric fundic mucosa *in vitro*. *Am. J. Physiol.*, **233**, E1–E12.

22. O'Brien, P. and Bushell, M. (1980). The role of acid–base status in the response of the isolated amphibian gastric mucosa to back diffusion of H^+. *Gastroenterology*, **79**, 439–46

23. Cheung, L.Y., Porterfield, G. (1979). Protection of the gastric mucosa against acute ulceration by intravenous infusion of sodium bicarbonate. *Am. J. Surg.*, **137**, 106–10

24. Kivilaakso, E., Barzilai, R., Schiessel, R., Crass, R. Silen, W. (1979). Ulceration of isolated amphibian gastric mucosa. *Gastroenterology*, **77**, 31–7

25. Bushell, M. and O'Brien, P. (1982). Acid–base imbalance and ulceration in the cold restrained rat. *Surgery*, **91**, 318–22

26. Lucas, C.W., Sugawa, C., Riddle, J., Rector, J., Rector, F., Rosenberg, B., Walt, A.J. (1971). Natural history and surgical dilemma of 'stress' gastric bleeding. *Arch. Surgery*, **102**, 266–72

27. Bowen, J.C., Fairchild, R.B. (1984). Oxygen in gastric mucosal protection. In Allen, A., Flemström, G., Garner, A., Silen, W., Turnberg, L. (eds) *Mechanisms of Mucosal Protection in the Upper Gastrointestinal Tract*, pp. 259–66. (New York: Raven Press)

28. Menguy, R., Desbaillets, L., Masters, Y.F. (1974). Mechanism of stress ulcers: I. Influence of hypovolemic shock on energy metabolism in gastric mucosa. *Gastroenterology*, **66**, 46–55

29. Kivilaakso, E., Ahonen, J., Aronsen, K-F., Hockerstedt, K., Kalima, T., Lempinen, M., Suoranta, H., Vernerson, E. (1982). Gastric blood flow, tissue gas tension and microvascular changes during hemorrhage-induced stress ulceration in the pig. *Am. J. Surg.*, **143**, 322–30

30. Menguy, R. and Masters, Y.F. (1974). Mechanism of stress ulcer. Differences between the antrum, corpus and fundus with respect to the effects of complete ischemia on gastric mucosal energy metabolism. *Gastroenterology*, **66**, 509–16

31. Sato, N., Kamada, T., Motoaki, S., Kawano, S., Hiroshi, A. and Hagihara, B. Measurement of hemoperfusion and oxygen sufficiency in gastric mucosa *in vivo*. *Gastroenterology*, **78**, 814–19

32. Martin, B.K. (1963). Accumulation of drug actions in gastric mucosal cells. *Nature (London)*, **198**, 896–7

33. O'Brien, P.E., Schultz, C. and Gannon, B. The protective effect of the synthetic prostaglandin Enprostil on the gastric microvasculature after ethanol injury in the rat. *Am. J. Med.*, **81**, 12–17

34. Guth, P.H., Paulsen, G., Nagata, H. (1984). Histologic and microcirculatory changes in alcohol-induced gastric lesions in the rat: effect of prostaglandin cytoprotection. *Gastroenterology*, **87**, 1083–90

35. Pihan, G., Majzoubi, I., Haudenschild, C., Trier, J., Szabo, S. (1986). Early microcirculatory stasis in acute gastric mucosal injury in the rat and prevention by 16,16-dimethyl prostaglandin E_2 or sodium thiosulphate. *Gastroenterology*, **91**, 1415–26

36. Augur, N. (1970). Gastric mucosal blood flow following damage by ethanol, and acid or aspirin. *Gastroenterology*, **58**, 311–20

37. Cheung, L.Y., Moody, F.G., Reese, R.S. (1975). Effect of aspirin, bile salt and ethanol on canine gastric mucosal blood flow. *Surgery*, **77**, 786–92

38. Whittle, B.J.R. (1977). Mechanisms underlying gastric mucosal damage induced by indomethacin and bile-salts, and the actions of prostaglandins. *Br. J. Pharmacol.*, **60**, 455–60

39. O'Brien, P. and Silen, W. (1973). Effects of bile salts and aspirin on the gastric mucosal blood flow. *Gastroenterology*, **64**, 246–53

40. Miller, T., Henagan, J. and Log, T. (1983). Impairment of aminopyrine clearance in aspirin-damaged canine gastric mucosa. *Gastroenterology*, **85**, 643–9

41. Guslandi, M. (1986). Mucosal blood flow and gastric protection – effect of neurohormonal and pharmacological agents. *Int. J. Clin. Pharmacol. Ther. Toxicol.*, **3**(24), 143–7

42. Kauffman, G.L., Arues, D. and Grossman, M.I. (1980). Intravenous indomethacin and aspirin reduce basal gastric mucosal blood flow in dogs. *Am. J. Physiol.*, **238**, G131–4
43. Gerkens, J.F., Shand, D.G., Flexner, C., Nies, A.S., Oates, J.A. and Data, J.L. (1977). Effect of indomethacin and aspirin on gastric blood flow and acid secretion. *J. Pharmacol. Exptl. Ther.*, **203**, 646–52
44. Harjola, P. and Sivula, A. (1966). Gastric ulcer following experimentally induced hypoxia and haemorrhagic shock: *in vivo* study of pathogenesis in rabbits. *Ann. Surgery*, **163**, 21–8
45. Gaskill, H.V., Sirinek, K.R. and Levine, B.A. (1983). Focal mucosal ischemia is a precursor to stress-mediated gastric mucosal ulceration. *Surg. Gastroenterol.*, **2**, 225–30
46. McGreevy, J.M. and Moody, F.G. (1981). Focal microcirculatory changes during the production of aspirin-induced gastric mucosal erosions. *Surgery*, **89**, 337–41
47. Ashley, S.W., Sonnenschein, L.A. and Cheung, L.Y. (1985). Focal gastric mucosal blood flow at the site of aspirin-induced ulceration. *Am. J. Surg.*, **149**, 53–9 May 22–23
48. Szabo, S., Trier, J.S., Brown, A. and Schnoor, J. (1985). Early vascular injury and increased vascular permeability in gastric mucosal injury caused by ethanol in the rat. *Gastroenterology*, **88**, 228–36
49. Robins, P.G. (1980). Ultrastructural observations on the pathogenesis of aspirin-induced gastric erosions. *Br. J. Exptl. Path.*, **61**, 497–503
50. Robert, A. (1981). Prostaglandins and the gastrointestinal tract. In Johnson, L.R. (ed.) *Physiology of the Gastrointestinal Tract*, pp. 1407–34. (New York: Raven Press)
51. Robert, A., Nezamis, J.E., Lancaster, C. and Hanchar, A.J. (1979). Cytoprotection by prostaglandins in rats: Prevention of gastric necrosis produced by alcohol, HCl, NaOH, hypertonic NaCl, and thermal injury. *Gastroenterology*, **77**, 433–43
52. Miller, T.A. (1983). Protective effects of prostaglandins against gastric mucosal damage: current knowledge and proposed mechanisms. *Am. J. Physiol.*, **245**, G601–G623
53. Hawkey, C.J. and Rampton, D.S. (1985). Prostaglandins and the gastrointestinal mucosa: are they important in its function, disease, or treatment? *Gastroenterology*, **89**, 1162–88
54. Lacy, E.R. and Ito, S. (1983). Microscopic analysis of ethanol damage to rat gastric mucosa after treatment with a prostaglandin. *Gastroenterology*, **83**, 619–25
55. Gaskill, H.V., Sirinek, K.R. and Levine, B.A. (1982). Prostacyclin increases gastric mucosal blood flow via cyclic AMP. *J. Surg. Res.*, **33**, 140–5
56. Main, I.H.M. and Whittle, B.J.R. (1973). The effects of E and A prostaglandins on gastric mucosal blood flow and acid secretion in the rat. *Br. J. Pharmacol.*, **49**, 428–36
57. Konturek, S.J., Robert, A., Hanchar, A.J. and Nezamis, J.E. (1980). Comparison of prostacyclin and prostaglandin E_2 on secretion, gastrin release and mucosal blood flow in dogs. *Dig. Dis. Sci*, **25**, 673–79
58. Gerkens, J.F., Gerber, J.G., Shand, D.G. and Branch, R.A. (1978). Effect of PGI_2, PGE_2 and 6-keto PGF_1 on canine gastric blood flow and acid secretion. *Prostaglandins*, **16**, 815–23
59. Jacobson, E.D. (1970). Comparison of prostaglandin E_1 and norepinephrine on the gastric mucosal circulation. *Proc. Soc. Exptl. Biol. Med.*, **133**, 516–19
60. Miller, T.A., Henagan, J. and Robert, A. (1980). The effect of 16,16-dimethyl prostaglandin E_2 on resting and histamine-stimulated canine gastric mucosal blood flow. *Dig. Dis. Sci.*, **25**, 561–7
61. Wilson, D.E. and Levine, R.A. (1972). The effect of prostaglandin E_1 on canine gastric acid secretion and gastric mucosal blood flow. *Am. J. Dig. Dis.*, **17**, 527–32
62. Main, I.H.M. and Whittle, B.J.R. (1973). The effects of E and A prostaglandins on gastric mucosal blood flow and acid secretion in the rat. *Br. J. Pharmacol.*, **49**, 428–36
63. Holm-Rutili, L. (1986). Effects of prostaglandin E_1, E_2 and 16,16-dimethyl-E_2 on gastric mucosal microcirculation and basal acid output in the rat. *Acta Physiol. Scand.*, **127**, 313–21
64. Holm-Rutili, L. and Obrink, K.J. (1985). Rat gastric mucosal microcirculation *in vivo*. *Am. J. Physiol.*, **248**, G741–G746
65. Leung, F.W., Robert, A. and Guth, P.H. (1985). Gastric mucosal blood flow in rats after administration of 16,16-dimethyl prostaglandin E_2 at a cytoprotective dose. *Gastroenterology*, **88**, 1948–53

66. Guth, P.H. and Paulsen, G. (1979). Prostaglandin cytoprotection does not involve interference with aspirin absorption. *Proc. Soc. Exptl. Biol. Med*, **162**, 128–30
67. Robert, A. Lancaster, C., Davis, J.P., Field, S.O., Wickrema Sinha, A.J., Thornburgh, B.A. (1985). Cytoprotection by prostaglandins occurs in spite of penetration of absolute ethanol into the gastric mucosa. *Gastroenterology*, **88**, 328–33
68. Arvidsson, S., Falt, K. and Haglund, U. (1984). Acute gastric mucosal ulceration in septic shock. An experimental study on pathogenic mechanisms. *Acta Chir. Scand.*, **150**, 541–7
69. Bowen, J.C. (1979). Persistent gastric mucosal hypoxia and interstitial edema after hemorrhagic shock: prevention with steroid therapy. *Surgery*, **85**, 268–74
70. Varhaug, J-E., Svanes, K., Svanes, C. and Lekven, J. (1984). Gastric blood flow determination: intramural distribution and arteriovenous shunting of microspheres. *Am. J. Physiol.*, **247**, G468–G479
71. Schiessel, R.J., Matthews, A., Barzilai, A., Merhav, A. and Silen, W. (1980). PGE$_2$ stimulates gastric chloride transport: possible key to cytoprotection. *Nature (London)* **283**, 671–73
72. Terano, A., Mach, T., Stachura, J., Tarnawski, A. and Ivey, K.J. (1984). Effect of 16,16-dimethyl prostaglandin E$_2$ on aspirin induced damage to rat gastric epithelial cells in tissue culture. *Gut*, **25**, 19–25
73. Barzilai, A., Schiessel, R., Kivilaakso, E., Matthews, J.B., Fleischer, L.A., Bartzokis, G. and Silen, W. (1980). Effect of 16,16-dimethyl prostaglandin E$_2$ on ulceration of isolated amphibian gastric mucosa. *Gastroenterology*, **78**, 1508–12
74. Garner, A., Flemström, G. and Heylings, J.R. (1979). Effects of anti-inflammatory agents and prostaglandins on acid and bicarbonate secretion in the amphibian isolated gastric mucosa. *Gastroenterology*, **77**, 451–7
75. Guth, P.H., Paulsen, G. and Foroozan, P. (1975). Experimental gastric ulcer due to ischemia in rats. *Am. J. Dig. Dis.*, **20**, 824–34
76. Silen, W. and Skillman, J.J. (1974). Stress ulcer, acute erosive gastritis and the gastric mucosal barrier. In Stollerman, G.H. (ed.) *Advances in Internal Medicine*, p. 195–212 (Chicago: Year Book Medical Publishers)
77. Butterfield, W.C. (1975). Experimental stress ulcers: a review. In Nyhus, L.M. (ed.) *Surgery Annual*, chap. 7, pp. 261–278. (NY: Appleton Century Crofts)
78. Lev, R., Molot, M.D., McNamara, J.J. and Stremple, J.F. (1971). 'Stress' ulcers following war wounds in Vietnam: a morphological and histochemical study. *Lab. Invest.*, **25**, 491–502
79. Goodman, A. and Osborne, M. (1972). An experimental model and clinical definition of stress ulceration. *Surg., Gynecol. Obstet.*, **134**, 563–71
80. Moody, F. and Aldrete, J. (1971). Hydrogen permeability of canine gastric secretory epithelium during formation of acute superficial erosions *Surgery*, **70**, 154–60
81. Granger, D.N., Hollwarth, M.E. and Parks, D.A. (1986). Ischemia-reperfusion injury: role of oxygen-derived free radicals. *Acta Physiol. Scand.*, **548**, 47–63
82. Cochran, T., Skpanko, J., Moore, C. and Saik, R. (1983). Dimethylsulfoxide protection against gastric stress ulceration. *Curr. Surg.*, **40**, 435-7
83. Itoh, M. and Guth, P. (1985). Role of oxygen-derived free radicals in hemorrhagic shock-induced gastric lesions in the rat. *Gastroenterology*, **88**, 1162–7

11
Enhancing mucosal defence and repair mechanisms

A. GARNER

INTRODUCTION

Inhibition of gastric acid secretion has proved to be an extremely effective pharmacological approach in the management of human peptic ulcer disease. This is reflected by the success of cimetidine and ranitidine, which have become the world's two top selling drugs, and by the plethora of other antisecretory agents which have entered clinical trials over recent years. Efficacy of anti-secretory therapy largely reflects retardation of wound healing by the acidic environment which prevails in the upper gastrointestinal tract. Hyperacidity does not, however, provide an aetiologic basis for the disease since gastric and most duodenal ulcer patients secrete normal or less than normal amounts of acid. Two possible causes of ulceration are failure of mechanisms which normally enable gastroduodenal mucosa to resist intraluminal acid and pepsin, or failure of mechanisms which normally enable the epithelium to rapidly repair superficial damage. Potentially, therefore, drugs which seek to enhance either mucosal protection or repair represent attractive alternatives to inhibiting acid secretion, particularly in view of concerns over the consequences of long-term therapy with antisecretory drugs. Thus, a number of potent, long-acting inhibitors of acid secretion have induced tumours in the stomachs of laboratory animals during toxicological evaluation[1], while diseases associated with hypo-chlorhydria such as pernicious anaemia, or surgery aimed at reducing intra-luminal acidity increase susceptibility to gastric cancer[2,3].

The ability of gastric and duodenal mucosa to resist autodigestion has been

225

a source of intrigue for more than two centuries but, despite intensification of basic research effort, the underlying mechanisms are not fully understood[4,5]. Lack of a unifying hypothesis of mucosal protection has hampered the search for drugs which act by mechanisms other than inhibiting acid secretion and the majority of protective drugs in current use were developed with little knowledge of their mode of action. Prostaglandins represent the most recent attempt to introduce a new class of antiulcer drug which combine antisecretory and protective actions. However, these agents have proved somewhat disappointing clinically and it would appear that efficacy can be explained solely on the basis of antisecretory activity[6]. In comparison with the study of acid secretion and even mucosal protection, mechanisms of healing of gastric and duodenal mucosal lesions have received much less attention. Recent descriptions of rapid re-epithelialization of the stomach following superficial injury have served to focus attention on one aspect of mucosal repair (see Chapter 8). While this process is clearly distinct from the repair of a chronic ulcer, it is possible that ulcers develop as a result of failure of superficial repair mechanisms.

The aims of this chapter are broadly two-fold: firstly, to review the actions of current protective drugs since it is only by understanding their activity that rational improvements in design can be contemplated and secondly, to describe proposed mechanisms of protection and repair in order that an appreciation can be gained of the prospects of developing novel antiulcer drugs.

PROTECTIVE DRUGS

These agents may be considered to act by enhancing protective mechanisms owing to a specific pharmacological action or by reducing the autolytic activity of luminal contents due to adsorption of HCl, proteolytic enzymes and bile acids within the lumen or at the mucosal surface. Adherence of insoluble particles to the mucosa may also induce liberation of biologically-active transmitters as a result of a counter-irritant response. Indeed, stimulation of mucosal prostaglandin production has been claimed for all of the agents in this category but whether this is anything more than an epiphenomenon has not been established.

Carbenoxolone

This compound is a synthetic derivative of glycyrrhizic acid, a constituent of liquorice, sold in the U.K. as Biogastrone® and Duogastrone® (Winthrop). Carbenoxolone was the first antiulcer drug to be actively promoted on the basis of absent antisecretory activity and demonstrated that peptic ulcers could be healed by mechanisms other than reducing luminal acidity. Actions of carbenoxolone which have been claimed to account for antiulcer activity include increasing the life-span of surface epithelial cells and stimulating mucus glycoprotein biosynthesis as well as elevating mucosal prostaglandin levels[7,8]. Potentially severe side-effects resulting from sodium retention and hypokalaemia limit the use of carbenoxolone. Deglycyrrhizinized liquorice products (e.g. Caved-S®, Tillots) are free of these undesirable effects but have lower efficacy as antiulcer drugs in man.

Bismuth salts

Interest in bismuth containing compounds has been revived with the introduction of the complex salt tripotassium dicitratobismuthate, marketed as De-Nol® (Gist-Brocades). Of particular interest has been the finding of a significantly lower relapse rate in patients treated with this drug. A summary of clinical trial data[9] reveals that De-Nol produces comparable rates of healing to cimetidine or ranitidine but relapse rates 12 months after healing are consistently lower compared with H_2-receptor antagonists in both gastric (40% versus 60%) and duodenal (64% versus 87%) ulcer patients. The compound has been reported to protect the mucosa of laboratory animals against acute gastric lesions induced by various noxious agents and to increase mucosal production of prostaglandins[10]. However, a potentially more important finding concerns the activity of De-Nol against *Campylobacter pylori* in humans[11]. These curved bacilli colonize the surface mucus layer in the stomach and have been implicated in the pathogenesis of gastritis, for which the evidence is good, and duodenal ulcer, for which the evidence is more tenuous[12]. *Campylobacter pylori* is moderately sensitive to bismuth salts *in vitro* and can be eradicated *in vivo*, a response which is proposed as a basis for the lowered relapse rate (see Chapter 5).

Sucralfate

Sucralfate is an aluminium salt of sulphated sucrose discovered by the Japanese company Chugai and sold under a number of trademarks including Antepsin® (Ayerst) in the U.K. and Carafate® (Marion) in the U.S.A. A large number of endoscopically-controlled trials have demonstrated sucralfate to be as effective as cimetidine in peptic-ulcer healing but, as with antisecretory therapy, subsequent recurrence is not influenced[13,14]. Sucralfate has low aqueous solubility and can be seen to form a white coating over the mucosal surface following oral administration. The drug was originally considered to act by inhibiting pepsin and by forming a protective barrier as a result of binding to exposed protein in the ulcer base. It remains a distinct possibility that local reaction to adherence of insoluble particles to the ulcer crater in some way promotes wound repair. Although sucralfate has minimal buffering capacity, it is also possible that local neutralization and adsorption of acid and pepsin at the ulcer site contributes to therapeutic activity. In common with other agents in this class, sucralfate induces local prostaglandin biosynthesis and protects against several forms of chemical injury in experimental animals[15,16]. These actions are blocked by non-steroidal anti-inflammatory agents, but the doses used have generally been far in excess of those required to specifically inhibit cyclooxygenase and the role of endogenous prostaglandin production in the overall mechanism of action of sucralfate remains an open question. The significance of enhanced prostaglandin formation for the healing of chronic peptic ulcers in man is similarly complicated not least by the lack of anti-secretory activity of sucralfate, an action in sharp contrast to that of exogenous prostaglandins which depend on inhibition of acid secretion to exert a therapeutic effect.

Prostaglandins

Numerous synthetic prostaglandins are currently in clinical development and two analogues, misoprostil (Cytote®, Searle) and enprostil (Gardrin®, Syntex) have been marketed in some countries. Initial interest in prostaglandins arose from the finding that members of the E series were extremely potent inhibitors of acid secretion. However, this property has been rather overshadowed by interest generated in the observation that prostanoids inhibited formation of acute mucosal haemorrhagic lesions by a mechanism independent of anti-secretory activity[17]. Numerous publications, reviews and symposia have addressed the mechanism of this so-called 'cytoprotective' action[18,19]. Current opinion favours the vasculature as the principal site of action with maintenance of blood flow and prevention of stasis as the principal mechanism of action of prostaglandins in preventing acute, chemically-induced gastric mucosal damage[20]. Although stimulation of gastroduodenal bicarbonate secretion and mucus release have been widely reported[21,22], these actions are unlikely to contribute to protection against acute damage induced by exogenous chemicals such as concentrated ethanol, acid or alkali. To date, the promise of synthetic prostaglandins has not generally been translated into clinical success with most trials reporting a high incidence of side effects (e.g. diarrhoea and abdominal cramp) and indicating that acute ulcer healing is due simply to inhibition of acid secretion[6].

Acid inhibitors

Interest generated in the phenomenon of 'cytoprotection' has prompted studies to determine whether this property is a feature of drugs designed to act on the parietal cell and hitherto regarded as acting solely by lowering luminal H^+ ion concentration. There are numerous reports in the literature that cimetidine protects the gastric mucosa of experimental animals against acute chemical injury. Similar findings have appeared extending the observations to other H_2-receptor antagonists, other classes of antisecretory agent, and antacids. Unfortunately, interpretation of these studies has been almost exclusively based on inhibition of acute damage in animals assessed by gross macroscopic appearance of the stomach. The dangers of such an approach have been emphasized in the literature on repeated occasions[23-25]. Studies using in vitro systems have reported a direct protective effect of the H^+–K^+-ATPase antagonist, omeprazole, on gastric epithelial cells in culture[26]. In addition to simple bulk neutralization, a direct action of certain cations (e.g. Ca, Mg, Al, Bi) on the epithelium may contribute to the antiulcer action of antacids as well as protective drugs. In the case of duodenal ulcer healing, however, it seems unlikely that mechanisms other than inhibition of acid output are relevant in view of the excellent correlation between therapeutic efficacy and antisecretory activity of a wide range of drugs[27].

IMPROVING CURRENT AGENTS

At present histamine H_2-receptor antagonists dominate the anti-ulcer market and protective drugs are unquestionably regarded as second-line therapy by the vast majority of prescribers. Current agents have no advantages over cimetidine or ranitidine in terms of healing response or pain relief and by comparison with H_2-receptor antagonists, all protective drugs suffer in terms of dose frequency, palatability and/or side-effect profile. There is also a theoretical risk of toxicity owing to absorption of aluminium or bismuth although this is unlikely to occur during short-term use. Since the mechanism(s) of action of protective drugs are not established, no rationale exists on which to base the search for improved activity and any improvements which are contemplated will probably be minor and involve, for example formulation changes and reductions in dose frequency. A major opportunity does exist for therapy which prolongs remission. Results comparing De-Nol with H_2-receptor antagonists suggest this is achievable although it cannot be totally discounted that healing with antisecretory agents in fact accelerates the process of recurrence by increasing parietal cell mass or sensitivity to agonists or even promoting bacterial colonization. Association of ulcer healing by De-Nol with disappearance of *Campylobacter pylori* has prompted clinical evaluation of antibiotics in combination with antiulcer drugs[11,28]. Preliminary findings that De-Nol plus an antibacterial agent reduces relapse over the following 12 months to a level comparable with that achieved by continuous treatment with an H_2-receptor antagonist offers the promise that the natural history of ulcer disease can be favourably modified by a single healing course without resort to maintenance therapy. Should these observations be confirmed, development of antimicrobial agents specifically targetted at *Campylobacter* organisms and the stomach could become attractive for treating gastritis and peptic ulcer.

A large number of compounds discovered by screening of acute gastric injury in animal models are under development but there is no way of predicting whether such agents will be clinically superior to existing anti-ulcer drugs. Many of these compounds are purported to induce prostaglandin generation although this may simply reflect the non-specific liberation of inflammatory mediators consequent upon mild irritation of the mucosa. A more specific approach to elevating mucosal eicosanoids is to stimulate local biosynthesis or inhibit metabolic inactivation. One such drug, sufalcone (Solon®, Taisho), is claimed to act by inhibiting the enzyme 15-hydroxy-prostaglandin-dehydrogenase responsible for degradation of prostaglandins[29]. Current analogues of the E-series prostaglandins do not seem to offer any advantage over established ulcer healing drugs and are unlikely to challenge the dominance of H_2-receptor antagonists even if longer acting derivatives, devoid of abortifacient potential and diarrhoeogenic side-effects, were available. It is possible that other conditions (e.g. motility disorders and adjunct therapy with anti-arthritic drugs) or even indications outside of the gastrointestinal tract, will provide the major clinical outlet for prostaglandins. Nevertheless, their combination of antisecretory activity with inhibition of gastrin release remains an attractive profile, particularly for long-term dosing. Indeed, these aspects of the activity profile of prostaglandins may be more worthwhile points of emphasis than protection against acute damage in designing future molecules for clinical use.

DEFENCE AGAINST ACID AND PEPSIN

In the stomach, pre-epithelial neutralization of H^+ ions in the mucus–bicarbonate barrier acts as a first line of defence against acid[30] (see Chapter 7). The mucus gel layer also provides a barrier to high-molecular-weight substances such as pepsin by virtue of a gel exclusion effect (see Chapter 6). Interaction between luminal H^+ and HCO_3^- produced by the epithelium gives rise to a standing pH gradient adjacent to the mucosa[31]. A neutral surface microenvironment is maintained at luminal pH 2–3 but the gradient is acidified and juxtamucosal pH falls when luminal acidity exceeds about 20 mM HCl. However, gastric mucosa presents a relatively impermeable barrier to H^+ ions by virtue of the high resistance of paracellular shunt pathways and low permeability of the apical cell membranes. In addition, mechanisms exist for disposal of H^+ ions and maintenance of acid–base balance in both the interstitial and intracellular compartments as a consequence of mucosal perfusion with HCO_3^--rich blood derived from the parietal cell alkaline tide and operation of membrane Na^+/H^+ and Cl^-/HCO_3^- exchangers[32,33]. Extracellular surface neutralization of acid is a proportionately more important mechanism of mucosal protection in the duodenum where rates of epithelial HCO_3^- secretion are considerably higher and where luminal pH[34] rarely falls below pH2. Adequate blood flow is also essential in order to maintain a HCO_3^- source since the main mechanism of duodenal HCO_3^- secretion is transcellular transport. The other major protective mechanism in the proximal duodenum is clearance of acid as a result of motility which transfers the luminal contents distally for bulk neutralization by pancreatic secretions.

Gastrointestinal epithelium has a high proliferative rate with exfoliated cells being continually replaced as a result of mitotic activity. A distinct mechanism for short-term maintenance of epithelial continuity has been identified in the stomach which is extremely rapid and does not necessitate cell division. This process has been termed 'restitution' by Silen and Ito[35] to distinguish it from repair of more severe lesions such as peptic ulcers. Healing of these chronic lesions necessitates tissue rebuilding and follows a course of events similar to that described for wound repair[36]. In contrast, restitution occurs in response to acute superficial injury which can be widespread but does not extend beyond the lamina propria. Damage and subsequent shedding of interfoveolar necrotic cells is followed by migration of viable epithelial cells from the gastric pits across the bare basal lamina. Experimentally, loss of surface cells and subsequent restitution can be induced by transient exposure of the mucosa to, for example, hyperosmolar salt or absolute ethanol. Since superficial exfoliation is also induced by food ingestion, short-term loss of barrier function in the upper gastrointestinal tract is a common occurrence which does not inevitably lead to development of haemorrhagic erosions unless the process of restitution is compromised. Indeed, failure of this process may underlie other gastro-intestinal disorders since rapid re-epithelialization occurs throughout the intestinal tract.

ENHANCING PROTECTIVE MECHANISMS

A therapeutic approach to ulcer disease based on enhancing currently-identified protective mechanisms would be aimed at preventing the formation or recurrence of mucosal lesions rather than healing a preformed ulcer. This contention is reinforced by the fact that synthetic prostaglandins, which enhance many of the processes regarded as important in mucosal protection, only produce acceptable rates of acute ulcer healing at antisecretory dose levels. Therapy which does not influence gastric acid secretion is attractive for maintenance of remission although many uncertainties and problems can be envisaged in developing a drug solely for this indication. Experimental and clinical evaluation of agents for essentially prophylactic use, which may not necessarily be active in acute phases of a disease are notoriously difficult, expensive and time-consuming. In the case of peptic ulcer disease, if mechanisms of protection in stomach and duodenum are different then treatments are likely to be specific for a particular location necessitating precise diagnosis. Furthermore, since an appropriate laboratory model in which to initially detect and then evaluate agents influencing ulcer relapse does not exist, approaches will be hypothesis-based and, therefore, high risk. A number of potential approaches can, however, be identified as the basis for discovering novel therapeutic entities which do not act either by inhibiting acid secretion or by the largely ill-defined mechanisms of current protective drugs.

Attempts to directly stimulate protective elements, e.g. mucus and bicarbonate secretions or blood flow, are susceptible to problems associated with all agonists such as tachyphylaxis. A stimulant of mucus release would provide a thicker barrier against luminal pepsin but would only be effective if accompanied by a compensatory increase in biosynthesis. The alternative approach of inhibiting peptic activity has met with little clinical success although this may reflect in part low binding affinity rather than failure of the approach *per se*. Increased thickness of the surface mucus layer would also provide a better unstirred layer for surface neutralization of acid by HCO_3^- secreted from the mucosa. A stimulant of HCO_3^- secretion (*viz.* a 'pharmacological antacid') provides a further approach which is supported by findings that alkaline secretion is inhibited by ulcerogens and increased by prostaglandins[37,38]. The likely clinical utility of this approach to maintenance therapy could be assessed with prostaglandins although the fact that prostanoids also inhibit pancreatic secretion and hence bulk neutralization[39] suggests that they do not represent the ideal therapeutic modality with which to test the hypothesis.

Increasing the resistance of cells to damage or reducing the inflammatory response are widely pursued goals throughout therapeutics which are equally applicable to the treatment of peptic ulcer and associated conditions. Approaches which attempt to protect mucosal cells and limit inflammatory reactions include calcium antagonists, free-radical scavengers, lipoxygenase inhibition and leucotriene antagonists[25,40]. Finally, disturbances of motility and gastric emptying have long been implicated in the aetiology of peptic ulcer disease. Increased understanding of the role of neuropeptides in regulating motor responses and other aspects of gastrointestinal function offers the possiblity that yet further targets for therapeutic intervention will be identified in the near future.

ENHANCING REPAIR PROCESSES

Healing of a chronic ulcer is essentially a problem of wound repair and influencing this process is thus an entirely different proposition from enhancing protective mechanisms. Rapid re-epithelialization is a physiological response to superficial cell exfoliation. Although failure of this process may be a contributory factor in progression from acute damage to chronic ulceration, the fact that biopsy sites heal rapidly in ulcer patients and ulcers tend to recur at the same site both imply that the precise anatomical location is significant, reflecting for example an area of suboptimal vascularization. Protection against acute damage involves yet another series of reactions and it is perhaps not surprising that agents designed for optimal activity in models of chemical injury fall short of expectation in clinical ulcer-healing trials.

Wound healing is a pathophysiological function which is essential for survival. In common with other wounds, a chronic ulcer generates a fully developed inflammatory response in which events such as cell division, collagen synthesis and angiogenesis are necessary for recovery[41,42]. These processes are regulated by intermediates of the inflammatory reaction such as chemotactic substances and by endogenous growth factors such as epidermal growth factor (EGF) and PDGF. The local microcirculation has an important role in wound repair since it delivers phagocytes to limit infection, nutrients for growth and oxygen, which is also capable of up-regulating rates of healing and organization within the wound. In the upper gastrointestinal tract these responses are retarded by autolytic secretions present in the lumen. The success of anti-secretory therapy seems largely due to raising intraluminal pH during the (nocturnal) period when motility and neutralizing secretions are reduced and ingested food is not available for buffering and adsorbing HCl or pepsin.

Speeding up the wound healing response provides another potential approach to ulcer therapy. If a concomitant increase in vascularization of the ulcerated area was also achieved, then a favourable influence on subsequent recurrence of the disease might be anticipated. Wound healing relies largely on normal growth mechanisms and is thus connected with the action of growth factors. In addition to mitogens, migratory factors involved in controlling the translocation of cells may also have a role in gastrointestinal protection and repair. Of the various growth factors identified, urogastrone or EGF is of particular interest since this peptide combines mitogenic activity with a potent but short-acting antisecretory response[43]. EGF has also been shown to have a protective action against mucosal damage in animals[44]. Whether other factors

233

will be identified as important in gastroduodenal mucosal repair or even shown to be deficient in ulcer patients remains an area for future work. The fact that long-term administration of trophic agents could conceivably lead to dysplasia by a mechanism similar to that occurring in response to the endogenous hypergastrinaemia induced by long-acting antisecretory agents presents a problem for toxicological evaluation of mitogens. Furthermore, growth factors are large peptides and would be expected to display poor systemic stability and poor bioavailability after oral administration. Some of these difficulties may be overcome with a slow release depot similar to that developed for the LHRH agonist Zoladex® (ICI) which is formulated in a biodegradable polymer and released over a period of a month[45].

FUTURE PROSPECTS

The therapeutic success of H_2-receptor antagonists reflects their efficacy, acute safety and convenience. There is little stimulus to develop more effective antisecretory agents unless the problem of gastric tumourogenicity can be overcome. The unpredictable clinical efficacy of mucosal protective agents makes this approach equally high risk and it is difficult to foresee any agent challenging the dominance of H_2-receptor antagonists in the immediate future. However, given the possible adverse effects of continuous administration of inhibitors of acid secretion, agents which enhance mucosal protection could eventually assume importance as drugs of choice for maintaining remission in those individuals requiring continuous therapy. Present antiulcer drugs do not cure the disease and there would seem little prospect of attaining this goal with current therapeutic strategies. In the absence of any clues as to the (environmental) factors responsible for ulceration, reduction in relapse rate represents a convenient means of monitoring real advances in drug therapy.

Drug therapy of peptic ulcer disease bears many parallels to that of hypertension where ion channel and enzyme inhibitors have joined beta-receptor blockers and fragmented the market. In the short-term, it is likely that new developments in ulcer therapy will take the form of further antisecretory drugs albeit acting via a mechanism other than H_2-receptor blockade, improved formulations of existing drugs, and possibly combinations of different drugs. In the future, increased understanding of basic epithelial function offers the possibility of agents acting on processes which control cytoplasmic pH, intracellular volume, membrane permeability or fluidity, and permeability of paracellular shunts or vascular endothelium. Certainly advances in fields which are traditionally unrelated to peptic ulcer research, including growth regulation and wound healing, vascular disorders and angiogenesis, inflammation, surface immunity and molecular biology could provide a more profitable basis for longer-term research and drug discovery. Otherwise gastroenterologists will be armed with a plethora of drugs to heal ulcers but nothing to cure the disease[40].

ACKNOWLEDGEMENT

The excellent secretarial assistance of Mavis Brightwell in preparation of this manuscript is most gratefully acknowledged.

REFERENCES

1. Wormsley, K.G. (1984). Assessing the safety of drugs for the long-term treatment of peptic ulcers. *Gut*, **25**, 1416–23
2. Ruddell, W.S.J., Bone, E.S., Hill, M.J. and Walters, C.L. (1978). Pathogenesis of gastric cancer in pernicious anaemia. *Lancet*, **i**, 521–3
3. Caygill, C.P.J., Hill, M.J., Kirkham, J.S. and Northfield, T.C. (1986). Mortality from gastric cancer following gastric surgery for peptic ulcer. *Lancet*, **i**, 929–31
4. Harmon, J.W. (ed.) (1981). *Basic Mechanisms of Gastrointestinal Mucosal Cell Injury and Protection*. (Baltimore: Williams & Wilkins)
5. Allen, A., Flemström, G., Garner, A., Silen, W. and Turnberg, L.A. (eds.) (1983). *Mechanisms of Mucosal Protection in the Upper Gastrointestinal Tract*. (New York: Raven Press)
6. Lauritsen, K. and Rask-Madsen, J. (1986). Prostaglandins and clinical experience in peptic ulcer disease. *Scand. J. Gastroenterol.*, **21** (Suppl. 125), 174–80
7. Lipkin, M. (1970). Carbenoxolone sodium and the rate of extrusion of gastric epithelial cells. In Baron, J.H. and Sullivan, F.M. (eds.) *Carbenoxolone Sodium*, pp. 11–17 (London: Butterworths)
8. Peskar, B.M., Holland, A. and Peskar, B.A. (1976). Effect of carbenoxolone on prostaglandin synthesis and degradation. *J. Pharm. Pharmac.*, **28**, 146–8
9. Pickard, R. (1985). Clinical review of colloidal bismuth subcitrate. In Axon, A.T.R. and Benyon, J.S.E. (eds.) *Pathogenesis and the Treatment of Peptic Ulcer Disease*, pp. 55–70 (Amsterdam: Excerpta Medica)
10. Konturek, S.J., Radecki, T., Piastucki, I. and Drozdowicz, D. (1986). Advances in the understanding of the mechanism of cytoprotective action by colloidal bismuth subcitrate. *Scand. J. Gastroenterol.*, **21** (Suppl. 122), 6–10
11. McNulty, C.A.M. (1987). The treatment of *Campylobacter* infections in man. *J. Antimicrob. Chemother.*, **19**, 281–4
12. Marshall, B.J. and Warren, J.R. (1984). Unidentified curved bacilli in the stomach of patients with gastritis and peptic ulceration. *Lancet*, **i**, 1311–15
13. Marks, I.N., Lucke, W., Wright, J.P. and Gridwook, A.H. (1981). Ulcer healing and relapse rates after initial treatment with cimetidine or sucralfate. *J. Clin. Gastroenterol.*, **3** (Suppl. 2), 163–5
14. Solhaug, J.H., Carling, L., Glise, H., Hallerbaak, B., Hallgren, T., Kagevi, I., Svedberg, L.E. and Wahlby, L. (1987). Ulcer recurrences following initial ulcer healing with sucralfate or cimetidine. *Scand. J. Gastroenterol.*, **22** (Suppl. 127), 77–80
15. Ligumsky, M., Karmeli, F. and Rachmilewitz, D. (1984). Sucralfate stimulation of gastric PGE_2 synthesis: possible mechanism to explain its effective cytoprotective properties. *Gastroenterology*, **86**, 1164
16. Hollander, D., Tarnawski, A., Krause, W.J. and Gergely, H. (1985). Protective effect of sucralfate against alcohol-induced gastric mucosal injury in the rat. *Gastroenterology*, **88**, 366–74
17. Robert, A., Schultz, J.R., Nezamis, J.E. and Lancaster, C. (1976). Gastric antisecretory and antiulcer properties of PGE_2, 15-methyl PGE_2 and 16,16-dimethyl PGE_2. *Gastroenterology*, **70**, 359–70
18. Miller, T.A. (1983). Protective effects of prostaglandins against gastric mucosal damage: current knowledge and proposed mechanisms. *Am. J. Physiol.*, **245**, G606–23

19. Cohen, M.N. (ed.) (1986). *Biological Protection with Prostaglandins*, Vol. 2. (Boca Raton: CRC Press)

20. Pihan, G., Majzoubi, D., Haudenschild, C., Trier, J.S. and Szabo, S. (1986). Early microcirculatory stasis in acute gastric mucosal injury in the rat and prevention by 16,16-dimethyl prostaglandin E$_2$ or sodium thiosulfate. *Gastroenterology*, **91**, 1415–26

21. McQueen, S., Hutton, D., Allen, A. and Garner, A. (1983). Gastric and duodenal surface mucus gel thickness in rat: effects of prostaglandins and damaging agents. *Am. J. Physiol.*, **245**, G388–93

22. Smeaton, L.A., Hirst, B.H., Allen, A. and Garner, A. (1983). Gastric and duodenal HCO$_3^-$ transport *in vivo*: influence of prostaglandins. *Am. J. Physiol.*, **245**, G751–9

23. Garner, A. (1977). Assessment of gastric mucosal damage: comparative effects of aspirin and fenclofenac on the gastric mucosa of the guinea pig. *Toxicol. Appl. Pharmacol.*, **42**, 477–86

24. Lacy, E.R. and Ito, S. (1982). Microscopic analysis of ethanol damage to rat gastric mucosa after treatment with a prostaglandin. *Gastroenterology*, **83**, 619–29

25. Silen, W., Walsh, J.H., Garner, A., Robert, A., Pfeiffer, C.J. and Szabo, S. (1986). Lessons from experimental ulcers: 'take-home messages' from the 5th International Conference on Experimental Ulcer. *Dig. Dis. Sci.*, **31**, 1265–8

26. Romano, M., Razandi, M. and Ivey, K.J. (1987). Omeprazole directly protects human gastric epithelial cells *in vitro*. *Clin. Res.*, **35**, 128A

27. Hunt, R.H., Howden, C.W., Jones, D.B., Burget, D.W. and Kerr, G.D. (1986). The correlation between acid suppression and peptic ulcer healing. *Scand. J. Gastroenterol.*, **21** (Suppl. 125), 22–9

28. Marshall, B.J., Goodwin, C.S., Warren, J.R., Blincow, E.D., Blackbourn, S., Phillips, M., Waters, T.E. and Sanderson, C.R. (1986). Prospective double-blind study of supplementary antibiotic therapy for duodenal ulcer associated with *Campylobacter pyloridis* infection. *Dig. Dis. Sci.*, **31** (Supplement: Abstracts of the World Congress of Gastroenterology, São Paulo), 1505

29. Muramatsu, M., Tanaka, M., Suwa, T., Fujita, A., Otomo, S. and Aihara, H. (1984). Effect of 2'-carboxymethoxy-4,4'-bis(3-methyl-2-butenyloxy)chalcone (SU-88) on prostaglandin metabolism in hog gastric mucosa. *Biochem. Pharmacol.*, **33**, 2629–33

30. Allen, A. and Garner, A. (1980). Mucus and bicarbonate secretion in the stomach and their possible role in mucosal protection. *Gut*, **21**, 249–62

31. Ross, I.N., Bahari, H.M.M. and Turnberg, L.A. (1981). The pH gradient across mucus adherent to rat fundic mucosa *in vivo* and the effect of potential damaging agents. *Gastroenterology*, **81**, 713–8

32. Kivilaakso, E. and Silen, W. (1979). Pathogenesis of experimental gastric mucosal injury. *New Engl. J. Med.*, **301**, 364–9

33. Machen, T.E. and Paradiso, A.M. (1987). Regulation of intracellular pH in the stomach. *Ann. Rev. Physiol.*, **49**, 21–35

34. Flemström. G., Garner, A., Nylander, O., Hurst, B.C. and Heylings, J.R. (1982). Surface epithelial HCO$_3^-$ transport by mammalian duodenum *in vivo*. *Am. J. Physiol.*, **243**, G348–58

35. Silen, W. and Ito, S. (1985). Mechanism for rapid re-epithelialization of the gastric mucosal surface. *Annu. Rev. Physiol.*, **47**, 217–29

36. Edwards, L.C. and Dunphy, J.E. (1958). Wound healing: injury and normal repair. *New Engl. J. Med.*, **259**, 224–233

37. Garner, A., Flemström, G. and Heylings, J.R. (1979). Effects of anti-inflammatory agents and prostaglandins on acid and bicarbonate secretions in the amphibian isolated gastric mucosa. *Gastroenterology*, **77**, 451–7

38. Rees, W.D.W., Gibbons, L.C. and Turnberg, L.A. (1983). Effects of non-steroidal antiinflammatory drugs and prostaglandins on alkali secretion by rabbit gastric fundus *in vitro*. *Gut*, **24**, 784–9

39. Case, R.M., Garner, A. and Uddin, K.K. (1983). Simultaneous determination of duodenal and pancreatic bicarbonate transport: differential effects of secretin and prostaglandin E$_2$ in the cat *in vivo*. *J. Physiol.*, **340**, 36–7P

40. Garner, A. (1986). Future opportunities for drug therapy in peptic ulcer disease. *Scand. J. Gastroenterol.*, **21** (Suppl. 125), 203–9
41. Wormsley, K.G. (1983). Duodenal ulcer: does pathophysiology equal aetiology? *Gut*, **24**, 775–80
42. Hunt, T.K. (1984). Can repair processes be stimulated by modulators of cell growth factors, angiogenic factors etc. without adversely affecting normal processes? *J. Trauma*, **24**(9) (suppl.), S39–46
43. Bower, J.M., Camble, R., Gregory, H., Gerring, E.L. and Willshire, I.R. (1975). The inhibition of gastric acid secretion by epidermal growth factor. *Experientia*, **31**, 825–6
44. Konturek, S.J., Radecki, T., Brzozowski, T., Piastucki, I., Dembinski, A., Dembinski-Kiec, A., Zmuda, A., Gryglewski, R. and Gregory, H. (1981). Gastric cytoprotection by epidermal growth factor *Gastroenterology*, **81**, 438–43
43. Hutchinson, F.G. and Furr, B.J.A. (1985). Biodegradable polymers for the sustained release of peptides. *Biochem. Soc. Trans.*, **13**, 520–3

Index

241